# The Aging Criminal

# The Aging Criminal:

## *Neurodegeneration Behind Bars*

Edited by

Adonis Sfera and Carolina Osorio

**Cambridge Scholars** Publishing

The Aging Criminal: Neurodegeneration Behind Bars

Edited by Adonis Sfera and Carolina Osorio

This book first published 2025

Cambridge Scholars Publishing

Lady Stephenson Library, Newcastle upon Tyne, NE6 2PA, UK

British Library Cataloguing in Publication Data
A catalogue record for this book is available from the British Library



ISBN: 978-1-0364-4266-8
ISBN (Ebook): 978-1-0364-4267-5

*To our patients and staff at Patton State Hospital*

This book is based on original research conducted by clinicians at Patton State Hospital and beyond and discusses outcome improvement in severe mental illness. The views expressed in this book are those of the author and do not necessarily reflect the opinions of Cambridge.

# TABLE OF CONTENT

# About the Editors

Carolina Osorio, M.D., completed her psychiatric residency at Loma Linda University and geriatric fellowship at UCLA, Semel Institute of Neuroscience and Human Behavior. She has been involved in University private practice, teaching, and research as an assistant professor of psychiatry, director for the geriatric psychiatry didactics for psychiatric residents, and spirituality and psychiatry committee member. Dr. Osorio is involved in the World Health Organization training for trainers on Problem Management Plus (PM+). Individual psychological help for adults impaired by distress in communities exposed to adversity in Latin America and Caribbean regions. She is now working as an attending psychiatrist at DSH-Patton.

Dr. Sfera graduated from medical school in 1980 and has been practicing medicine for over forty years. From 1984 to 1989, Dr. Sfera worked in analytical psychotherapy research at the Carl Gustav Jung Institute of Los Angeles, where he participated in the production of a documentary entitled "A Matter of Heart" on the life and work of Swiss psychiatrist C.G. Jung.

In 1998, Dr. Sfera completed a psychiatry residency and a consultation and liaison psychiatry fellowship at the University of Southern California in Los Angeles. Dr. Sfera worked at USC as a principal investigator in schizophrenia research.

In 1999, Dr. Sfera started a schizophrenia research institute named South Coast Clinical Trials in Anaheim, California. During this time, he wrote over 100 articles and book chapters on biological psychiatry, herbal medicine, and lifestyle medicine. Since 2006, Dr. Sfera has been the chief of professional education for the California Department of State Hospitals at Patton.

# INTRODUCTION

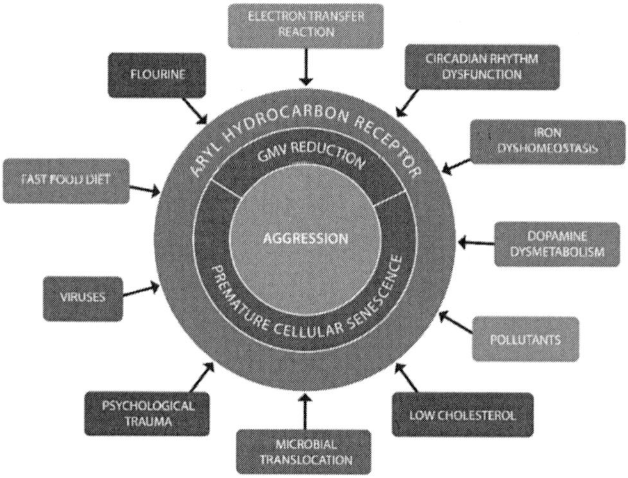


## Visual Abstract

## Highlights

- Reduced brain gray matter volume (GMV) is a significant driver of aggressive behaviors in patients with severe mental illness (SMI).
- Without neuroprotecting agents, schizophrenia (SCZ), dementia, as well as most antipsychotic drugs, reduce GMV.
- State hospitals continue to exist because the outcomes of chronic mental illness are marginally affected by the available treatments.
- SMI has been associated with premature cellular/neuronal senescence, which disrupts biological barriers and allows gut microbes to migrate into host tissues, including the brain.

- Aryl hydrocarbon receptor (AhR), activated by intestinal microorganisms and or their molecules, drives cellular senescence, disrupting plasma and mitochondrial membranes.
- More than other dementias, behavioral variant frontotemporal dementia (bvFTD) predisposes to violence and is challenging to differentiate from SMI.
- Biochemical and biophysical treatments, including polyphenols, membrane lipid replacement (MLR), mitochondrial transplantation, and brain gamma wave entrainment, are potential novel interventions that could improve outcomes in SMI.

Forensic hospitals are large public institutions for the treatment of patients with severe mental illness (SMI) and a history of criminal violations. In the past, individuals with chronic schizophrenia (SCZ) and schizophrenia-like disorders (SLDs) lived, on average, 15-20 years shorter than the general population and rarely developed late-life neurodegenerative disorders. However, improved medical care over the past decades has led to unprecedented longevity in this population, which, at the same time, has increased the prevalence of dementia (1).

## Sustained recovery in SMI

The very existence of State hospitals is proof of the concept that sustained recovery is rare in most patients with SMI. Indeed, according to the newest studies, only 13.5% of patients with SCZ or SLDs achieve complete recovery (return to the premorbid level of functioning) after the first psychotic episode (2). Full-time employment after the first psychotic outbreak, an indirect measure of recovery, has been averaging 10-20% and has remained in that range for the past 100 years (3). Instead of returning to the premorbid level of functioning, most SCZ patients adhere to medications and achieve partial recovery, as evidenced by the amelioration of positive symptoms and improvement in their activities of daily living (ADLs).

## *Antipsychotic drugs, the good, the bad, and the ugly*

Antipsychotic drugs are highly productive for acute psychosis but less adequate, possibly even detrimental when administered for extended periods, as they contribute to GMV reduction, as demonstrated by numerous voxel-based morphometric studies using neuroimaging. Indeed, SCZ itself, as well as exposure to most first and second-generation antipsychotics, was associated with a reduction of GMV, an established driver of aggressive behavior (4)(5)(6). This raises the question of iatrogenic aggression, as documented in akathisia-induced violence.

Maintaining homeostasis and preventing GMV reduction can be attained by the concomitant administration of antipsychotic drugs with neuroprotective, electron-donating agents, including dopamine (DA) D1 receptor agonists or acetylcholine (ACh) muscarinic agonists, such as PF-6294 and xanomeline respectively (7)(8)(9)(10)(11)(12)(13). As these compounds protect the gray matter and gut barrier, they are likely beneficial for patients with SMI (14)(15).

Together, these findings suggest that acute psychosis and chronic schizophrenia (SCZ) or schizophrenia-like disorders (SLDs) may be different conditions that require different approaches. The natural and synthetic neuroprotective electron-donor agents are discussed in detail in the following chapters.

## *Forensic detainees with SMI*

Inefficient mental health policies implemented over the past 4 to 6 decades swell the number of state and federal detainees over the age of 55, from 3% in 1991 to 15% in 2021. In addition, over 61,000 older adults with dementia are estimated to die in prison each year (16). Moreover, incarcerated individuals age at a much faster rate compared to the general population, suggesting that the psychological stress of life in captivity promotes premature cellular/neuronal senescence and accelerated brain aging. Indeed, it is estimated that each year spent in prison takes away two years of an individual's life expectancy. At the same time, age-related diseases, including dementia, appear much earlier in prisoners than in nonincarcerated people, probably due to increased activation of stress and inflammatory pathways (17). Taken together, the early occurrence of age-related diseases and increased healthcare expenditures highlight the need for novel solutions and treatment models for forensic psychiatric patients (18)(19).

Neurocognitive disorders in older forensic detainees are inadequately studied and often challenging to differentiate from the underlying SMI (20)(21)(22). However, this differentiation is essential as diagnosing dementias early is of the essence because antipsychotic drugs can precipitate cardiovascular or cerebrovascular adverse events in patients with neurocognitive disorders. This raises a dilemma unknown to the previous generation clinicians: continuing antipsychotic drugs may have detrimental effects while discontinuing treatment with these agents may increase the risk of violent behavior and injuries (23).

The discovery of chlorpromazine in the 1950s has revolutionized psychiatry and contributed to the deinstitutionalization of people with SMI. Subsequently, homelessness and incarceration of individuals with SCZ and SLDs increased dramatically, suggesting that symptomatic relief rarely translates into sustained recovery (2)(3). In addition, for the past 70 years, the dopamine (DA) hypothesis has been the critical working model in SCZ. This paradigm has contributed to the development of numerous antipsychotic drugs that can effectively clear psychotic symptoms but cause marginal outcome improvement (3).

### *The cells of righteousness and wrath*

During the past decades, there was limited research on the quantifiable pathological changes in SCZ, including premature cellular/neuronal, senescence, GMV reduction, attenuation of gamma oscillations on electroencephalogram (EEG), and lipid damage in plasma or mitochondrial membranes.

The forensic psychiatric population is comprised of two major subgroups: 1) career criminals with a life-long history of SMI who are getting older and develop dementia, and 2) a smaller category of first-time offenders after the age of 55 with behavioral variant frontotemporal (bvFTD) dementia. The latter subgroup exhibits a preference for criminal violations and is difficult to distinguish from SCZ and SLDs, as cognition may remain intact for an extended period (24)(25)(26).

Von Economo neurons (VENs) are large, bipolar cells implicated in empathy and emotional intelligence, which bvFTD selectively targets. Reduced number of VENs and subsequent impulsivity, apathy, loss of empathy, and decreased fear of consequences may encourage the patient to engage in criminal violations, including homicide (27).

We surmise that VENs are preferentially targeted by frontotemporal lobar degeneration, the bvFTD pathology, because of their large cell surface and increased vulnerability to lipid peroxidation and ferroptosis. VENs, more numerous in the right hemisphere than the left, are found in the anterior cingulate cortex (ACC) and anterior insular cortex (AIC), areas associated with insight as well as gastrointestinal (GI) inflammation (27). VENs are large neurons in superior mammals, including humans, great apes, elephants, and dolphins.

In the 1990s, bvFTD was poorly defined. Over the past two decades, a wealth of data became available, linking AIC and ACC to interoception insight and "gut feeling" or intuition, processes altered in SCZ and dementia. However, despite the progress in this area, few forensic psychiatrists are familiar with bvFTD, and this disorder is often missed or construed as SCZ or bipolar disorder, resulting in risky treatments and inadequate admission in State hospitals. This is unfortunate as these institutions promote the recovery model, which does not apply to patients with neurodegenerative disorders. Instead, patients with dementia should be referred to palliative care facilities. In a previous article, we recommended these facilities and screening for bvFTD in first offenders after age 55.

### *AhR-driven premature aging and barrier permeability*

Accelerated aging is a well-documented feature of SCZ and SLDs, but its role in the pathogenesis of these illnesses remains unclear (28). Cellular senescence, the source of organismal aging, is an anticancer program marked by proliferative arrest, resistance to apoptosis, active metabolism, and a toxic secretome that can spread senescence to neighboring healthy cells. Senescent cells, including neurons and glia, undergo lipidomic changes in plasma and organelle membranes. These changes are primarily oxidative and lead to the loss of membrane cholesterol and an increase in ceramide, altering the biophysical properties as well as nutrient intake and neurotransmission (29)(30)(31).

At the level of the intestinal barrier and blood-brain barrier (BBB), senescent cells alter permeability, facilitating the translocation of microbes and their components into the systemic circulation from where they can reach the brain (32)(33). This may explain the high comorbidity between SCZ and the disorders of increased gut permeability, such as human immunodeficiency virus (HIV) infection or inflammatory bowel disease (IBD), conditions marked by microbial migration from the gut into the host tissues (34). It has been established that senescent brain cells, including microglia and astrocytes, may promote neurodegeneration by becoming neurotoxic, engaging in the aberrant phagocytosis of healthy neurons and synapses (35).

Throughout this book, we discuss several articles derived from the presentations at the Annual Forensic Conferences at Patton State Hospital in San Bernardino County, California. These presentations highlight novel ideas, concepts, and models for treating chronic SMI with superimposed dementia.

## References

1. Glick ID, Zamora D, Davis JM, Suryadevara U, Goldenson A, Kamis D. Are Patients With Schizophrenia Better Off With Lifetime Antipsychotic Medication?: Replication of a Naturalistic, Long-Term, Follow-Up Study of Antipsychotic Treatment. J Clin Psychopharmacol. 2020 Mar/Apr;40(2):145-148. doi: 10.1097/JCP.0000000000001171. Erratum in: J Clin Psychopharmacol. 2020 Jul/Aug;40(4):430. PMID: 32142495.
2. Jääskeläinen E, Juola P, Hirvonen N, McGrath JJ, Saha S, Isohanni M, Veijola J, Miettunen J. A systematic review and meta-analysis of recovery in schizophrenia. Schizophr Bull. 2013 Nov;39(6):1296-306. doi: 10.1093/schbul/sbs130.

3. Richard Warner. Recovery from schizophrenia: psychiatry and political economy. Routledge, London EC4P 4EE. 1994. Second Edition. 366 pp. ISBN 0-415-09260-4. ISBN 0415-09261-2
4. Vita A, De Peri L, Deste G, Sacchetti E. Progressive loss of cortical gray matter in schizophrenia: a meta-analysis and meta-regression of longitudinal MRI studies. Transl Psychiatry. 2012 Nov 20;2(11): e190. Doi: 10.1038/tp.2012.116. Erratum in: Transl Psychiatry. 2013;3:e275. PMID: 23168990
5. Guo F, Zhu YQ, Li C, Wang XR, Wang HN, Liu WM, Wang LX, Tian P, Kang XW, Cui LB, Xi YB, Yin H. Gray matter volume changes following antipsychotic therapy in first-episode schizophrenia patients: A longitudinal voxel-based morphometric study. J Psychiatr Res. 2019 Sep;116:126-132. doi: 10.1016/j.jpsychires.2019.06.009.
6. Chester DS, Lynam DR, Milich R, DeWall CN. Physical aggressiveness and gray matter deficits in the ventromedial prefrontal cortex. Cortex. 2017 Dec;97:17-22. doi: 10.1016/j.cortex.2017.09.024. Epub 2017 Oct 7.
7. Jones-Tabah J, Mohammad H, Paulus EG, Clarke PBS, Hébert TE. The Signaling and Pharmacology of the Dopamine D1 Receptor. Front Cell Neurosci. 2022 Jan 17;15:806618. doi: 10.3389/fncel.2021.806618.
8. Martini ML, Ray C, Yu X, Liu J, Pogorelov VM, Wetsel WC, Huang XP, McCorvy JD, Caron MG, Jin J. Designing Functionally Selective Noncatechol Dopamine D1 Receptor Agonists with Potent In Vivo Antiparkinsonian Activity. ACS Chem Neurosci. 2019 Sep 18;10(9):4160-4182. doi: 10.1021/acschemneuro.9b00410.
9. Shekhar A, Potter WZ, Lightfoot J, Lienemann J, Dubé S, Mallinckrodt C, et al. Selective muscarinic receptor agonist xanomeline as a novel treatment approach for schizophrenia. Am J Psychiat. 2008;165:1033–1039.
10. Singh A. Xanomeline and Trospium: A Potential Fixed Drug Combination (FDC) for Schizophrenia-A Brief Review of Current Data. Innov Clin Neurosci. 2022 Oct-Dec;19(10-12):43-47.
11. Lewis AS, Picciotto MR. Regulation of aggressive behaviors by nicotinic acetylcholine receptors: Animal models, human genetics,

and clinical studies. Neuropharmacology. 2020 May 1;167:107929. doi: 10.1016/j.neuropharm.2019.107929

12. Yohn SE, Weiden PJ, Felder CC, Stahl SM. Muscarinic acetylcholine receptors for psychotic disorders: bench-side to clinic. Trends Pharmacol Sci. 2022 Dec;43(12):1098-1112. doi: 10.1016/j.tips.2022.09.006.
13. Uwada J, Nakazawa H, Muramatsu I, Masuoka T, Yazawa T. Role of Muscarinic Acetylcholine Receptors in Intestinal Epithelial Homeostasis: Insights for the Treatment of Inflammatory Bowel Disease. Int J Mol Sci. 2023 Mar 30;24(7):6508. doi: 10.3390/ijms24076508.
14. Cheadle GA, Costantini TW, Bansal V, Eliceiri BP, Coimbra R. Cholinergic signaling in the gut: a novel mechanism of barrier protection through activation of enteric glia cells. Surg Infect (Larchmt). 2014 Aug;15(4):387-93. doi: 10.1089/sur.2013.103.
15. Chen ZR, Huang JB, Yang SL, Hong FF. Role of Cholinergic Signaling in Alzheimer's Disease. Molecules. 2022 Mar 10;27(6): 1816. doi: 10.3390/molecules27061816.
16. Onah ME. The Patient-to-Prisoner Pipeline: The IMD Exclusion's Adverse Impact on Mass Incarceration in United States. Am J Law Med. 2018 Mar;44(1):119-144. doi: 10.1177/0098858818763818. PMID: 29764321.
17. Bureau of Justice Statistics: https://csat.bjs.ojp.gov/quick-tables
18. 8. Greene M, Ahalt C, Stijacic-Cenzer I, Metzger L, Williams B. Older adults in jail: high rates and early onset of geriatric conditions. Health Justice. 2018 Feb 17;6(1):3. doi: 10.1186/s40352-018-0062-9.
19. Ahalt C, Trestman RL, Rich JD, Greifinger RB, Williams BA. Paying the price: the pressing need for quality, cost, and outcomes data to improve correctional health care for older prisoners. J Am Geriatr Soc. 2013 Nov;61(11):2013-9. doi: 10.1111/jgs.12510. PMID: 24219203; PMCID: PMC3984258.
20. Adamowicz DH, Lee EE. Dementia among older people with schizophrenia: an update on recent studies. Curr Opin Psychiatry. 2023 May 1;36(3):150-155. doi: 10.1097/YCO.0000000000000861.

21. Kerssens CJ, Krudop WA, Prins ND, van Berckel BN, Rozemuller A, Seeley WW, Scheltens P, Stek ML, Pijnenburg YA. Schizophrenia as a mimic of behavioral variant frontotemporal dementia. Neurocase. 2016 Jun;22(3):285-8. doi: 10.1080/13554794.2016.1187178
22. Bhanji NH, Tempier R. Managing schizophrenia during the stable phase: is there consensus among practice guidelines? Can J Psychiatry. 2002 Feb;47(1):76-80. PMID: 11873712.
23. Buckley NA, Sanders P. Cardiovascular adverse effects of antipsychotic drugs. Drug Saf. 2000 Sep;23(3):215-28. doi: 10.2165/00002018-200023030-00004. PMID: 11005704.
24. Mendez MF. The unique predisposition to criminal violations in frontotemporal dementia. J Am Acad Psychiatry Law. 2010;38(3):318-23.
25. Diehl-Schmid J, Perneczky R, Koch J, Nedopil N, Kurz A. Guilty by suspicion? Criminal behavior in frontotemporal lobar degeneration. Cogn Behav Neurol. 2013 Jun;26(2):73-7.
26. Seeley WW. Anterior insula degeneration in frontotemporal dementia. Brain Struct Funct. 2010 Jun;214(5-6):465-75. doi: 10.1007/s00429-010-0263-z.
27. Koren T, Yifa R, Amer M, Krot M, Boshnak N, Ben-Shaanan TL, Azulay-Debby H, Zalayat I, Avishai E, Hajjo H, Schiller M, Haykin H, Korin B, Farfara D, Hakim F, Kobiler O, Rosenblum K, Rolls A. Insular cortex neurons encode and retrieve specific immune responses. Cell. 2021 Nov 24;184(24):5902-5915.e17. doi: 10.1016/j.cell.2021.10.013.
28. Papanastasiou E, Gaughran F, Smith S. Schizophrenia as segmental progeria. J R Soc Med. 2011 Nov;104(11):475-84. doi: 10.1258/jrsm.2011.110051.
29. Zhuo, C., Zhao, F., Tian, H., et al. Acid sphingomyelinase/ceramide system in schizophrenia: implications for therapeutic intervention as a potential novel target. Transl Psychiatry 12, 260 (2022). https://doi.org/10.1038/s41398-022-01999-7
30. Wi JH, Heo CH, Gwak H, Jung C, Kim SY. Probing Physical Properties of the Cellular Membrane in Senescent Cells by

Fluorescence Imaging. J Phys Chem B. 2021 Sep 16;125(36):10182-10194. doi: 10.1021/acs.jpcb.1c05403

31. Sikora E, Bielak-Zmijewska A, Dudkowska M, Krzystyniak A, Mosieniak G, Wesierska M, Wlodarczyk J. Cellular Senescence in Brain Aging. Front Aging Neurosci. 2021 Feb 25;13:646924. Doi: 10.3389/fnagi.2021.646924.
32. Stehle JR Jr, Leng X, Kitzman DW, Nicklas BJ, Kritchevsky SB, High KP. Lipopolysaccharide-binding protein, a surrogate marker of microbial translocation, is associated with physical function in healthy older adults. J Gerontol A Biol Sci Med Sci. 2012 Nov;67(11):1212-8. doi: 10.1093/gerona/gls178.
33. Branca JJV, Gulisano M, Nicoletti C. Intestinal epithelial barrier functions in aging. Ageing Res Rev. 2019 Sep;54:100938. doi: 10.1016/j.arr.2019.100938. Epub 2019 Jul 29. PMID: 31369869.
34. Qian, L., He, X., Gao, F. et al. Estimation of the bidirectional relationship between schizophrenia and inflammatory bowel disease using the Mendelian randomization approach. Schizophr 8, 31 (2022). https://doi.org/10.1038/s41537-022-00244-w
35. Brown, G., Neher, J. Microglial phagocytosis of live neurons. Nat Rev Neurosci 15, 209–216 (2014). https://doi.org/10.1038/nrn3710

# CHAPTER 1

# NEURODEGENERATION AND CRIMINAL VIOLATIONS

Along with the "graying" of the population at large, incarcerated individuals living with severe mental illness (SMI) also age and develop dementia prematurely. It is estimated that over 61,000 older adults with dementia are predicted to die in detention each year (1). In addition, incarcerated individuals age at a much faster rate compared to the general population, suggesting that loss of freedom predisposes to accelerated aging. Indeed, it is estimated that each year spent in captivity may decrease life expectancy by two years. Moreover, age-related diseases, including dementia, start earlier in incarcerated individuals (2).

Aside from the fact that correctional institutions are poorly equipped for the treatment of geriatric pathology, age-related complications have led to increased healthcare expenditures, highlighting the need for novel solutions and concepts (2)(3).

Age-related pathology is not different in State hospitals compared to other institutions that house patients with SMI and a history of criminal violations. The very existence of these facilities is proof of the concept that sustained recovery is rare in most patients with SMI. According to the newest data, only 13.5% of SCZ patients achieve complete recovery (premorbid level of functioning without relapse) after the first psychotic episode (4). Employment, another measure of recovery, is around 10-20% at any time after the first psychotic outbreak (5). Instead of sustained recovery, most SCZ patients undergoing antipsychotic treatment achieve symptomatic improvement as well as some degree of independence in the activities of daily living (ADLs).

Antipsychotic drugs are highly productive for acute psychosis but inadequate, possibly even detrimental, for the patients in the "stable" phase of SCZ (6) (Fig.1).

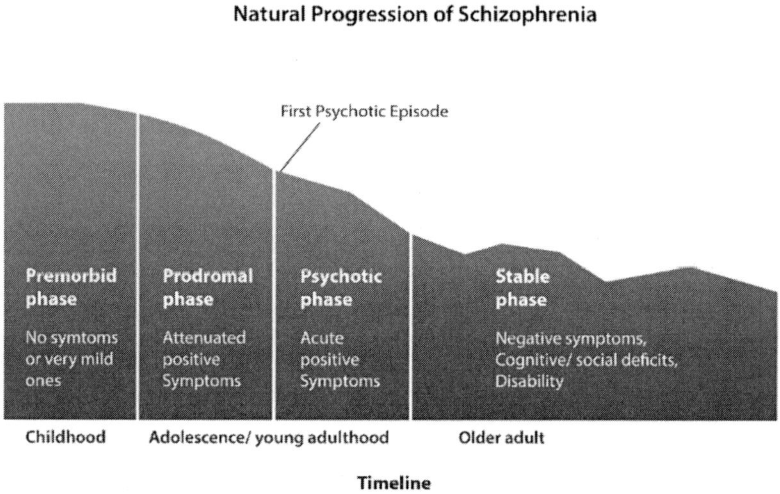


**Fig. 1 SCZ is most likely a neurodevelopmental disorder starting "in utero." There are usually no or very few symptoms in the initial premorbid phase. The following prodromal phaseis marked by behavioral changes but no overt psychosis. Acute positive symptoms, multiple hospitalizations, and frequent nonadherence to medication characterize the psychotic phase. The "stable" SCZ phase, beginning around the age of 50, is characterized by negative and cognitive symptoms, significant disability, and poor response to medications. As patients get older, cognitive disorders usually begin during this phase.**

Both SCZ and most antipsychotic drugs have been associated with GMV reduction, which is more pronounced when patients with SMI develop superimposed dementia. Indeed, numerous neuroimaging studies have documented GMV loss triggered by first and second-generation antipsychotic drugs, suggesting that these agents should be administered with neurotrophic compounds, such as dopamine D1 receptor agonists or acetylcholine (ACH) agonists (7-13). This is important as GMV loss is the chief driver of aggression in neuropsychiatric disorders, raising the question of iatrogenic-induced violence (14)(15)(16).

A novel, quantum psychopharmacological concept divides antipsychotic drugs into electron donors and acceptors. DA antagonists accept electrons, while agonists and DA itself give electrons away (17)(18). Electron acceptors promote GMV reduction, while donors, like DA, prevent brain atrophy. This is important as neuroimaging studies showed most DA-blocking antipsychotics to deplete the gray matter. This highlights the fact that DA (and its agonists) are indispensable for maintaining gray matter integrity (19)(20). Indeed, lower DA levels reflect higher gray matter loss. The partial DA receptor agonists, including aripiprazole, aripiprazole, cariprazine, and lumateperone, may preserve the GMV. However, more studies are needed to establish the biophysical properties of these agents (21). The same applies to ACh agonists, which exert antipsychotic properties, preserve the GMV, and give electrons away (20)(22)(23).

DA itself and several antipsychotic drugs are activators of AhR, a transcription factor that is also the master regulator of cellular senescence. In addition, AhR controls the growth of dendrites and dendritic spines, which comprise the bulk of GMV (24)(25). SCZ has been associated with premature cellular/neuronal senescence, a property that triggers GMV reduction. In the gut, AhR-induced cellular senescence increases the barrier permeability, facilitating microbial translocation into the host tissues and organs (26)(27). Like bacteria, commensal viruses, known as the virome, dwell in the gut and other organs. Interestingly, a virome was recently identified in the brain, linking viruses to premature neuronal senescence, GMV loss, and aggressive behavior (28). Indeed, virus-induced cellular senescence (VIS) has been documented during the COVID-19 pandemic, linking the virome to GMV reduction (29).

The pathway from AhR activation to premature cellular senescence, GMV loss, and aggressive behavior is likely comprised of the following steps:

1. Exogenous and endogenous ligands activate AhR, inducing cellular/neuronal senescence.
2. In the gut, intestinal epithelial cells (IECs) senescence disrupt the gut barrier, enabling microbial translocation from the GI tract into the systemic circulation.

3. SCZ and dementia are characterized by immune activation in response to translocated gut bacteria and viruses.
4. Deficient gut interleukin-22 (IL-22) increases intestinal permeability, enhancing microbial translocation. For this reason, human recombinant IL-22 may be therapeutic.
5. SCZ and dementias are comorbid with inflammatory bowel disease (IBD), emphasizing the critical role of microbial migration in these pathologies.
6. SCZ and dementias are characterized by upregulated peripheral blood translocation markers, further emphasizing the role of microbes.
7. bacterial and viral molecules in the brains of patients with SCZ and dementia further support microbial translocation in these pathologies.

Von Economo neurons (VENs) are large, spindle-shaped cells with a single dendrite that reside in layer five of the insular cortex (IC) and anterior cingulate cortex (ACC). VENs are part of the brain salience network (SN), a neuronal assembly associated with emotional intelligence, empathy, and morality (30) (see next chapter). Due to their large cell membrane surface, VENs are susceptible to the lipid bilayer's peroxidation, explaining why these cells are preferentially affected in bvFTD and possibly in SCZ (31). As cognition is often intact in the initial phase of bvFTD, this condition is frequently misdiagnosed as SCZ, bipolar disorder, or major depression, triggering inadequate treatment and placement in forensic rather than palliative facilities (32).

A recent transcriptomic study of human VENs has implicated dysfunctional VENs in SMI (33). For example, adrenoceptor alpha 1A (ADRA1A), gamma-aminobutyric acid (GABA) type A receptor, GABA subunit theta (GABRQ), and vesicular monoamine transporter 2 (VMAT2) are VEN signatures identified in SCZ and dementia (34). As VMAT2 provides neuroprotection from both endogenous and exogenous toxicants, loss of this protein may activate AhR via ligands, such as DA and serotonin (5HT) (35) (Fig.2). Indeed, dysfunctional VMAT2 was associated with excessive fear, linking monoamines to fearful traumatic experiences (36). Indeed, aggression and violent behaviors were previously associated with monoamine oxidase A (MAOA), a gene that implicates dysfunctional DA and 5-HT in this pathology (37)(38)(39). This may explain why, compared to AD, in which 10% of patients exhibit criminal behavior,50% of bvFTD patients commit crimes criminality, including homicide (40)(41)(42)(43).

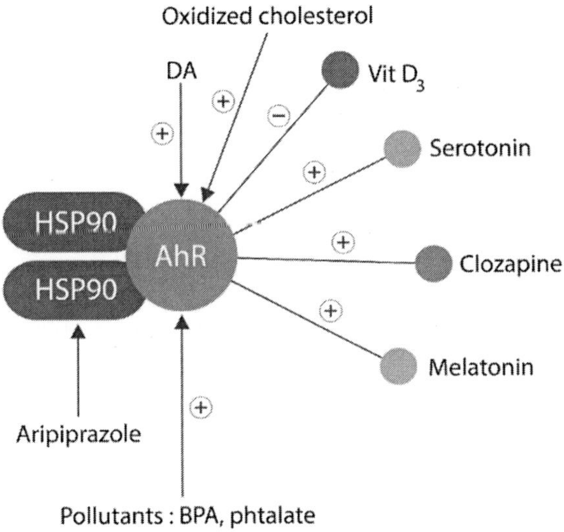


**AhR is a sensor for endogenous and exogenous molecules, including DA, serotonin (5-HT), vitamin D, melatonin, cholesterol, pollutants, bisphenol A, and phthalate. In the cytosol, AhR is stabilized by two heat shock protein 90 (HSP90) molecules. When attached to HSP90, AhR is inactive as it cannot enter the nucleus and act as a transcription factor. Aripiprazole enhances the HSP90 bond with AhR, probably explaining why it does not induce GMV loss.**

From the judiciary perspective, bvFTD is highly challenging as these patients can often appreciate right and wrong but cannot adaptively act on this assessment (see attached paper).

## Dementia and the criminal justice system

Over 6 million older Americans are currently living with neurocognitive disorders, and a small percentage of this population violates social norms and engages in criminal behavior, including homicide (44). For example, according to the most extensive dataset, 20% of individuals living with bvFTD commit murder (45).

In AD, criminal violations are less common. However, some individuals enter the criminal justice system and get incarcerated or admitted to State hospitals. Indeed, between 1993 and 2013, the "graying" of the population throughout the country has contributed to a 400% increase in the number of State prison inmates over the age of 55, suggesting a direct correlation between longevity and the prevalence of dementia (46)(47).

State hospitals and prisons are ill-equipped for the treatment of patients with age-related diseases who may not be independent in their activities of daily living (ADLs). In addition, these institutions operate on a recovery model, which does not apply to patients with neurocognitive disorders who are rarely restored to competency. Since more adequate palliative care facilities are not currently available, individuals with dementing illnesses will continue to inundate the prisons and State Hospitals for the foreseeable future.

The criminal justice system for the elderly with dementia requires changes in two specific areas:

1. Development of public, private, or hybrid palliative institutions specialized for patients with dementia.
2. The sequence of events from the arrest to sentencing and incarceration requires a system of diverting dementia patients away from the criminal justice system.

The interaction of patients with dementia with the criminal justice system, from arrest through incarceration, has not been adequately studied, and few professionals can navigate this system with confidence. Along these lines, in 2022, the Commission on Law and Aging released a study on people with dementia in the criminal justice system. This report, based on a nationwide survey of legal professionals, healthcare workers, and correctional staff, has concluded that:

1. A growing number of persons with dementia come to the attention of law enforcement, and this number is likely to increase over the next decade.
2. There are few screening tools available to law enforcement to assess the presence or absence of dementia in arrestees.
3. People living with dementia (PLWD) who are deemed incompetent to stand trial should not be committed to State hospitals for restoration of capacity.
4. Strategies to divert people with dementia from entering the criminal justice system are needed.
5. Palliative care units in State hospitals or prisons are urgently needed as individuals with criminal violations are ineligible for placement in the community.

Should individuals with dementia who commit crimes be protected in the same manner as people living with SCZ who may be deemed “not guilty because of insanity”? Since “not guilty because of dementia” does not exist, people with cognitive disorders, especially bvFTD, may be trapped by the mental competency laws. For example, cases of dementia superimposed on the “stable phase” of SCZ are also referred to State hospitals, although they may never be restored to capacity. In California, the Murphy conservatorship is a legal avenue for these patients. This legal pathway refers to a court-ordered appointment of a guardian for an individual who cannot regain capacity and who is charged with a felony involving great bodily harm, death, or a severe threat to the physical well-being of another person. However, Murphy's conservatorship does not solve the placement issue in the community, as felons with or without a conservatorship are not eligible to reside in an outside facility. This situation is illustrated by the following case from Patton State Hospital:

*Murder at Del Rio*

*RB was an African-American female in her 70s who had chronic SCZ since the age of 30. RB resided at Del Rio Convalescent Center in Bel Gardens, California, a community approximately 25 miles East of Los Angeles. RB was on SCZ maintenance therapy, consisting of Haldol Decanoate monthly injection, and when agitated due to her auditory hallucinations, RB received rescue medication.*

*Ms. RB suffered from insomnia, and 2 or 3 nights per week, she would pace up and down the hallway, talking to herself. After an hour or two, RB would return to her room and sleep till the following day. As this behavior had been going on for many years, the staff viewed it as "normal" for this patient, and since RB rarely bothered anyone else, they seldom intervened.*

*One night in 1998, instead of walking back to her room, RB, unnoticed by the staff, entered another room where a bedridden 69-year-old lady with advanced dementia resided. The lady had her old purse on the pillow next to her. This purse was brought in by her family, hoping that it would remind the patient of the happier days in her life and bring her some joy. RB grabbed the purse and strangled the bedridden patient with the purse string. Next, RB proceeded to hit her victim in the forehead, causing a fracture that ultimately killed her.*

*After the police arrived to examine the scene, RB was transferred to Los Alamitos Medical Center, an acute local hospital with a geropsychiatric unit, where she stayed until admitted to Patton State Hospital.*

This case portrays an unprovoked homicide perpetrated by a patient with a long history of SCZ and superimposed late-life dementia. Although cruel, this crime lacked "men's rea" knowledge of wrongdoing. For this reason, instead of being jailed, JB was transferred to a state hospital under Cal. Pen. Code § 1370, incompetent to stand trial. RB never regained capacity and was placed on Murphy's conservatorship. In contrast to this case, the opposite is also problematic when the police, physicians, or judges surmise that an older individual has dementia and place them in a facility, therefore denying them freedom and access to their property. These incidents are sometimes initiated by the family members who consciously or unconsciously aspire to inherit early the property or financial assets of their loved one.

Here is a real case from our practice:

*"I need to talk to President Clinton."*

*FDW was a short, slim man in his mid-80s, a known sculptor from the post-WW2 era, famous for his statues depicting Marines in action. FDW had a successful career, an active social life, and no prior psychiatric history.*

*I met FDW in a nursing home in Anaheim, California, where I served as a psychiatric consultant. FDW was brought in by the police to West Anaheim Medical Center Emergency Room (ER) because he got lost and ran a red light. When approached by the officers, he "seemed confused, mumbling something about President Clinton." While in the ER, the social worker found that FDW was recently diagnosed with SCZ and had a conservatorship, which named his wife as conservator.*

*EB's laboratory studies showed mild to moderate dehydration but were otherwise unremarkable. The ER doctor diagnosed him with acute delirium superimposed on a mild cognitive impairment (MCI). The ER social worker called the wife, and it was established that she was FDW's third spouse, who was 45 years younger and was assigned to be his conservator. She agreed to transfer FDW to a nearby locked nursing home specializing in SCZ.*

*The next day, I was called by the nursing home staff and the primary physician to see FDW because "he is delusional and keeps asking staff to call President Clinton." He insisted he leave the facility "because I have a speech in San Diego, in front of the Marines." FDW held a paper with a phone number that he handed to staff members, asking them to call the President at that number. Thinking that FDW was "delusional," everyone in that facility ignored him.*

*During my interview with him, FDW was alert and oriented in all four spheres, including person, time, place, and reason for examination. He was unsure about the name of the nursing home he was in, but this was not surprising, considering that he had arrived there only 24 hours earlier. FDW was coherent, but he presented with mild word-finding difficulties, which he compensated for by talking slowly and using synonyms. He scored 29/30 on the mini-mental status exam (MMSE) and told me that because of his artwork, he developed a close relationship with the Marines, and every year on Memorial Day (the next day), he spoke in front of the Marine Corps. Asked about President Clinton, he said that presidents usually attend his Memorial Day speeches, and President Clinton called him to let him know that he would be present. He offered me the phone number to contact the President. I did not call but started to believe his story. There was no SCZ at all, and I never found out who or why diagnosed FDW with this condition (he might have had a delirium that was confounded with SCZ). Indeed, FDW's conservatorship papers listed SCZ as the primary diagnosis and dementia, possibly Alzheimer's type, as the secondary. After discussing the case with the primary physician, it was decided that FDW should be admitted to the geriatric psychiatry unit at West Anaheim Medical Center to complete a dementia workup. When neuroimaging and blood work came back normal, FDW was taken off the conservatorship, and the SCZ diagnosis was replaced with acute delirium; the clinical picture likely manifested when the police stopped him.*

This case illustrates how a misdiagnosed SCZ or dementia can deprive an older individual of both their freedom and property. Indeed, the criminal justice system lacks a consistent approach to screening older offenders for dementia. There are instances in which the police realize that the arrestee has a cognitive impairment but have no adequate place to bring the person except the nearest ER.

The following case mirrors societal stereotyping of older individuals as having dementia when making non-conventional choices. Although these concerns may be genuine and well-intentioned, they may affect the autonomy and freedom of aging people to actuate their property and finances according to their will.

Turbulence in *Leisure World*

*EB was a gentleman in his late 80s, a retired physicist known for participating in the Manhattan Project after WW2. EB was never married and had no children of his own. He lived alone in Leisure World, a retirement community in Southern California, and enjoyed traveling and interacting with friends. EB hired a Mexican lady to clean his home twice weekly a few years prior. In time, he became friends with this person. At 87, he decided that upon his death, he would leave his property and seven-figure life savings to this lady. He wrote his will to this effect and notarized it in Leisure World. However, the notary felt this could be inappropriate. He called the retirement community social worker, expressing his concerns that "EB may not be in his right mind" and that the lady may have coerced him to sell the property to her.*

*The social worker told EB that a psychiatric evaluation was necessary to make sure that he was competent and that the will would not be challenged by a potential relative who might come forward after his death. EB was initially upset but agreed to be evaluated. During the assessment, EB was calm, cooperative, and pleasant. He did not exhibit pathology, and his thought process was logical and sequential, with tight associations. His long and short-term memory were intact.*

*When asked about his decision to leave his property and finances to the lady helping him, he stated: "You know, a man doesn't go to his grave with a U-Haul; my house and money cannot go with me." He explained the rationale of leaving his property to a needy person vs. the government. He was not upset with the government, saying, "I gave them the atomic bomb of which I am not proud." He became tearful and apologized for sobbing. I felt that he had reached the stage of gerotranscendence, a cosmic communion with the infinite and a sense of detachment from this world and everything in it, including his possessions that he cared so much about when he was younger (48). This man was of sound mind, and his desire to give his property to someone in need after his death was reasonable.*

*EB was cleared of any psychiatric pathology, he did not have dementia, and he logically made his decisions; therefore, he was not coerced or incompetent to dispose of his belongings in the manner he desired.*

This book, aiming to steer controversy and open honest discussions, significantly contributes to neuropsychiatry. It prompts us to consider how much our discipline relies on unbiased data, steering clear of the influence of biased sources such as industry-sponsored studies. Along this line, we focus on microbial and viral translocation from the GI tract into the systemic circulation and its role in the etiopathogenesis of SMI. We delve deeper into the role of pathogen-induced premature cellular senescence and the brain virome on GMV loss, a key biomarker of aggressive behavior, violence, and criminality (8). Aside from GMV reduction, senescent brain cells contribute to lipid peroxidation, depletion of rapid rhythms on electroencephalogram (EEG), and neuronal death by ferroptosis.

# ARTICLE FOR CHAPTER 1: NEURODEGENERATION BEHIND BARS: FROM MOLECULES TO JURISPRUDENCE

## ADONIS SFERA[1], CAROLINA OSORIO[2], ROBERTO GRADINI[3] AND AMY PRICE[4]

*1 Department of Psychiatry, Patton State Hospital, Patton, CA, USA*
*2 Loma Linda University, Loma Linda, CA, USA*
*3 Department of Pathology, Sapienza University of Rome, Rome, Italy*
*4 Evidence Based Health Care, University of Oxford, Oxford, UK*

*Edited by:*

*Iliya Lefterov, University of Pittsburgh, USA*

*Reviewed by:*

*Mariana Dimitrova Arnaoudova, Medical University Varna, Bulgaria*
*Lyudmila Lozanova, Trakia University, Bulgaria*

**Keywords: frontotemporal dementia, m'Naughten rule, von Economo neurons, saience network, neurodegenerative disorders**

The prison population is aging and developing neurodegenerative disorders at a faster pace than the general population. Hidden among this group of recidivist, career criminals, there is a subpopulation of first offenders with frontotemporal dementia behavioral variant (bvFTD). The pathological hallmark of this condition is frontotemporal lobar degeneration (FTLD), which early on spares cognition, yet predisposes to criminal violations. From the neurobiological perspective, bvFTD originates in a large-scale brain network in charge of motivation and concern, the salience network (SN). From the judiciary perspective, bvFTD is challenging because patients often retain the "appreciation" of right and wrong, yet may be organically incapable to act accordingly. Equally challenging are the dispositions in regards to bvFTD patients: return to the community, risking further violations, vs. incarceration with dismal punitive or rehabilitative benefit. In this article, we advocate for screening of all first offenders who are 55 years of age or older via neuropsychological testing and/or positron emission tomography (PET) and should bvFTD be diagnosed, their placement in, yet to be developed, palliative programs in state or private facilities.

## Introduction

It is estimated that 40,000 inmates with dementia are currently incarcerated in U.S. prisons with forecasted increases topping a quarter of a million persons by 2050 (1). The reasons for the graying of prison population are multiple, including longer incarceration periods, mandatory prison sentences, and an increase in the number of older first offenders (2). It is also believed that people in prison age at a faster rate than the general population (3). The category of older first offenders has increased steadily over the past two decades. According to the Human Rights Watch report, the number of persons over 60 years of age entering state prisons as new court commitments grew by 109% between 1995 and 2009 (4). Recent studies demonstrate that 54% of bvFTD patients commit criminal acts (5) and since this condition represents 5–6% of all dementias, it is possible that it accounts for the large numbers of older first offenders entering prisons. Moreover, up to 51% of bvFTD patients are misdiagnosed at the initial evaluation because the symptoms resemble psychiatric conditions and are missed by routine cognitive testing (6). In this opinion article, we emphasize a multidisciplinary approach to bvFTD; we believe that input from disciplines such as neurobiology, psychology, psychiatry, forensic psychiatry, and jurisprudence could help us comprehend better this complex disorder.

## Neurobiology of the Salience Network

### *The Network*

It has been known for almost a century that frontotemporal lesions lead to anti-social acts (7). The reason for this condition is not entirely clear, but it has been hypothesized that the anterior insular cortex (AIC) and anterior cingulate cortex (ACC), especially in the right hemisphere, harbor pro-social cognition, such as the sense of fairness and playing by the rules and that lesions in these nodes result in criminal violations (8). Currently, this represents the working hypothesis attempting to explain why 54% of patients with bvFTD are involved in criminal behavior, compared to only 12% of patients with Alzheimer's disease (5).

Recent studies demonstrated that AIC and ACC in the right hemisphere are in charge of implementing and adjusting mental models to social contexts, for example, concern for the rule of law and civilized behavior (9). Patients with bvFTD may understand legal and societal rules, however, they seem to present with dissociation between the knowledge of wrongfulness of acts and the concern for avoiding them.

The pathology in bvFTD consists of FTLD, which originates in the ACC and AIC, mainly in the right brain hemisphere. This focal lesion represents the starting point of a unique trail leading, via psychological and anthropological domains, to jurisprudence. Functional neuroimaging studies combined with brain network analysis place these nodes in the SN, which is one of the large-scale brain intrinsic connectivity networks (ICN) (10, 11). It is involved in selecting and attributing salience to external or internal stimuli. Three ICNs have implications for bvFTD: the central executive network (CEN), the SN, and the default mode network (DMN) (12) (Table 1).

In addition to its cortical areas, SN comprises subcortical nodes, such as amygdala, ventral tegmental area, substantia nigra, and the thalamus (13). Together the cortical and subcortical components of action (SMA) system, which translates selected thoughts and ideas into action. This process may function as a filter that prioritizes informational input by tagging it with various degrees of salience (14). Input raising enough concern and requiring immediate physical or mental action is prioritized and enacted.

Neuroimaging studies demonstrate AIC activation during risk evaluation, suggesting the insula may play a role in human concern about obstacles in reaching targets (15). The ACC activates during evaluation of prediction models or reward related activities, suggesting a connection between anticipation, motivation, and action (16). Direct stimulation of ACC triggers motivation and readiness to act: in case reports of direct electrical stimulation of the ACC, patients reported having a sensation of imminent challenge coupled with a determined attitude to overcome it (17). Ability to abide by the rule of law or the societal code of conduct requires mental operations such as risk evaluation, prediction of behavioral outcome, and motivation to avoid negative outcomes, capabilities, which patients with bvFTD do not possess.

**Table 1 | The three major ICNs and their implications in bvFTD.**

| **CN** | **Cortical location** | **Function** | **Social context** |
|---|---|---|---|
| CEN | Dorsolateral prefrontal cortex (DLPFC), supramarginal gyrus | Planning, working memory, direction of attention | Outer reality, task, actions, problem-solving |
| DMN | Posterior cingulate cortex, medial prefrontal cortex, medial temporal lobe, and angular gyrus | Self-related mental activity, including autobiographical, self-monitoring, and social functions | Inner reality, thoughts, ideas, societal rules, self, and the community |
| SN | Anterior cingulate cortex (ACC) and frontoinsular cortex (FIC) | Detection and orientation to salient external stimuli and internal events | Self-related mental activity, including autobiographical, self-monitoring, and social functions |

## *The Cells*

At the cellular level, the SN is home to von Economo neurons (VENs). VENs are large projection neurons with equally large axons and high conduction speed, qualities, which enable them to integrate multiple signals from distant brain areas (18, 19). Recent studies demonstrate that FTLD originates and preferentially targets VENs in the right ACC and AIC. Interestingly, there are 30% more VENs in the right hemisphere (20). Since empathy and social intelligence are impaired in bvFTD, it is believed that these qualities are lateralized in the SN of the right hemisphere, containing more VENs (21). The right hemisphere is known to participate in social intelligence, which includes the need for affiliation with peers, while the left contributes to individuation, competition, and differentiation from the group (22, 23). In bvFTD, the VENs population of ACC is reduced by an average of 53–74% and most surviving VENs are severely altered (18, 24). Interestingly, suicide completers have a higher number of VENs, suggesting that over-attribution of saliency may overwhelm this network (20). The role of VENs' in salience processing is further suggested by the fact that these neurons express high levels of disruption in schizophrenia 1 (DISK 1) protein, known to be associated with the ability to shift attention (25).

### *The Molecules*

At the molecular level of VENs, bvFTD was shown to target either the DNA-binding protein TDP-43 or the microtubules associated tau protein (MAPT) (26, 27). Tau protein is known to be a microtubule (MT) stabilizer, while TDP-43 forms cytoplasmic mRNP granules that are transported via MTs to distal neuronal compartments (28). MTs were demonstrated essential in information processing and memory encoding

(29). For example, hyper-phosphorylation of tau, which is known to impair MT assembly and structure also impairs cognition (30). VENs are known by their large diameter axons, which may contain the highest proportion of MTs in the CNS. The loss of VENs in FTLD may be secondary to the loss of MTs, and thus constitute the reason that these neurons are preferentially targeted by this neurodegenerative process. In addition, biophysical evidence documents the ability of MTs to process information by accessing logic gates in transistor-like fashion, as well as by the ability to reorganize their molecular structures in response to electromagnetic fields (31–33). Taken together, these capabilities of MTs suggest a role in information and saliency processing.

## Psychology and Anthropology

From a psychological perspective, the loss of MTs and VENs may manifest as impaired social cognition. Psychological traits engendered by the SN and lost in bvFTD include: detection of deception, empathy, detection of social error, motivation, risk prediction, recognition of error, awareness, insight, risky decisions, rapid intuition, detecting malevolent intentions in others, viewing faces of allies.

Anthropologically, the human civilization was ultimately engendered by the human brain. Over time, the SN may have sharpened human attention and concentration, enabling symbolic representation, which is the stepping stone of civilization (34, 35). By affecting the same brain networks that contributed to the development of human civilization, FTLD may regress the thought process to a pre-symbolic stage that dominated human thinking prior to the existence of the civil society and the rule of law. For example, this stage may have been depicted by Aeschylus (456 BC) in "Oresteia" trilogy, which chronicles the House of Atreus, disintegrating under a curse consisting of a primeval cycle of blood-revenge. This curse is reversed by the implementation of a civil society based on the rule of law (36).

## Jurisprudence and the Salience Network

Disturbed individuals who commit crimes remain dilemmas for society since ancient times. Plato, for example, believed that such individuals were not responsible for their acts the way others were and should not be punished by the same means (37).

The majority of patients with dementia do not engage in violent acts, however, about a third are aggressive, presenting with agitation, paranoia, wandering, and sexual disinhibition. These behaviors can bring them into conflict with the criminal justice system (38). In bvFTD assessing competency to stand trial (CST) and determining culpability and suitable sentencing is especially challenging because these defendants are sometimes able to appreciate the wrongfulness of their acts and might understand societal rules, but may be organically incapable of regulating their behavior (39). Currently, in the US, the M'Naughte rule (United States

Code, Title 18, Section 17) defines legal incapacity of a defendant as being "unable to appreciate the nature and quality of the wrongfulness of his acts." According to M'Naughten rule, patients with bvFTD would not qualify to plead "not guilty by reason of insanity" (5). A similar situation is encountered in the assessment of the capacity to stand trial (CST). The legal standard for CST is "whether the individual has sufficient present ability to consult with his lawyer with a reasonable degree of rational understanding and whether he has a rational as well as factual understanding of the proceedings against him (40, 41)." Frequently psychiatric reviews leave these accused in legal limbo, waiting to regain competency in facilities embracing recovery models (42).

In the case of Alzheimer's disease, studies demonstrate that 30–50% of criminal defendants older than 60 are incompetent to stand trial (IST) (43), but no similar studies have been completed in bvFTD.

We are in need of a modern system for placement of individuals with neurodegenerative disorders. Such a system, based on the palliative model, would benefit elderly offenders diagnosed with dementia, while at the same time help decongest correctional facilities not designed to accommodate patients with neurodegeneration.

We recommend task forces at both federal and state levels to study the issue of palliative placement of incarcerated dementia patients as well as screening first offenders 55 years of age or older for bvFTD. The screening should follow the criteria of the 2011 International Behavioral Variant Frontotemporal Dementia Criteria Consortium (BVFDC). These criteria consist of six clinical hallmarks, including: disinhibition, apathy/inertia, loss of sympathy/empathy, perseverative/compulsive

behaviors, hyperorality, and dysexecutive neuropsychological profile. According to BVFDC, at least three of these features must be present for the diagnosis of "possible" bvFTD. "Probable" bvFTD requires the presence of functional disability and characteristic neuroimaging in addition to clinical symptoms. "Definite" diagnosis of bvFTD needs either documentation of FTLDby histopathological confirmation or a pathogenic mutation (44).

## Conclusion

The difficulty in distinguishing symptoms of bvFTD from antisocial personality disorder or psychosis constitutes the reason individuals with this condition can be found in correctional institutions. FTLD of the structures comprising the SN renders these defendants organically incapable of concern with social norms or the rule of law. This interesting observation offers a unique glimpse in the mechanisms the brain uses in selecting salient stimuli from the background noise of irrelevant input.

The criminal justice system and the correctional institutions were not designed to accommodate persons with dementia. Most forensic psychiatric programs are founded on the recovery model geared toward the mentally ill expected to regain CST and is not adequate for individuals with neurodegenerative disorders. Appropriate care of these patients requires the development of preventative programs for screening and placement in palliative care facilities.

## References

1. Bureau of Justice Statistics: https://csat.bjs.ojp.gov/quick-tables
2. Greene M, Ahalt C, Stijacic-Cenzer I, Metzger L, Williams B. Older adults in jail: high rates and early onset of geriatric conditions. Health Justice. 2018 Feb 17;6(1):3. doi: 10.1186/s40352-018-0062-9.
3. Ahalt C, Trestman RL, Rich JD, Greifinger RB, Williams BA. Paying the price: the pressing need for quality, cost, and outcomes data to improve correctional health care for older prisoners. J Am Geriatr Soc. 2013 Nov;61(11):2013-9. doi: 10.1111/jgs.12510. PMID: 24219203; PMCID: PMC3984258.
4. Jääskeläinen E, Juola P, Hirvonen N, McGrath JJ, Saha S, Isohanni M, Veijola J, Miettunen J. A systematic review and meta-analysis of recovery in schizophrenia. Schizophr Bull. 2013 Nov;39(6):1296-306. doi: 10.1093/schbul/sbs130.
5. Marwaha S, Johnson S. Schizophrenia and employment a review. Soc Psychiatry Psychiatr Epidemiol. 2004 May;39(5):337-49. doi: 10.1007/s00127-004-0762-4.

6. Lieberman JA, Small SA, Girgis RR. Early Detection and Preventive Intervention in Schizophrenia: From Fantasy to Reality. Am J Psychiatry. 2019 Oct 1;176(10):794-810.
doi: 10.1176/apps. app.2019.19080865.
7. Chester DS, Lynam DR, Milich R, DeWall CN. Physical aggressiveness and gray matter deficits in the ventromedial prefrontal cortex. Cortex. 2017 Dec;97:17-22.
doi: 10.1016/j.cortex.2017.09.024.
8. 23. Deng MY, McAlonan GM, Cheung C, Chiu CP, Law CW, Cheung V, et al. A naturalistic study of grey matter volume increase after early treatment in anti-psychotic naive, newly diagnosed schizophrenia. Psychopharmacology (Berl) 2009;206:437–446. doi: 10.1007/s00213-009-1619-z.
9. Girgis RR, Diwadkar VA, Nutche JJ, Sweeney JA, Keshavan MS, Hardan AY. Risperidone in first-episode psychosis: a longitudinal, exploratory voxel-based morphometric study. Schizophr Res. 2006;82:89–94. doi: 10.1016/j.schres.2005.10.019.
10. Vita A, De Peri L, Deste G, Barlati S, Sacchetti E. The Effect of Antipsychotic Treatment on Cortical Gray Matter Changes in Schizophrenia: Does the Class Matter? A Meta-analysis and Meta-regression of Longitudinal Magnetic Resonance Imaging Studies. Biol Psychiatry. 2015 Sep 15;78(6):403-12.
Doi: 10.1016/j.biopsych.2015.02.008.
11. Liu X, Liu Z, Wu Z, Ren J, Fan Y, Sun L, Cao G, Niu Y, Zhang B, Ji Q, et al. Resurrection of endogenous retroviruses during aging reinforces senescence. Cell. 2023 Jan 19;186(2):287-304.e26. doi: 10.1016/j.cell.2022.12.017.
12. Crowner ML, Douyon R, Convit A, Gaztanaga P, Volavka J, Bakall R. Akathisia and violence. Psychopharmacol Bull. 1990;26(1):115-7. PMID: 1973544.
13. Li, C.-T., Chou, K.-H., Su, T.-P., Huang, C.-C., Chen, M.-H., Bai, Y.M., & Lin, C.-P. (2013). Gray matter abnormalities in schizophrenia patients with tardive dyskinesia: A magnetic resonance imaging voxel-based morphometry study. PLoS ONE, 8(8), Article e71034. https://doi.org/10.1371/journal.pone.0071034

14. Chester DS, Lynam DR, Milich R, DeWall CN. Physical aggressiveness and gray matter deficits in the ventromedial prefrontal cortex. Cortex. 2017 Dec;97:17-22. doi: 10.1016/j.cortex.2017.09.024.
15. Zhang YD, Zhou JS, Lu FM, Wang XP. Reduced gray matter volume in male adolescent violent offenders. PeerJ. 2019 Sep 3;7:e7349. doi: 10.7717/peerj.7349.
16. Hofhansel L, Weidler C, Votinov M, Clemens B, Raine A, Habel U. Morphology of the criminal brain: gray matter reductions are linked to antisocial behavior in offenders. Brain Struct Funct. 2020 Sep;225(7):2017-2028. doi: 10.1007/s00429-020-02106-6
17. Kawczak P, Bober L, Bączek T. Activity evaluation of some psychoactive drugs with the application of QSAR/QSPR modeling methods. Med Chem Res. 2018;27(10):2279-2286. doi: 10.1007/s00044-018-2234-5.
18. Martínez A, Ibarra IA, Vargas R. A quantum chemical approach represents a new perspective concerning agonist and antagonist drugs in schizophrenia and Parkinson's. PLoS One. 2019 Dec 12;14(12):e0224691. doi: 10.1371/journal.pone.022469
19. Kurose S, Kubota M, Takahata K, Yamamoto Y, Fujiwara H, Kimura Y, Ito H, Takeuchi H, Mimura M, Suhara T, Higuchi M. Relationship between regional gray matter volumes and dopamine D2 receptor and transporter in living human brains. Hum Brain Mapp. 2021 Aug 15;42(12):4048-4058. doi: 10.1002/hbm.25538.
20. Rogeau, A., Nordio, G., Veronese, M. et al. The relationship between glutamate, dopamine, and cortical gray matter: A simultaneous PET-MR study. Mol Psychiatry 27, 3493–3500 (2022). https://doi.org/10.1038/s41380-022-01596-6
21. Lai CH, Wu YT, Chen CY, Hou YC. Gray matter increases in fronto-parietal regions of depression patients with aripiprazole monotherapy: An exploratory study. Medicine (Baltimore). 2016 Aug;95(34): e4654. doi: 10.1097/MD.0000000000004654
22. Goode-Romero G, Dominguez L, Martínez A. Electron Donor-Acceptor Properties of Different Muscarinic Ligands: On the Road to Control Schizophrenia. J Chem Inf Model. 2021 Oct 25;61(10): 5117-5124. doi: 10.1021/acs.jcim.1c00780

23. Garzón B, Lövdén M, de Boer L, Axelsson J, Riklund K, Bäckman L, Nyberg L, Guitart-Masip M. Role of dopamine and gray matter density in aging effects and individual differences of functional connectomes. Brain Struct Funct. 2021 Apr;226(3):743-758. doi: 10.1007/s00429-020-02205-4
24. Kim HY, Huang BX, Spector AA. Phosphatidylserine in the brain: metabolism and function. Prog Lipid Res. 2014 Oct;56:1-18. doi: 10.1016/j.plipres.2014.06.002.
25. Kimura E, Kubo K, Matsuyoshi C, Benner S, Hosokawa M, Endo T, Ling W, Kohda M, Yokoyama K, Nakajima K, Kakeyama M, Tohyama C. Developmental origin of abnormal dendritic growth in the mouse brain induced by in utero disruption of aryl hydrocarbon receptor signaling. Neurotoxicol Teratol. 2015 Nov-Dec;52(Pt A):42-50. doi: 10.1016/j.ntt.2015.10.005.
26. Lau, V., Ramer, L. & Tremblay, MÈ. An aging, pathology burden, and glial senescence build-up hypothesis for late-onset Alzheimer's disease. Nat Commun 14, 1670 (2023). https://doi.org/10.1038/s41467-023-37304-3
27. Eckers, A., Jakob, S., Heiss, C. et al. The aryl hydrocarbon receptor promotes aging phenotypes across species. Sci Rep 6, 19618 (2016). https://doi.org/10.1038/srep19618
28. Dang X, Hanson BA, Orban ZS, Jimenez M, Suchy S, Koralnik IJ. Characterization of the brain virome in human immunodeficiency virus infection and substance use disorder. PLoS One. 2024 Apr 17;19(4):e0299891. doi: 10.1371/journal.pone.0299891.
29. Lee, S., Yu, Y., Trimpert, J. et al. Virus-induced senescence is a driver and therapeutic target in COVID-19. Nature 599, 283–289 (2021). https://doi.org/10.1038/s41586-021-03995-1
30. Seeley WW, et al. Distinctive neurons of the anterior cingulate and frontoinsular cortex: a historical perspective. Cereb. Cortex. 2012;22:245–250. doi: 10.1093/cercor/bhr005.
31. Hunter P. The basis of morality. Psychologists, anthropologists, and biologists are uncovering the bigger picture of the development of empathy and altruism. EMBO Rep. 2010 Mar;11(3):166-9. doi: 10.1038/embor.2010.19.

32. Brüne M, et al. Von Economo neuron density in the anterior cingulate cortex is reduced in early-onset schizophrenia. Acta Neuropathologica. 2010;119:771–778. doi: 10.1007/s00401-010-0673-2.
33. Dijkstra AA, Lin L-C, Nana AL, Gaus SE, Seeley WW. Von Economo neurons and fork cells: a neurochemical signature linked to monoaminergic function. Cereb. Cortex. 2016;28:131–144. doi: 10.1093/cercor/bhw358.
34. Guillot TS, Miller GW. Protective actions of the vesicular monoamine transporter 2 (VMAT2) in monoaminergic neurons. Mol Neurobiol. 2009 Apr;39(2):149-70. doi: 10.1007/s12035-009-8059-y.
35. Narboux-Nême, N., Sagné, C., Doly, S. et al. Severe Serotonin Depletion after Conditional Deletion of the Vesicular Monoamine Transporter 2 Gene in Serotonin Neurons: Neural and Behavioral Consequences. Neuropsychopharmacol 36, 2538–2550 (2011). https://doi.org/10.1038/npp.2011.142
36. Branco RC, Burkett JP, Black CA, Winokur E, Ellsworth W, Dhamsania RK, Lohr KM, Schroeder JP, Weinshenker D, Jovanovic T, Miller GW. Vesicular monoamine transporter 2 mediates fear behavior in mice. Genes Brain Behav. 2020 Jun;19(5):e12634. Doi: 10.1111/gbb.12634.
37. Kolla NJ, Bortolato M. The role of monoamine oxidase A in the neurobiology of aggressive, antisocial, and violent behavior: A tale of mice and men. Prog Neurobiol. 2020 Nov;194:101875. doi 10.1016/j.pneurobio.2020.101875.
38. Sohrabi S. The criminal gene: the link between MAOA and aggression (REVIEW). BMC Proc. 2015 Jan 14;9(Suppl 1):A49. doi: 10.1186/1753-6561-9-S1-A49.
39. McSwiggan S, Elger B, Appelbaum PS. The forensic use of behavioral genetics in criminal proceedings: Case of the MAOA-L genotype. Int J Law Psychiatry. 2017 Jan-Feb;50:17-23. doi: 10.1016/j.ijlp.2016.09.005.
40. Haußmann R, Krug C, Noppes F, Brandt M, Lange J, Donix M. Delinquentes Verhalten im Rahmen more frontotemporal Demenzen und der Alzheimer-Erkrankung [Criminal behavior in frontotemporal

dementia and Alzheimer's disease]. Nervenarzt. 2022 Jan;93(1):59-67. German. Doi: 10.1007/s00115-021-01070-8.

41. Liljegren M, Naasan G, Temlett J, Perry DC, Rankin KP, Merrilees J, Grinberg LT, Seeley WW, Englund E, Miller BL. Criminal behavior in frontotemporal dementia and Alzheimer's disease. JAMA Neurol. 2015 Mar;72(3):295-300. doi: 10.1001/jamaneurol.2014.3781.
42. Talaslahti T, Ginters M, Kautiainen H, Vataja R, Elonheimo H, Erkinjuntti T, Suvisaari J, Lindberg N, Koponen H. Criminal Behavior in the Four Years Preceding Diagnosis of Neurocognitive Disorder: A Nationwide Register Study in Finland. Am J Geriatr Psychiatry. 2021 Jul;29(7):657-665. doi: 10.1016/j.jagp.2020.11.011.
43. Hatem Z, Amina G, Yosr H, et al: Homicide révélateur d'une démence [Homicide revealing dementia]. Revue Maghrebine de Neurosciences 4:1–4, 2009
44. Tali Elsayed Sundakov-Krumins, Sean Lubbe, Anne Pamela Frances Wand; Homicide and Dementia: A Systematic Review. Dement Geriatr Cogn Disord 19 April 2022; 51 (1): 1–17. https://doi.org/10.1159/000521878
45. Schier E, Baird A, Kennett J. Dataset of published Australian of homicide in which the accused had a diagnosis of dementia. 2020. https://doi.org/10.17632/wn8kr5htsg
46. Brindle N, Kennedy M, Walsh C, Alderson B. The Interface between Dementia and the Criminal Justice System. In: A Clinician's Brief Guide to Dementia and the Law. Cambridge University Press; 2023:144-150.
47. Persons Living with Dementia in the Criminal Legal System. American Bar Association Commission on Law and Aging in collaboration with NASMHPD Research Institute, 2022. https://www.americanbar.org/news/abanews/aba-news-archives/2022/06/dementia-in-the-criminal-justice-system/
48. Jewell AJ. Tornstam's notion of gerotranscendence: re-examining and questioning the theory. J Aging Stud. 2014 Aug;30:112-20. doi: 10.1016/j.jaging.2014.04.003.

# CHAPTER 2

# NEUROSCIENCE IN THE COURTROOM

Neuroscience has made significant strides in the US courtrooms as neuroimaging, initially used to provide information about the victim, can now be utilized for identifying potential pathology in perpetrators (1)(2). Usually, when a central nervous system (CNS) lesion is located, the testifying neuroscientist is asked to decide whether a person is meant to break the law. In the US jurisprudence, a crime consists of a subjective component, "men's rea," and an objective one, "actus reus." The presence of both usually leads to a guilty verdict, while one component alone does not meet the "beyond reasonable doubt" criterion.

In 1966, Charles Joseph Whitman, known as the "Texas Tower Sniper," was a 25-year-old University of Texas student and ex-marine. He climbed to the top of the University of Texas Clock Tower and went on a shooting spree, killing 14 people and wounding another 33. After being shot by the police, an autopsy revealed that Whitman had a brain tumor located above his amygdala. The autopsy concluded that the cancer did not influence Whitman's behavior during the shooting. However, others believed that this pathology may have increased impulsivity to the level of violence, especially as Whitman visited several university doctors in 1965 and was prescribed psychotropic medications (3). The unanswered question is: should Whitman have survived, would the presence of the tumor convinced the jury that Whitman was not responsible for the crime because of insanity?

Along this line, a more common neuroimaging marker, brain atrophy, was sufficient to persuade a jury that John W. Hinckley Jr. was not responsible for his crime. On March 30th, 1981, John W. Hinckley Jr shot President Ronald Reagan and three other people (4). His infatuation with actress Jodie Foster and his plan to assassinate a president to impress her led his defense team to argue that John W. Hinckley Jr had undiagnosed SCZ. Hinckley Jr.'s attorneys based this hypothesis on a computerized axial tomography

(CAT) scan showing brain atrophy, a pathology more common in patients with SCZ compared to the general population. This convinced the jury that John W. Hinckley Jr was "not guilty because of insanity."

Another jury rejected a similar hypothesis in the case of *People v. Weinstein,* a man who in 1992 threw his former wife out of a 12-story building, trying to make her death look like a suicide (5). In this case, a CAT scan showed a large cyst impinging on Weinstein's brain. Still, the Court did not accept it as an attenuating circumstance because the prosecution presented cases of individuals with identical or similar pathologies who had not engaged in criminal activity.

These real-life vignettes illustrate how neuroscience can influence judicial decisions by deciding whether the defendant intended to break the law.

Over the past two decades, the US Supreme Court based three separate decisions on neuroscientific findings: in 2002, the justices opined that executing an intellectually disabled or legally insane person is a violation of the Eighth Amendment's ban on cruel and unusual punishment. In 2005, the Supreme Court cited neuroscience in establishing that the prefrontal cortex of juveniles is not fully developed. Therefore, those under the age of 18 cannot receive the death penalty. Again, in 2012, the Supreme Court applied the same reasoning when it decided that juveniles could not receive life imprisonment without the possibility of parole (6).

## Not guilty because of dementia?

Not guilty because of insanity is a well-known plea in which the defendant claims mental illness or incapacity at the time of the offense (7). This plea does not apply to people with dementia because, unlike SCZ patients, they are believed incapable of learning new information to recover and cooperate with the courts. However, certain dementias that primarily affect executive function and leave cognition intact, such as bvFTD, may lead the forensic evaluator to believe that the defendant could be capable of standing trial and be sent to prison rather than a facility specialized in dementia.

The following case involves a psychiatrist who practiced in Riverside County, California. Joel Stanley Dreyer, a respected psychiatrist, worked in the community for 40 years, was diagnosed with bvFTD at the age of 62 but continued working until the age of 72. In 2010, Dr. Dreyer was convicted of prescribing, selling, and distributing large amounts of addictive painkillers and benzodiazepines. As a result, one person died of an overdose, and Dr. Dryer's license was revoked. Despite the opinion of experts that Dreyer suffered from bvFTD, he was sentenced to 10 years in a prison/medical facility. In 2012, a higher court overturned the sentence, holding that the judge should have ordered a special competency hearing during the trial (United States v. Dreyer, 705 F.3d 951 [9th Cir. 2013]). However, Dr. Dreyer served his entire sentence because he could not secure 50% of the votes in the United States Court of Appeals for the Ninth Circuit. The trial judge based her sentence on the opinion of the prison psychiatrist, who did not dispute that Dreyer had bvFTD but declared him competent. (https://story.californiasunday.com/joel-dreyer-criminal-psychiatrist/).

Due to frequently preserved cognitive function, patients with bvFTD are usually misdiagnosed as SCZ or bipolar disorder. This happened in the following case from Patton State Hospital (PSH). Ms. KS (initials changed) was a 68-year-old Caucasian female, divorced elementary school teacher who lived alone before her admission at PSH.

Ms. KS did not have a psychiatric history until the age of 56, when she purchased a gun and shot her neighbor in the shoulder. When interviewed, KS stated that she attacked the neighbor because he was spying on her and came into her house at night. Ms. KS was diagnosed with SCZ and admitted to PSH. Throughout her hospital stay, she was treated with several antipsychotic drugs with poor response. She remained unaware of wrongdoing, and her poor insight, apathy, and impulsivity were documented during her six-year stay at PSH. Because of inadequate progress, Ms. KS never met the criteria for transfer to the conditional release program (CONREP) and could not be discharged.

In 2014, Ms. KS became more forgetful, required more assistance with the activities of daily living (ADL), and changed her food preferences. For example, she asked for ice cream daily, although she had told staff in the past that she never liked ice cream. In time, she became more apathetic and often refused to get out of bed. The internal medicine consultant performed a dementia workup, but the laboratory studies came back normal, except for mild anemia and a vitamin D level of 29.3 nmol/L. Vitamin B12 and folate were WNL. In addition, Ms. KS scored 25/30 on the mini-mental status exam (MMSE) and 23/30 on the Montreal Cognitive Assessment (MoCA), revealing altered executive function. A neuropsychology consultant was called, and after a battery of tests, bvFTD was diagnosed. At that point, the treatment team petitioned the Court, arguing that Ms. KS did not benefit from being hospitalized at PSH as she was not expected to recover. The Court agreed with the team and ordered placement in a facility specialized for dementia.

This case was reported by Reuters in 2015:
(https://www.reuters.com/article/us-crime-dementia-idUSKBN0KE1Q020150105/).

State hospitals house patients with a lifelong history of SMI and criminal violations, frequently associated with substance use and comorbid antisocial personality disorder (APD). Aside from this group of carrier criminals, there is a subpopulation of older first offenders without significant psychiatric history. Patients with bvFTD are usually found in this group and are often diagnosed with SCZ, bipolar disorder, or major depressive disorder (MDD).

Compared to AD, in which approximately 6% of patients break the law, in bvFTD, 33%-50% of patients engage in criminal offenses (8)(9). Moreover, since this condition deteriorates over time, incarceration is not an adequate placement for people with dementia. Jails and prisons are ill-equipped to address medical complications associated with neurocognitive disorders (10). Moreover, as attorneys and judges may not be familiar with the clinical presentation and mental status of patients with dementia, there is an acute need for specialized courts that would be able to balance safety, placement, sentencing, and ethical considerations (11).

Currently, in many jurisdictions, the standard procedure for patients with dementia consists of a commitment to a state hospital for determining the potential for "restoration of competence to stand trial." Suppose the state hospital treatment teams determine that the patient cannot be restored to competency because of the severity of dementia. In that case, the patient may be sent back to prison, and the cycle will be repeated. State hospitals are not prepared for the treatment of patients with dementia as they cannot learn new information and usually show little progress. Furthermore, placement in outside facilities is problematic not only because of prohibitive costs but also because there is potential for violence. For this reason, new courts, laws, and standards of practice are needed for patients with dementia (11)(12).

## Dementia and homicide

People living with dementia, especially bvFTD, may engage in law-breaking and violence, including homicide. Caregivers and family usually report personality changes preceding overt antisocial behaviors. These may include apathy, impulsivity, aggression, lack of empathy, and newly acquired food preferences (13).

We present a homicide case from the late 1990s admitted at PSH.

RB (initials changed) is a 67-year-old female with life-long SCZ who started exhibiting symptoms of dementia in her late 50s. She was diagnosed with possible AD and lived in a large nursing home, twenty miles East of Los Angeles, California, which specialized in the treatment of older patients with SMI. Ms. RB was known to wander up and down the hallways at night but was never aggressive. One night in 1997, Ms. RB entered the room of a bedridden patient and strangled her to death with the straps of a handbag. Ms. RB was found unable to stand trial because of neurocognitive impairment and was transferred to PSH, where she died four years later.

This case illustrates an instance of homicide in a patient with lifelong SCZ and superimposed dementia. As the possibility of bvFTD was never entertained in this case and neuroimaging was not performed, Ms. RB may have had bvFTD rather than AD, as violent behavior is more common in the former (14).

A more recent case occurred in New Mexico on Thanksgiving Day, 2022, when Karlan Denio, a 62-year-old man diagnosed with bvFTD two years earlier, killed, dismembered, and disemboweled his wife on the bedroom floor. After the crime, Mr. Danio went to bed and was found sound asleep when the police arrived. Despite being diagnosed with bvFTD, Mr. Danio was charged with murder and transferred to a state hospital. (https://lawandcrime.com/crime/new-mexico-man-allegedly-dismembered-and-disemboweled-his-wife-just-before-guests-were-scheduled-to-arrive-for-thanksgiving-dinner/).

Another example of possible bvFTD and homicide is the case of George Weller. He was an 86-year-old man who, on July 16, 2003, plowed his 1992 Buick LeSabre over a crowd of people at the Farmer's Market in Santa Monica, California, killing ten and injuring over 70 individuals, including a child. His lack of remorse, when interviewed by the police suggests that he likely had bvFTD.
(https://www.nytimes.com/2006/11/21/us/21sentence.html)

Mr. Weller was convicted of 10 counts of vehicular manslaughter with gross negligence and could have been sentenced to up to 18 years in prison; however, due to the defendant's failing health, he did not receive a prison sentence.

Dementia due to infectious or metabolic causes can also lead to homicide. A case report presents a state hospital patient with dementia caused by vitamin B-12 deficiency and syphilis who shot his ex-wife dead with his gun (15). Along this line, a study from Sweden examined secondary causes of dementia vis-à-vis violence and homicide. The study looked at various primary illnesses, including head trauma, stroke, infection, cardiovascular disease, and epilepsy, concluding that secondary dementia can lead to violence and homicide (16). In this regard, a recent study of 15 688 participants over 32 years validated the above by identifying infection as the most common cause of secondary dementia (17).

## Dementia-related homicide (mercy murders)

Providing care to a spouse with dementia is challenging, exhausting, and depressing. Witnessing progressive deterioration, personality changes, and hostility toward loved ones often leads to caregiver burnout and the belief that death would be preferable to living with pain, confusion, and unawareness of one's family or surroundings. These feelings are further exacerbated when, during a lucid moment, the patient asks the spouse to help them die.

Cara and Ray Laird were husband and wife for over six decades and lived in Seal Beach, California. When they were younger, they took an oath: if one gets disabling dementia to the point that the quality of life is no longer acceptable, the more functional spouse would kill the other one. Cara developed AD and got worse over the following five years; she could not talk, she was disabled and bedridden, unaware of her surroundings. She spent days in a row chewing on her pillow; she could not sleep and yelled during the night. Finally, she had difficulties swallowing and developed several bouts of aspiration pneumonia, which she survived. One day, Ray came to the nursing home and stayed in his wife's room. When the staff went to lunch, and there were few people around, he shot his wife in the head with a pillow, ending her life. Ray, who was 86 at that time, was arrested and taken to jail until his day in court. The couple's two daughters testified that Ray had done the right thing and that they were aware of the covenant between their parents. The Court released Mr. Laird but ordered him to reside in a retirement facility and see a psychiatrist twice a month. The judge thought that Ray would get depressed as he would realize the magnitude of his crime. However, Mr. Laird did not and continued to state that he had done the right thing. He died three years later.

The following case we present could have been adjudicated as an assisted suicide, but the husband took full responsibility, stating that he killed his wife at her request.

Pam Kruspe, a 61-year-old female, was married for 42 years to Stephen Kruspe, an ex-marine. Because of advanced AD, Pam resided at Parkside Inn assisted living facility in Boynton Beach, Florida. Her husband visited with her every day, and during a lucid moment, she said to him: "I want you to kill me." On March 27, 2017, Mr. Kruspe shot his wife dead outside the facility. He called the police, telling them what he had done. Interestingly, Pam's DNA was found on the gun, suggesting that the husband may have helped Pam to commit suicide, a lesser crime with lower prison time. Due to the pandemic, the trial was postponed many times. Finally, Stephen Kruspe had his day in court. He pleaded guilty to killing his wife, denied that Pam pulled the trigger, and was sentenced to 20 years in prison. He refused to plead "assisted suicide," which would have carried a shorter sentence and took full responsibility for himself.

## The neuro-moral network

Neuroscientists have established that the fundamental moral principles, including fairness or not harming others, are innate to the human brain and likely located in the ventromedial prefrontal cortex (VMPC), anterior cingulate cortex (ACC), and anterior insular cortex (AIC) (also known as the fronto-insular cortex), more in the right hemisphere than the left (18). Hereditary or acquired pathology in these areas has been associated with the hallmarks of sociopathy, such as lack of empathy, impulsivity, and deviant and violent behaviors (19)(20).

Acquired sociopathy, measured by deficits in solving moral dilemmas, was reported with pathologies altering the neuro-moral network, including traumatic brain injuries (TBI), strokes, or tumors (21)(22)(23)(24). Moral dilemmas are challenging scenarios without obvious or straightforward solutions, often requiring compromising one's ethical principles to help others. Table 1. provides examples of moral dilemmas in which information processing occurs in the neuro-moral network (VMPC, AIC, and ACC).

A unique type of acquired sociopathy caused by neurodegeneration has been documented in bvFTD (25). The pathology in bvFTD consists of frontotemporal lobar degeneration (FTLD), primarily affecting the right hemisphere. Functional neuroimaging studies and brain network analysis have identified salience network (SN) pathology in bvFTD. SN is one of the three intrinsic connectivity networks (ICN), which also includes the default network (DN) and central executive network (CEN) (26)(27). The SN is the switch that can shift attention from CEN to DMN and vice-versa (Table 2).

Within the SN, AIC processes information related to concerns about overcoming the obstacles to reach goals (28). The ACC was shown to process information related to anticipation, reward, prediction, and readiness to act (29)(30). The ability to abide by the rule of law or the societal code of conduct requires adequate functioning of the SN to evaluate risk, acquire motivation, and predict the outcomes.

**Table 1 Examples of moral dilemmas reflecting information processing in the neuro-moral network**

| Moral Dilemmas |
|---|
| You are at the wheel of a runaway trolley, quickly approaching a fork in the tracks. On the tracks to the left is a group of five railway workmen. On the tracks going to the right is a single railway workman. If you do nothing, the trolley will proceed to the left, causing the deaths of the five workers. The only way to avoid the deaths of these workmen is to hit a switch on your dashboard that will cause the trolley to proceed to the right, causing the death of the single workman. Would you hit the switch to avoid the deaths of the five workers? |
| Enemy soldiers have taken over your village. They have orders to kill everyone. You have hidden in the basement of a large house along with other people. Outside, you hear the voices of soldiers who have come to search the house. Your baby begins to cry loudly. You cover his mouth to block the sound. If you remove your hand from his mouth, the soldiers will hear his crying and will kill you, your baby, and the other people hiding in the basement. To save yourself and the others, you must smother your child to death. Would you smother your child to save yourself and other people? |
| A working individual is the caregiver for their mother, who has cancer. On the one hand, they want to provide proper care and miss work, but on the other, they fear losing their job. The individual is torn between two responsibilities. If they lose their job, they will not have the resources. |

**Table 2. Intrinsic connectivity networks (ICN), their location, physiological, and social function**

| ICN | Cortical location | Function | Social context |
|---|---|---|---|
| CEN | dorsolateral prefrontal cortex (DLPFC), supramarginal gyrus | Planning, working memory, direction of attention | Outer reality, task, actions, problem-solving |
| DMN | posterior cingulate cortex, medial prefrontal cortex, medial temporal lobe, and angular gyrus | self-related mental activity, including autobiographical, self-monitoring, and social functions | Inner reality, thoughts, ideas, societal rules, self and the community |
| SN | anterior cingulate cortex (ACC) and frontoinsular cortex (FIC) | detection and orientation to salient external stimuli and internal events | Switches the focus of concern back and forth from the inner to the outer reality |

The SN information processing required for solving moral dilemmas is believed to occur in the von Economo neurons (VENs) residents of AIC and ACC (31). VENs are selectively targeted in bvFTD, suggesting that these cells play a crucial role in empathy, concern for others, and solving moral dilemmas (32).

VENs were first described by Constantin von Economo in 1926 as cells with a unique, elongated corkscrew-like soma in the layer Vb of AIC and ACC (33). VENs are large projection neurons with long axons capable of integrating signals from multiple, distant brain areas, indicating participation in the neuro-moral network (34). Indeed, these cells, implicated in empathy and social intelligence, are only present in superior mammals, such as African great apes, elephants, and dolphins, and in much larger numbers in humans (35). In bvFTD, the VENs population is 53% to 74% lower compared to healthy controls, emphasizing that these neurons are selectively targeted by FTLD, promoting acquired sociopathy (32). Aside from bvFTD, VEN pathology has been associated with SCZ, in which numerous lysosomal aggregates were detected in VENs, likely indicating that impaired autophagy leads to the selective elimination of these neurons (36).

Novel studies found that gut inflammations are recorded in the insular cortex, an area that also regulates the cardiovascular system, especially heart rate variability (HRV) (37)(38). Since HRV is altered in inflammatory bowel disease (IBD) and inflammatory markers are elevated in sociopathy, this pathology may be triggered by VEN loss (39). Moreover, HRV may likely comprise a biomarker of both bvFTD and IBD (40)(41).

# Article for Chapter 2: Frontotemporal Dementia Behavioral Variant as an Acquired Psychopathy

Adonis Sfera[1], Imran Hassan[1] and Peter Bota[2]

*1 Department of Psychiatry, Loma Linda University, Patton State Hospital, University of California Riverside, United States of America*
*2 Medical student California University of Science and Medicine, United States of America*



## Abstract

Frontotemporal dementia behavioral variant (bvFTD) is a Young Onset Dementia (YOD) in which the symptoms of executive dysfunction occur before the age of

65. This neurodegenerative disorder is unique as the memory can remain intact for many years, making it difficult to differentiate from schizophrenia, antisocial personality disorder, or bipolar pathology.

Late onset criminal behavior was demonstrated in over 50% of patients with bvFTD. Lawbreaking occurs late in life and frequently criminal violation, including homicide, may comprise the first sign of pathology. The change in personality occurs very slowly, over several years, and family members rarely suspect a dementing condition. They often describe the patient as careless, calloused, selfish, and without remorse, changes that take place gradually, making it difficult to pinpoint the exact onset. Moreover, as they exhibit no cognitive impairment, bvFTD patients are often convicted for their crime or admitted to psychiatric hospitals.

**Keywords:** Insular Cortex • Von Economo Neurons (VENs) • Criminal Violations • Psychotropic Drugs • Early Onset Dementia

## Introduction

### *Executive Dysfunction Without Memory Loss*

The early stages of bvFTD are often marked by executive dysfunction without significant memory loss, a characteristic that may be confounded with psychiatric pathology [1]. Patients with this YOD may exhibit initial neurodegenerative manifestations in their 40s and 50s and frequently these consist of criminal violations, which may often include homicide [2,3]. Indeed, compared to Alzheimer's Disease (AD), in which approximately 12% of patients engage criminal conduct, individuals with bvFTD may exhibit unlawful behaviors in up to 50% of cases [4,5].

### *Von Economo Neurons, The Empathy Cells*

At the cellular level, bvFTD, is marked by a selective loss of Von Economo Neurons (VENs), comprising approximately 193,000 large cells located in the Anterior Insular Cortex (AIC) and Anterior Cingulate Cortex (ACC). VENs are the "empathy cells" which process the higher brain functions, including self-awareness, social cognition, morality, and emotional intelligence [5,6]. Selective loss of these neurons in bvFTD may result in personality changes and criminal behavior.

Historically, post-traumatic psychopathy was first described in Phineas Gage, a British railroad worker who in 1848 sustained a traumatic brain injury in which a metal rod (which measured 3 ft 7 in. in length and 1.25 in. in diameter) was propelled by an explosion through his left cheek and head, damaging the AIC and ACC. Although he regained consciousness immediately, permanent psychopathic traits were the long-term consequences.

Despite the fact that TDP-43 accumulation and aggregation are well-established in bvFTD, here, we focus on VENs as loss of these cells, especially in the right hemisphere, has been associated with impulsivity, criminal behavior and difficulties in solving moral dilemmas (Table 1 provides examples of moral dilemmas processed by the AIC and ACC).

We surmise that, due to their size, VENs are selectively targeted by the frontotemporal lobar degeneration as they are more susceptible to plasma membrane lipid peroxidation and mitochondrial loss.

In the following section, we present four real case vignettes to illustrate the basic features of bvFTD, with the intention to educate clinicians in State hospitals and correctional institutions to recognize this condition and differentiate it from psychiatric disorders.

| | |
|---|---|
| 1 | You are at the wheel of a runaway trolley quickly approaching a fork in the tracks. On the tracks going to the left is a group of five railway workmen. On the tracks going to the right is a single railway workman. If you do nothing, the trolley will proceed to the left, causing the deaths of the five workmen. The only way to avoid the deaths of these workmen is to hit a switch on your dashboard that will cause the trolley to proceed to the right, causing the death of the single workman. Would you hit the switch to avoid the deaths of the five workmen? |
| 2 | Enemy soldiers have taken over your village. They have orders to kill everyone. You have hidden in the basement of a large house along with other people. Outside you hear the voices of soldiers who have come to search the house. Your baby begins to cry loudly. You cover his mouth to block the sound. If you remove your hand from his mouth the soldiers will hear his crying and will kill you, your baby, and the other people hiding in the basement. To save yourself and the others you must smother your child to death. Would you smother your child in order to save yourself and the other people? |
| 3 | A working individual is the caregiver for their mother who has cancer. On the one hand, they want to provide proper care and miss work, but on the other they fear losing their job. The individual is torn between two responsibilities. If they lose their job, they would not have resources to take care of the mother, while if they miss work less, they would not be able to provide quality care. |

## Case Presentation

### *Case 1: The Teacher Who Shot Her Neighbor*

Ms. KS (initials changed), a Caucasian female, age 68, divorced, retired elementary school teacher, lived alone prior to her admission to Patton State Hospital. Ms. KS did not have a psychiatric history until the age of 56 when she purchased a gun and shot her neighbor in the shoulder. She stated that she attacked the man because he was spying on her and intruded into her house during the night. She was convicted of attempted murder and sent to prison, where her condition deteriorated, prompting transfer to our forensic institution. KS was diagnosed with SCZ and admitted as a forensic detainee.

During her hospital stay, KS was treated with various antipsychotic drugs with minimal symptomatic relief. She was unaware that she did anything wrong and her poor insight and impulsivity were documented during her six years of hospital stay. Because of poor insight, KS never met criteria for the Conditional Release Program (CONREP).

In 2014, KS became more forgetful, required assistance with most Activities of Daily Living (ADLs), and exhibited a change in her dietary preferences. For example, she asked for ice cream daily, although earlier in her life she detested ice cream. In time, KS became more apathetic and often refused to get out of bed. The internal medicine consultant performed a dementia workup, but the laboratory studies came back normal, except for mild anemia, and a vitamin D level of 29.3 nmol/L. KS scored 25/30 on Mini Mental Status Exam (MMSE) and when a Montreal Cognitive Assessment (MoCA) was administered, the score was 23/30, consistent with executive dysfunction. Neuropsychology consult was called, and after a battery of tests, bvFTD was diagnosed.

With this information, the treatment team petitioned the Court, arguing that KS did not benefit from hospitalization in a forensic institution as she was not expected to recover. The judge agreed with the treating clinicians and ordered placement in a facility for palliative care specialized in dementia.

Due to the numerous clinical and legal ramifications (discussed below), this case was featured in the mass media at the time:

- https://www.reuters.com/article/us-crime-dementia idUSKBN0KE1Q020150105/
- https://www.foxnews.com/health/breaking-the-law-may-be-a-sign-of-dementia
- https://clbb.mgh.harvard.edu/when-frontotemporal-dementia-leads-to-crime-prosecution-or-protection/

### *Case 2: The Attorney with a Sweet Tooth*

An outpatient we treated in 2013, was a 72 years old, retired attorney, arrested because he stole chocolate from a grocery store while casually conversing with the owner. When confronted, he replied: "what's the problem, I have a sweet tooth". According to the family, the patient came across as careless and indifferent of his children and the spouse, being either apathetic or angry and irritable. For example, when he learned that his son-in-law died unexpectedly, he reacted by saying "let's go out to eat". His eating habits had changed dramatically, according to his wife, consuming mostly sweets which previously he had avoided. When told to eat more nutritious food, he often became angry.

### *Case 3: The Psychiatrist Turned a Drug Dealer*

Dr. Joel Stanley Dreyer was a well-respected psychiatrist who had his practice in Riverside, California. In 1990s, Dr. Dreyer was diagnosed with bvFTD but continued to practice psychiatry, and in 2010 was convicted for prescribing, selling, and distributing large amounts of addictive painkillers and benzodiazepines. As a result of careless prescribing, one person died of an overdose and Dr. Dreyer was convicted and served ten years in prison despite having been diagnosed with bvFTD prior to his crime. This case emphasizes that some jurisdictions do not recognize bvFTD as an attenuating circumstance. The court ruling was based on the testimony of the prison psychiatrist who did not challenge the diagnosis of bvFTD but stated that since not all individuals with this disorder engage in criminal behavior, "direct causality" between Dr. Dreyer's crime and bvFTD could not be established. A detailed history of this case can be found at the link below:
https://story.californiasunday.com/joel-dreyer-criminal-psychiatrist/

### *Case: 4 The Buick LeSabre Murderer*

On July 16, 2003, Mr. GRW, an 83 years old man crashed his Buick LeSabre in an open-air market in Santa Monica, California, killing 10 and injuring 63 individuals. Despite the catastrophic event he caused, GRW did not express remorse, showed indifference, callousness, and lack of empathy. In the court, he appeared apathetic, angry, and unapologetic, stating that he was sorry the dead and injured could not "enjoy the value of their purchases". No psychiatric evaluation was ordered because there was no previous history, however, criminal behavior may often represent the first symptom of bvFTD. Despite never being diagnosed with a neurodegenerative disorder, people who knew GRW noticed a drastic personality change in the years prior to this event, indicative of bvFTD. His neighbors, friends, and his pastor, described GRW as caring, pleasant, and friendly individual. He had been married for over 60 years, was compassionate, involved in peoples' lives, and after retirement, volunteered with various civic organizations. Although GRW was never officially diagnosed with bvFTD, this case illustrates the difficulty clinicians encounter because this "dementia without cognitive impairment" affects the executive function, leaving memory intact for many years. Indeed, shortly before his crime, GRW was able to pass his DMV license renewal test, suggesting that his memory was unaffected. Since in California drivers who are 70 years or older must renew their driver's license in person, GRW did not raise a red flag with the DMV worker.

## Discussion

Since bvFTD comprises 2.7% of all dementias and in early stages, patients retain their cognitive abilities, this condition is often misdiagnosed as schizophrenia, major depressive, or bipolar disorder, and frequently admitted to psychiatric institutions [5,6]. Patients with bvFTD respond poorly to antipsychotic drugs, are often labeled "treatment resistant", and prescribed additional psychotropics [7]. Moreover, as criminal behavior is frequently the initial manifestation of bvFTD, clinicians rarely suspect this condition when examining an incarcerated individual [8,9]. However, there are several characteristics of this illness which should prompt the clinician to think of a neurodegenerative condition. These include absence of psychiatric history at a younger age, first legal violation after the age of 55, poor insight despite a previously successful career, sudden change in eating habits, altered sleep pattern, lack of empathy, and engaging in criminal acts despite the presence of witnesses.

## Conclusion

Although bvFTD is often thought of as a rare condition, it comprises the second most common cause of major cognitive disorder (after AD). Predisposition for criminal violations is the main characteristic that singles out this condition from other dementias. Moreover, due to the preservation of cognitive abilities for a longer time, neurocognitive disorders are rarely suspected by either the family or the clinicians.

Education and differentiation of bvFTD from psychiatric disorders is necessary to ensure proper patient placement as well as adequate treatment.

## References

1. Vilares I, Wesley MJ, Ahn W-Y, et al. I am predicting the knowledge – recklessness distinction in the human brain. Proc. Natl Acad. Sci. USA 114(12), 3222–3227 (2017).
2. Cornwall W. Did you knowingly commit a crime? Brain scans could tell. Science Magazine, DC, USA (2017). tell
3. Metzl JM, MacLeish KT. Mental illness, mass shootings, and the politics of American firearms. Am J Public Health. 2015 Feb;105(2): 240-9. doi: 10.2105/AJPH.2014.302242.
4. Aono D, Yaffe G, Kober H. Neuroscientific evidence in the courtroom: a review. Cogn Res Princ Implic. 2019 Oct 22;4(1):40. doi: 10.1186/s41235-019-0179-y. PMID: 31641963; PMCID: PMC6805839.
5. People v. Weinstein, 156 Misc. 2d 34, 591 N.Y.S.2d 715 (Sup. Ct. 1992).
6. Siegel DM. The Supreme Court and the sentencing of juveniles in the United States: reaffirming the distinctiveness of youth. Child Adolesc Psychiatr Clin N Am. 2011 Jul;20(3):431-45. doi: 10.1016/j.chc.2011.03.011. PMID: 21683911.

7. Antar AY. Guilty or not guilty because of insanity? A comparative study of murderers referred for psychiatric examination by court order. Health Justice. 2023 Sep 5;11(1):35. doi: 10.1186/s40352-023-00230-z. PMID: 37668924; PMCID: PMC10478500.

8. Shinagawa S, Shigenobu K, Tagai K, Fukuhara R, Kamimura N, Mori T, Yoshiyama K, Kazui H, Nakayama K, Ikeda M. Violation of Laws in Frontotemporal Dementia: A Multicenter Study in Japan. J Alzheimers Dis. 2017;57(4):1221-1227. doi: 10.3233/JAD-170028. PMID: 28304308.

9. Haußmann R, Krug C, Noppes F, Brandt M, Lange J, Donix M. Delinquentes Verhalten im Rahmen more frontotemporal Demenzen und der Alzheimer-Erkrankung [Criminal behavior in frontotemporal dementia and Alzheimer's disease]. Nervenarzt. 2022 Jan;93(1):59-67. German. Doi: 10.1007/s00115-021-01070-8.

10. Williams BA, Goodwin JS, Baillargeon J, Ahalt C, Walter LC. Addressing the aging crisis in U.S. criminal justice health care. J Am Geriatr Soc. 2012 Jun;60(6):1150-6. doi: 10.1111/j.1532-5415.2012.03962.x.

11. Persons Living with Dementia in the Criminal Legal System. American Bar Association Commission on Law and Aging in collaboration with NASMHPD Research Institute and The University of Virginia and Faculty from The University of Michigan, May 2022

12. Arias, J. & Flicker, L. (2020). A Matter of Intent: A Social Obligation to Improve Criminal Procedures for Individuals with Dementia. The Journal of Law, Medicine, & Ethics, 48, 318-327.

13. Zago S, Scarpazza C, Difonzo T, Arighi A, Hajhajate D, Torrente Y, Sartori G. Behavioral Variant of Frontotemporal Dementia and Homicide in a Historical Case. J Am Acad Psychiatry Law. 2021 Jun;49(2):219-227. doi: 10.29158/JAAPL.200081-20.

14. Tali Elsayed Sundakov-Krumins, Sean Lubbe, Anne Pamela Frances Wand; Homicide and Dementia: A Systematic Review. Dement Geriatr Cogn Disord 19 April 2022; 51 (1): 1–17. https://doi.org/10.1159/000521878

15. Rayel MG, Land WB, Gutheil TG. Dementia as a risk factor for homicide. J Forensic Sci. 1999 May;44(3):565-7. PMID: 10408111.

16. Ekström, A., Kristiansson, M. & Björkstén, K.S. Dementia and cognitive disorder identified at a forensic psychiatric examination a study from Sweden. BMC Geriatr 17, 219 (2017). https://doi.org/10.1186/s12877-017-0614-1
17. Bohn B, Lutsey PL, Misialek JR, et al. Incidence of Dementia Following Hospitalization With Infection Among Adults in the Atherosclerosis Risk in Communities (ARIC) Study Cohort. JAMA Netw Open. 2023;6(1):e2250126. doi:10.1001/jamanetworkopen.2022.50126
18. Mendez MF. The neurobiology of moral behavior: review and neuropsychiatric implications. CNS Spectr. 2009 Nov;14(11):608-20. Doi: 10.1017/s1092852900023853. PMID: 20173686; PMCID: PMC3163302.
19. Markowitsch HJ. Neuroscience and crime. Neurocase. 2008;14:1–6.
20. Sener MT, Ozcan H, Sahingoz S, Ogul H. Criminal Responsibility of the Frontal Lobe Syndrome. Eurasian J Med. 2015 Oct;47(3):218-22. doi: 10.5152/eurasianjmed.2015.69. PMID: 26644774; PMCID: PMC4659527.
21. Li Y, Zhang T, Li W, Zhang J, Jin Z, Li L. Linking brain structure and activation in anterior insula cortex to explain the trait empathy for pain. Hum Brain Mapp. 2020 Mar;41(4):1030-1042. doi: 10.1002/hbm.24858.
22. Ying X, Luo J, Chiu CY, Wu Y, Xu Y, Fan J. Functional Dissociation of the Posterior and Anterior Insula in Moral Disgust. Front Psychol. 2018 Jun 1;9:860. Doi: 10.3389/fpsyg.2018.00860. PMID: 29910758; PMCID: PMC5992674.
23. de Oliveira-Souza R, Paranhos T, Moll J, Grafman J. Gender and Hemispheric Asymmetries in Acquired Sociopathy. Front Psychol. 2019 Mar 19;10:346. Doi: 10.3389/fpsyg.2019.00346. PMID: 30941065; PMCID: PMC6433972.
24. Sitaram R, Caria A, Veit R, Gaber T, Ruiz S, Birbaumer N. Volitional control of the anterior insula in criminal psychopaths using real-time fMRI neurofeedback: a pilot study. Front Behav Neurosci. 2014 Oct 14;8:344. doi: 10.3389/fnbeh.2014.00344. PMID: 25352793; PMCID: PMC4196629.

25. Liljegren M, Naasan G, Temlett J, et al. Criminal Behavior in Frontotemporal Dementia and Alzheimer Disease. JAMA Neurol. 2015;72(3):295–300. doi:10.1001/jamaneurol.2014.3781
26. Chiong W, Wilson SM, D'Esposito M, Kayser AS, Grossman SN, Poorzand P, et al. The salience network causally influences default mode network activity during moral reasoning. Brain (2013) 136(Pt 6):1929–41 10.1093/brain/awt066 [PMC free article] [PubMed] [CrossRef] [Google Scholar]
27. Seeley WW, Crawford RK, Zhou J, Miller BL, Greicius MD. Neurodegenerative diseases target large-scale human brain networks. Neuron (2009) 62(1):42–52 doi: 10.1016/j.neuron.2009.03.024
28. Bossaerts P. Risk and risk prediction error signal in the anterior insula. Brain Struct Funct (2010) 214(5–6):645–53 10.1007/s00429-010-0253-1
29. Ryan RM. Editor. The Oxford Handbook of Human Motivation. Oxford, UK: Oxford University Press; (2012). 371 p. [Google Scholar]
30. Parviziemail J, Rangarajan V, Shirer WR, Desai N, Greicius MD. The will to persevere is induced by electrical stimulation of the human cingulate gyrus. Neuron (2013) 80:1–9 doi: 10.1016/j.neuron.2013.10.057
31. Singleton, E.H., Pijnenburg, Y.A.L., Gami-Patel, P. et al. The behavioral variant of Alzheimer's disease does not show a selective loss of Von Economo and phylogenetically related neurons in the anterior cingulate cortex. Alz Res Therapy 14, 11 (2022). https://doi.org/10.1186/s13195-021-00947-9
32. Santillo AF, Nilsson C, Englund E. von Economo neurons are selectively targeted in frontotemporal dementia. Neuropathol Appl Neurobiol. 2013 Aug;39(5):572-9. doi: 10.1111/nan.12021. PMID: 23346995; PMCID: PMC3749467.
33. von Economo, C. (1926). Eine neue Art Spezialzellen des Lobus cinguli und Lobus insulae. Z. Ges Neurol. Psychiatr 100, 706–712. doi: 10.1007/bf02970950

34. Stimpson CD, Tetreault NA, Allman JM, Jacobs B, Butti C, Hof PR, et al. Biochemical specificity of von Economo neurons in hominoids. Am J Hum Biol (2011) 23(1):22–8 10.1002/ajhb.21135PMCID
35. Banovac I, Sedmak D, Judaš M, Petanjek Z. Von Economo Neurons Primate-Specific or Commonplace in the Mammalian Brain? Front Neural Circuits. 2021 Sep 1;15:714611. doi: 10.3389/fncir.2021.714611. PMID: 34539353; PMCID: PMC8440978.
36. Krause M, Theiss C, Brüne M. Ultrastructural Alterations of Von Economo Neurons in the Anterior Cingulate Cortex in Schizophrenia. Anat Rec (Hoboken). 2017 Nov;300(11):2017-2024. Doi: 10.1002/ar.23635
37. Chouchou F, Mauguière F, Vallayer O, Catenoix H, Isnard J, Montavont A, Jung J, Pichot V, Rheims S, Mazzola L. How the insula speaks to the heart: Cardiac responses to insular stimulation in humans. Hum Brain Mapp. 2019 Jun 15;40(9):2611-2622. doi: 10.1002/hbm.24548.
38. Olszewska DA, Lang AE. The Role of Insular Cortex in Gut-Inflammation Memory: What Does It Mean for Parkinson's Disease? Mov Disord. 2022 Apr;37(4):700-701. doi: 10.1002/mds.28975.
39. Segarra P, Poy R, Branchadell V, Ribes-Guardiola P, Moltó J. Psychopathy and heart rate variability: A new physiological marker for the adaptive features of boldness. Personal Disord. 2022 Sep;13(5):557-562. doi: 10.1037/per0000573.
40. Liu KY, Elliott T, Knowles M, Howard R. Heart rate variability about cognition and behavior in neurodegenerative diseases: A systematic review and meta-analysis. Ageing Res Rev. 2022 Jan;73:101539. doi: 10.1016/j.arr.2021.101539. Epub 2021 Dec 6. PMID: 34883203; PMCID: PMC8783051.
41. Kim KN, Yao Y, Ju SY. Heart rate variability and inflammatory bowel disease in humans: A systematic review and meta-analysis. Medicine (Baltimore). 2020 Nov 25;99(48):e23430. doi: 10.1097/MD.0000000000023430. PMID: 33235125; PMCID: PMC7710256.

# CHAPTER 3

# ARYL HYDROCARBON RECEPTOR, POLLUTANTS, AGGRESSION, AND MENTAL ILLNESS

Although aggression is evolutionally conserved and adaptive in the animal kingdom, especially when obtaining food and defending the territory, humans view this behavior as pathological. In the past three decades, a growing body of evidence has linked environmental pollutants to aggression, violence, SCZ, and neurodegenerative disorders (1)(2)(3)(4). For example, exposure to ozone or particulate matter in the air smaller than 2.5 μm (PM2.5) has been associated with criminal and aggressive behavior as well as SCZ and neurodegeneration (5)(6)(7)(8). Since both ozone and PM2.5 are AhR ligands, it is suggested that overactivation of this transcription factor may trigger violence and neuropathology. Interestingly, not only Alzheimer's disease (AD) and Parkinson's disease (PD) but also frontotemporal dementia has been associated with exposure to PM2.5 and other pollutants (9). Along this line, plasticizers, including bisphenol-A, are AhR ligands that disrupt several endocrine pathways, inducing premature cellular senescence and predisposing to SCZ (10)(11). Putting it all together, pollutants promote aggression, SCZ, and dementias by inducing premature cellular senescence and subsequent GMV depletion (12)(13)(14).

## AhR, cholesterol, and homicide

AhR is activated by numerous endogenous and exogenous molecules and oxides previously associated with violent behavior, including homicide (1)(15). In addition, the AhR chaperone, heat shock protein 90 (HSP90), regulates not only behavior but also pain (16)(17)(18).

Cholesterol, an AhR ligand, has been implicated in violent crime, including homicide (19)(20)(21)(22). Indeed, individuals with lower HDL cholesterol levels exhibit three times higher aggression compared to AD or SCZ patients with average cholesterol (23) (see Chapter 4).

## Dopamine and AhR

In the 1950s, when the DA hypothesis was developed, many characteristics of SCZ needed to be better defined. For example, autoantibodies against various human proteins, comorbidity with IBD, premature cellular senescence, higher prevalence in Northern regions, and association with pollutants were unknown. In time, the DA hypothesis was revised twice to incorporate genetic and epigenetic factors, toxic causes, and pathogens, highlighting the non-dopaminergic etiologies of SCZ and SLDs.

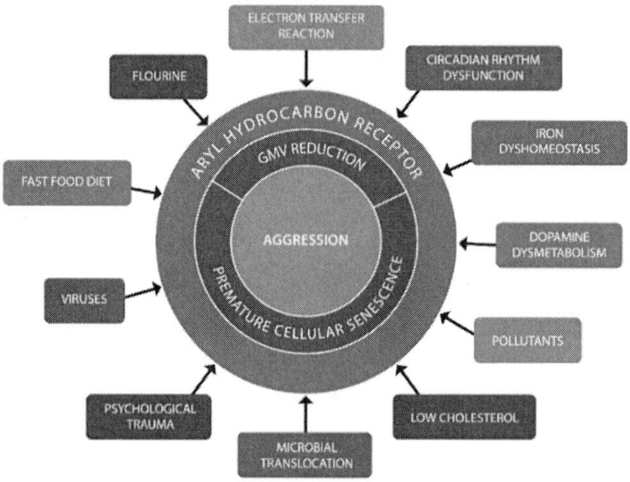


**Exogenous and endogenous factors activate AhR, reducing GMV and premature cellular senescence and promoting aggressive behavior.**

## AhR, cellular senescence, and SCZ

AhR, discovered in the 1970s, is the dioxin (2,3,7,8-tetrachlorodibenzo-p-dioxin) receptor found in many tissues and organs, including the gut and blood-brain barriers (BBB). It was later revealed that several AhR ligands are biomolecules implicated in neurodegeneration, SCZ, and SLDs. For example, gut microbes and their metabolites, pollutants, DA, clozapine, serotonin (5HT), melatonin, and carbidopa are AhR ligands, bringing this receptor into the neuropsychiatric arena (Fig. 1). On the other hand, aripiprazole, a ligand of HSP90, blocks AhR nuclear entry and the expression of SCZ risk genes.

AhR is also the master regulator of cellular senescence, a phenotype associated with SCZ and dementia, emphasizing the critical role of premature aging in these pathologies. Moreover, the senescent intestinal barrier has been associated with microbial migration from the GI tract (where microbiota is immunologically tolerated) into the systemic circulation (where commensals are vehemently attacked by host immunity) (24). Neurodegenerative and neuropsychiatric pathology in SCZ and dementia are likely triggered by the host's immune reaction to the translocated microbes and their molecules, which release proinflammatory cytokines and antibodies directed at microbial receptors. For example, gut microbes-derived lipopolysaccharide (LPS), a component of Gram-negative bacteria, was detected in the brains of patients with AD and SCZ, linking these pathologies to microbial migration through the GI barrier and BBB (25)(26). Another example of bacteria-induced psychosis is illustrated by the urinary tract infection (UTI)-mediated exacerbation or new onset of SCZ. As UTIs are usually caused by *Escherichia coli (E. coli*), the role of microbes in neuropathology is further emphasized (27).

### *Dopamine-independent antipsychotic drugs*

Muscarinic cholinergic receptor agonists comprise a novel class of DA-independent antipsychotic drugs, indicating that blocking DA neurotransmission may not be the only antipsychotic mechanism in existence. Indeed, like DA, acetylcholine (ACh) prevents GMV reduction and aggression. Moreover, DA is an AhR activator, while phenazines and phenothiazines inhibit AhR, ameliorating acute psychotic symptoms. Microbial phenazines are endogenous antipsychotic-like biomolecules generated by the gut microbiota for various physiological purposes. Moreover, vitamin D3 deactivates AhR, likely explaining the high prevalence of SCZ in Northern areas with less abundant sunshine.

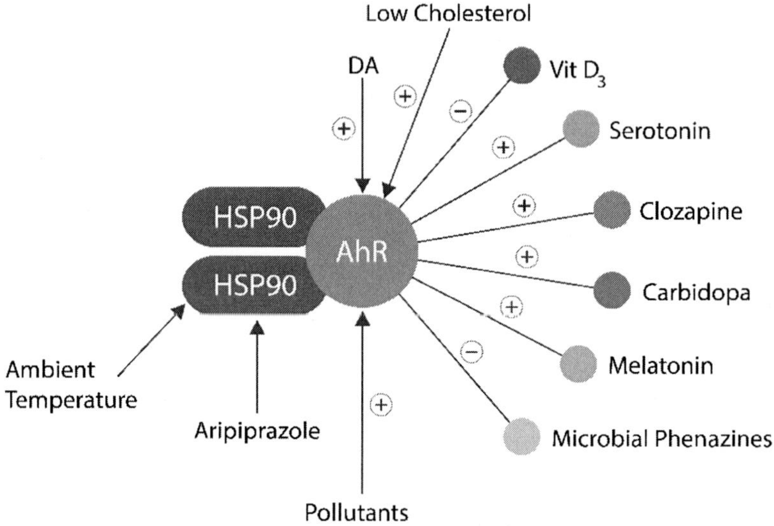


**Aryl hydrocarbon receptor (AhR) is a cytoplasmic protein stabilized by two molecules of HSP90. AhR ligands, dopamine, serotonin, clozapine, carbidopa, phenazines, pollutants, and cholesterol are relevant for neuropathology. When activated, AhR translocates to the nucleus, enabling the transcription of numerous genes, including those for cellular senescence and gray matter volume (GMV) loss.**

### *AhR antagonists as antipsychotics*

The antipsychotic properties of AhR antagonists comprise the proof of concept that excessive AhR activation can trigger psychosis. The following natural and synthetic AhR inhibitors were demonstrated to exert therapeutic properties in AD and SCZ (table).

*Quercetin* is a natural flavonoid and a negative allosteric modulator of gamma-aminobutyric A (GABA-A) receptors. This compound lowers prefrontal cortex inhibition, potentiating glutamatergic transmission, which is deficient in SCZ (28)(29)(30).

The indole alkaloid *alstonine*, polyphenols apigenin, and *luteolin* have been identified as plant-based remedies with antipsychotic properties (7)(8). For example, *luteolin* is currently in clinical trials for SCZ (NCT05204407) (31)(32)(33).

Synthetic compounds, including Sorafenib, 1,3-diketone, IK-175, and HBU651, are novel AhR antagonists developed primarily for cancer, but their profile suggests potential beneficial effects in AD and SCZ (1)(34)(35)(36)(37).

| Exogenous agonists | Endogenous agonists | Dietary antagonists | Synthetic antagonists |
|---|---|---|---|
| Benzotriazole UV stabilizer | Tryptophan photo metabolites and FICZ | Quercetin | Sorafenib |
| Plasticizers (Bisphenol) | Indoles | Apigenin | 1,3-diketone |
| Clozapine | D3 hydroxyderivatives | Luteolin | IK-175 |
| Carbidopa | DA | Alstonine | HBU651 |

**Endogenous and exogenous AhR agonists and antagonists**

# Article for Chapter 3: Six Decades of Dopamine Hypothesis: Is Aryl Hydrocarbon Receptor the New D2?

## Adonis Sfera [1,2,3]

*1. Paton State Hospital, 3102 Highland Ave, Patton, CA 92369, USA; adonis.sfera@dsh.ca.gov*
*2. School of Behavioral Health, Loma Linda University, 11139 Anderson St., Loma Linda, CA 92350, USA*
*3. Department of psychiatry, University of California, Riverside 900 University Ave, Riverside, CA 92521, USA*

### Abstract

In 1957, Arvid Carlsson discovered that dopamine, at the time believed to be nothing more than a norepinephrine precursor, was a brain neurotransmitter in and of itself. By 1963, postsynaptic dopamine blockade had become the cornerstone of psychiatric treatment as it appeared to have deciphered the "chlorpromazine enigma", a 1950s term, denoting the action mechanism of antipsychotic drugs. The same year, Carlsson and Lindqvist launched the dopamine hypothesis of schizophrenia, ushering in the era of psychopharmacology. At present, six decades later, although watered down by three consecutive revisions, the dopamine model remains in vogue. The latest emendation of this paradigm proposes that "environmental and genetic factors" converge on the dopaminergic pathways, upregulating postsynaptic transmission. Aryl hydrocarbon receptors, expressed by the gut and blood–brain barrier, respond to a variety of endogenous and exogenous ligands, including dopamine, probably participating in interoceptive awareness, a feed-back loop, conveying intestinal barrier status to the insular cortex. The conceptualization of aryl hydrocarbon receptor as a bridge, connecting vagal terminals with the microbiome, may elucidate the aspects of schizophrenia seemingly incongruous with the dopamine hypothesis, such as increased prevalence in urban areas, distance from the equator, autoantibodies, or comorbidity with inflammatory bowel disease and human immunodeficiency 1 virus. In this review article, after a short discussion of schizophrenia outcome studies and insight, we take a closer look at the action mechanism of antipsychotic drugs, attempting to answer the question: do these agents exert their beneficial effects via both dopaminergic and nondopaminergic mechanisms? Finally, we discuss potential new therapies, including transcutaneous vagal stimulation, aryl hydrocarbon receptor ligands, and restoring the homeostasis of the gut barrier.

**Keywords:** dopamine hypothesis; microbial translocation; antipsychotic drugs.

## 1. Introduction

The dopamine hypothesis (DH) of schizophrenia (SCZ), launched by Carlsson and Lindqvist in 1963, surmises that the postsynaptic blockade of dopamine (DA) receptors is responsible for the beneficial effect of antipsychotic drugs in SCZ and SCZ-like disorders [1]. Arvid Carlson's experiments with DA depletion by reserpine, followed by chlorpromazine inhibition of dopaminergic transmission, led to a better understanding of the pathology at work in Parkinson's disease (PD) and acute psychosis [2]. Carlsson and Lindqvist surmised that excessive DA activation of the postsynaptic DA type 2 receptors (D2R) in the central nervous system (CNS) triggered psychotic symptoms, while dopaminergic blockade of these receptors comprised the remedy [3]. This model was further substantiated by the 1970s observation that amphetamine enhanced dopaminergic signaling, often exacerbating psychotic symptoms [4]. However, the realization that antipsychotic drugs exert properties, seemingly unrelated to DA, such as antimicrobial, antiviral, antiproliferative, cell cycle arrest, autophagy activation, alteration of iron metabolism, DNA methylation, and telomere elongation, led to the third DH revision, which emphasized genetic and epigenetic input in dopaminergic transmission [5–10].

Aside from the antipsychotic drugs, several characteristics of SCZ itself may be incongruous with the DH, including increased prevalence in industrialized countries and urban areas, variance with latitude, autoantibodies, and high comorbidity with inflammatory bowel disease (IBD) and human immunodeficiency virus 1 (HIV-1) (Table 1). Moreover, excessive DA in the CNS would likely promote euphoria, motivation, and heightened alertness instead of hallucinations or delusions. Furthermore, DH equates acute psychosis with SCZ, an assumption not always shared by clinicians, many of whom conceptualize positive symptoms of SCZ as epiphenomena of this pathology [11].

**Table 1. DA-unrelated SCZ characteristics explained by translocated microbes/AhR activation.**

| DH-Discordant SCZ Features | Non-DA Mechanisms | References |
|---|---|---|
| Negative symptoms | Translocation of *Hafnei alvei, Pseudomonas aeruginosa, Morganella morganii, Pseudomonas putida, and Klebsiella pneumoniae* | [12–14] |
| Comorbidity with IBD | AhR/STAT3/IL-22-regulated intestinal permeability and microbiota translocation | [11,15,16] |
| Comorbidity with HIV | hR/STAT3/IL22-regulateted gut barrier permeability | [12,17,18] |
| Poor insight (anosognosia) | IC activation by gut Prevotella and Bacteroides abundance | [19–25] |
| Higher prevalence in urban areas | Pollutants are AhR ligands associated with SCZ and are more prevalent in industrialized countries and urban areas | [26–34] |
| Increasing prevalence with the distance from the equator | Sunlight-driven vitamin D derivatives and tryptophan light metabolites are AhR ligands | [35–39] |
| Autoantibodies | Gut microbes express molecules, including GABA and NMDA, which can elicit formation of antibodies upon translocation | [40–42] |

Aryl hydrocarbon receptor (AhR), a cytosolic transcription factor, initially described as the dioxin receptor, responds to numerous exogenous and endogenous ligands, inducing both immune tolerance of gut microbes as well as their prompt elimination upon translocation into host tissues [43,44]. In the cytosol, AhR is bound by two heat shock protein 90 (HSP90) chaperones, molecules recently identified as both SCZ and Parkinson's disease (PD) targets [45–52]. Other AhR ligands significant for SCZ include DA, carbidopa, clozapine, melatonin, serotonin, microbial phenazines, and various pollutants, linking endogenous and exogenous molecules to this pathology [53–56].

At the subcellular level, AhR, a signal transducer and activator of transcription 3 (STAT3) and interleukin 22 (IL-22), communicates with both the central cholinergic system and the microbiome, relaying the "gut status" to the insular cortex (IC) [57–59]. Impaired AhR signaling was associated with IBD and HIV, disorders highly comorbid with SCZ, marked by a dysfunctional gut barrier, suggesting that microbial translocation may be the common denominator of these pathologies [60,61]. For example, upregulated plasma levels of immunoglobulins M and/or A against Hafnei alvei, Pseudomonas aeruginosa,

Morganella morganii, Pseudomonas putida, and Klebsiella pneumoniae were found in SCZ patients with negative symptoms, further linking this disorder to microbial translocation [12]. Furthermore, poor insight or anosognosia, a characteristic SCZ feature, present in up to 98% of patients, was associated with intestinal-inflammation-induced IC pathology [62–65]. We hypothesize that gut barrier disruption enables the migration of microbes or their components into the host systemic circulation, eventually reaching the brain, generating neuroinflammation and psychotic symptoms. This model is based on the following findings:

1. In SCZ, IBD, and HIV-1, the blood microbiome exhibits an increased level and diversity of intestinal microbes, suggesting translocation from the gut [66–68].
2. Monocytosis and elevated microbial translocation markers, including lipopolysaccharide (LPS), LPS-binding protein (LBP),

and soluble CD14 (sCD14), were documented in SCZ, HIV, and IBD, indicating translocation [69–74].

3. Elevated cell-free DNA (cfDNA) in SCZ, HIV, and IBD likely reflects gut barrier and BBB disruption [75–77].
4. Various "autoantibodies" detected in SCZ, IBD, and HIV are likely conventional immunoglobulins elicited by the translocated microbes and/or their components [78–81].

In this review article, after a brief discussion of SCZ outcome studies and anosognosia, we discuss the action mechanism of antipsychotic drugs, interrogating the nondopaminergic actions of these agents. Finally, we discuss new therapies, including transcutaneous vagal stimulation, aryl hydrocarbon receptor ligands, and recombinant IL22-mediated gut barrier rehabilitation. Less emphasis will be placed on the SCZ topics discussed in other articles, such as premature cellular senescence, ferroptosis, DNA methylation, innate lymphoid cells (ILCs), and lactylation [82,83].

## 2. DH and SCZ Outcome Studies

SCZ is a complex, multifactorial, and partially understood disorder marked by episodic symptomatic relief intertwined with periods of exacerbation and relapse [84]. The outcome of this illness is variable and difficult to measure as the conceptualization of functional recovery may differ among people [84]. For example, phrases like improved social and cognitive functioning, greater autonomy to manage one's own life, remission of positive and negative symptoms, better quality of life, or reintegration into the community may raise different expectations in each involved party, including patients, families, clinicians, or consumer advocates, indicating that recovery in SCZ is a complex and often subjective process [85–90]. In contrast to recovery, remission is a more concrete outcome measure that requires six months of minimal symptomatology without a full return to the premorbid level of functioning [91]. Despite the fact that remission is more attainable than recovery, most clinicians and family members would agree that living independently, maintaining stable employment or going to school, living an optimistic and hopeful life, and dating or getting married are goals rarely accomplished by patients with chronic SCZ even when adherent to treatment [92–94]. For example, novel studies have shown that 33% of SCZ patients relapse during the first 12 months after an initial psychotic episode, 26% remain homeless at 2 years of follow-up, while 5 years after the first psychotic outbreak, only 10% are employed [95–97]. Recovery at 15 and 25 years of follow-up is marginally better, at 16%, indicating that sustained recovery in chronic SCZ is infrequent [98]. Indeed, only 13.5% of patients meet recovery criteria at any point in time after the first psychotic episode [99].

Surprisingly, longitudinal studies looking at the overall SCZ recovery rate during the 20th century found little change since 1900, and, according to some studies, a steadily deteriorating outcome [99–101]. Moreover, contrary to the expectations of most researchers and clinicians, the proportion of patients with "good" outcomes has not increased in the decades following the discovery of antipsychotic drugs [7,90,102,103]. For example, a large meta-analysis of 114 follow-up studies by Warner R. looked at the time period from 1900 to 1996 and found the following rates of complete recovery and employment [101] (pp. 74):

1. 1901–1920, 20% complete recovery, 4.7% employed;
2. 1921–1940, 12% complete recovery, 11.9% employed;
3. 1941–1955, 23% complete recovery, 4.1% employed;
4. 1956–1975, 20% complete recovery, 5.1% employed;
5. 1976–1995, 20% complete recovery, 6.9% employed.

These data led the author to conclude that "recovery rates for patients admitted following the introduction of the antipsychotic drugs are no better than for those admitted after the Second World War or during the first two decades of the twentieth century" (page 78). Moreover, the employment rate of patients with SCZ has been decreasing steadily over the past 50 years in industrialized countries, a finding congruent with Warner's recovery data [104,105]. Furthermore, unlike public hospitals for tuberculosis or leprosy, discontinued for over half a century, long-term state institutions for the treatment of SCZ and like disorders continue to exist, representing a proof of concept that sustained recovery from these illnesses remains unsatisfactory [90,100].

Neuroimaging SCZ studies correlate well with the recovery and employment data, showing progressive, treatment-independent cortical gray matter loss, suggesting that the evolution of this disorder toward disability, cognitive deficit, and early neurodegeneration may be undeterred by the available therapies [86,106–110]. However, several neuroimaging studies in SCZ patients treated with second-generation antipsychotic drugs found delayed rates of gray matter loss, indicating that more outcome studies are needed in patients on atypical antipsychotics [111,112].

Taken together, although there is no doubt that antipsychotic drugs are extremely effective for the treatment of acute psychosis, chronic SCZ is less amenable to recovery, a finding in line with Kraepelin's initial observations of steady progression to premature dementia [113]. In summary, the reasons DH may require further revisions include the following:

1. Continued need for long-term public institutions for the treatment of chronic mental illness.
2. DA blockers may not alter the progression of SCZ toward disability and cognitive deficit.
3. Several SCZ characteristics are difficult to reconcile with the DH.
4. Life-long gray matter loss occurs despite treatment with DA blockers.
5. Upregulated DA in the CNS would be expected to result in euphoria, increased motivation, and alertness rather than hallucinations or delusions.
6. Anosognosia, the most common symptom of SCZ, is infrequently influenced by DA-blocking treatments.

## 3. Insight vs. Anosognosia, Lessons from COVID-19 and HIV

Poor insight or anosognosia is a cardinal symptom of SCZ, occurring in up to 98% of patients, which may not respond adequately to antipsychotic drugs [19]. Insight has been associated with interoceptive awareness and perception of internal body cues, such as heartbeat, respiration, intestinal function, position of limbs, and "self" vs. "non-self", a process impaired in many neuropsychiatric conditions, including traumatic brain injury (TBI), stroke, and SCZ [20,21]. Novel studies have associated IC, an area previously implicated in SCZ, with both anosognosia and error awareness [22–25,63].

Communication between IC and vagus nerve (VN) was described more than three decades ago, and recent studies have not only confirmed the existence of this dialog but also found that transcutaneous auricular VN stimulation (taVNS) can enhance interoceptive awareness, suggesting potential application in SCZs [114,115]. Others have shown that gut microbiota can alter IC connectivity, indicating that this area specializes in processing GI tract interoceptive input [116]. Interestingly, a study found that risperidone can upregulate IC connectivity, suggesting that second-generation antipsychotic drugs may influence insight more than the first-generation compounds [117]. In this regard, recent studies have reported that GI tract inflammation activates IC, while electrical stimulation of IC exerts an anti-inflammatory GI tract response, suggesting a potential therapeutic strategy for IBD [62,118]. Along this line, a preclinical study found that memories of previous intestinal inflammations (induced in rodents by mixing dextran sodium sulfate (DSS) with drinking water) are stored in IC, and stimulation of this area, weeks or months later, can trigger intestinal inflammation in the absence of DSS [62,118]. This study is in line with other research data on interoceptive awareness and IC, likely pinpointing the neuroanatomical location of an "insight center" [64,118,119]. Indeed, functional neuroimaging and connectivity studies have demonstrated that the awareness of error, insight, and the position of limbs is regulated by the IC neuronal networks [120]. Moreover, neuroimaging studies in patients with Chron's disease are in line with preclinical data, linking IC connectivity to IBD [62,120,121]. Interestingly, activation of IC was shown to increase the abundance of gut Prevotella and Bacteroides species, indicating that insular neurons are capable of regulating microbiota composition [116].

### *3.1 Mononuclear Cells and Insight*

Novel data have shown that AhR, the master regulator of peripheral mononuclear cells, drives the differentiation of monocytes into dendritic cells vs. macrophages/microglia, therefore altering the peripheral blood level of these cell types [122].

Studies during the COVID-19 pandemic found that the SARS-CoV-2 virus can induce cognitive deficit of which the patients themselves were unaware, known as anosognosia for impaired memory. Moreover, anosognosia in these individuals was associated with peripheral monocytosis (defined as 7.35% or more of the total number of leukocytes), suggesting that infections can alter insight, while monocyte count could represent a biomarker for interoceptive awareness [123]. The correlation between monocytosis and anosognosia is not new or limited to COVID-19, as it was reported earlier in the context of HIV-associated neurocognitive disorder (HAND), a condition marked by impaired insight [124]. This is significant as monocyte levels are elevated in SCZ, highlighting a potential general marker of anosognosian neuropathology [125–127]. For example, a recent study found that patients in the preclinical phase of SCZ exhibited monocytosis and increased microbial translocation markers, further linking gut microbes with this pathology [128]. Moreover, upregulated blood monocytes were documented during the transition phase from mild cognitive impairment (MCI) to Alzheimer's disease (AD), connecting bacterial translocation with neurodegenerative disorders [129,130]. Indeed, microbes and LPS were found in AD brains, further linking bacteria to cognition and insight [131–133]. Along this line, peripheral monocytes were shown to infiltrate the CNS and differentiate into microglia, cells that under pathological circumstances can engage in the aberrant phagocytosis of healthy neurons, predisposing to neurodegeneration [134,135]. For example, SCZ-related cognitive deficit, probably including anosognosia, was associated with the engulfment of intact synapses and dendritic spines by abnormally activated microglia [136,137].

### *3.2 Cholinergic Anti-Inflammatory Pathway and Insight*

Discovered in 2000 by Borovikova et al. [138], the cholinergic anti-inflammatory pathway (CAP) is a brain-to-periphery neural loop mediated by alpha7 nicotinic acetylcholine receptors (α7nAChRs) expressed by neurons, immune cells, and intestinal epithelial cells (IECs) (Figure 1). CAP likely participates in interoceptive awareness and regulates intestinal permeability, reporting on the gut status, via VN, to the IC [138,139]. For example, addiction medicine studies have shown that both acetylcholine

(ACh) and nicotine can activate IC, ameliorating anosognosia, further linking insight to CAP [140–142]. Moreover, CAP likely mediates "cholinergic behavior" (addiction, emotion, and motivation) after activation by ACh or nicotine, probably linking tobacco use by SCZ patients to improved awareness and insight [143–149]. Indeed, nicotine was demonstrated to improve spatial neglect in stroke patients, suggesting that anosognosia is driven, at least in part, by the cholinergic pathways [150,151] (Figure 1).

Several novel studies have found that nicotine (and probably ACh) stimulates AhR via STAT3, engendering a "molecular interoceptive system" which connects to IC via VN [151]. Within this system, AhR receives input from the microbiome as well as the environment (via xenobiotics, toxins, and photo-metabolites) and relays these data to the CNS for processing and discernment, completing the interoceptive loop [152, 153].

At the subcellular level, phosphorylated STAT3 (pSTAT3) bridges the gap between ACh, AhR, and IL-22, which closes the interoceptive circuit by generating more pSTAT3 and repeating the cycle [17,122,154,155]. Indeed, the AhR/STAT3/IL-22 axis upregulates Bifidobacterium and Lactobacillus spp., microbes known for producing IL-10, upregulating pSTAT3 further (Figure 1).

The barrier-protective role of IL-22 surfaced during the 1980s HIV-1 epidemic, an infection known for disrupting the intestinal barrier, promoting microbial translocation [156,157]. IL-22 is regulated by AhR/STAT3 and is produced by several types of lymphocytes, including T helper (Th) 17 cells, $\gamma\delta$ T cells, natural killer cells (NKCs), and innate lymphoid cells (ILC) [158]. IL-22 plays a key role in preventing premature cellular senescence and thymic involution, a pathology documented in SCZ [159,160].

Taken together, interoceptive awareness is driven by the IC via CAP. At the subcellular level, the "molecular insight" is mediated by the AhR/STAT3/IL-22 axis, connecting the microbiome to the IC.

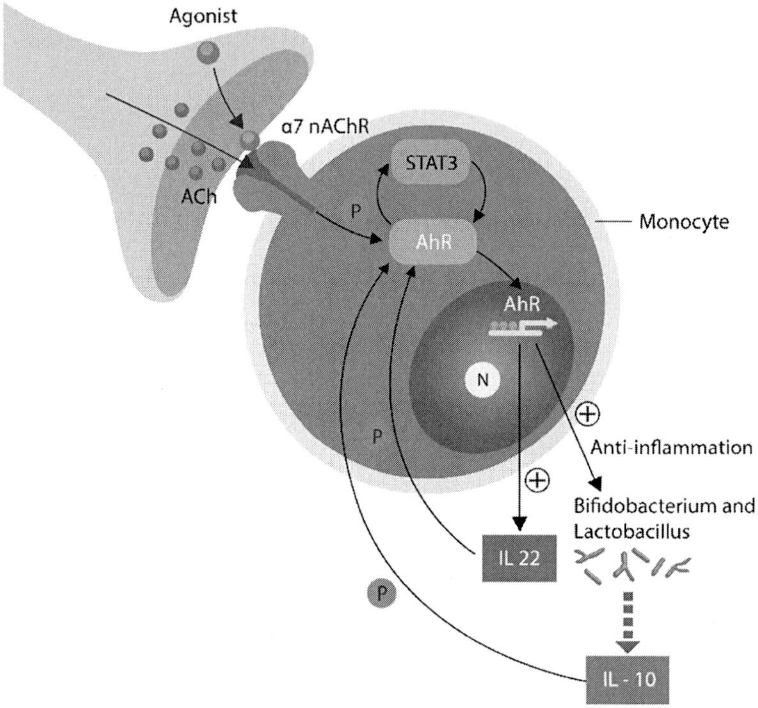


**Figure 1. Upregulated peripheral monocytes may reflect the status of IC-mediated interoceptive awareness. At the molecular level, insight is likely driven by α7nAChRs which connect CAP to the AhR/STAT3/IL-22 axis. Beneficial gut microbes *Bifidobacterium* and *Lactobacillus* release IL-10, a cytokine that provides feedback to the IC via STAT3 phosphorylation. IL-22 (related to IL-10) also phosphorylates STAT3, closing the feedback loop.**

## 4. DH-Incongruent SCZ Features

Antipsychotic drugs are extremely efficacious for the treatment of acute psychosis and will likely remain the gold standard of psychiatric practice worldwide for the foreseeable future. However, in patients with chronic SCZ, the response to these drugs is less substantial as roughly one out of every seven patients recover, indicating a likely etiopathogenetic difference between acute psychosis and chronic schizophrenia [102,161–163]. Moreover, unlike the discovery of antibiotics which rendered inpatient public institutions for communicable diseases obsolete, the advance of antipsychotic drugs produced a less dramatic effect and only at the expense of high rates of incarceration and homelessness [90,164–166].

The gut microbiome is separated from the rest of the body by a single layer of IECs that microbes cross routinely during development to "educate" the host immune system in tolerating commensal flora. However, translocation during adult life, depending on the species, triggers inflammation and immunogenicity [167].

### *4.1 Markers of Gut Barrier Dysfunction*

SCZ has been associated with microbial translocation, likely promoted by premature senescence and the accumulation of senescent, damaged cells at the gut barrier and BBB [13,168–170]. In SCZ, the pilling up of senescent cells is likely induced by accelerated tissue aging and/or impaired autophagy [171,172]. Aging cells are marked by short telomeres, replication arrest, active metabolism, and a detrimental secretome, known as senescence-associated secretory phenotype (SASP) that can spread senescence throughout the body [173]. In addition, senescent and defective cells can easily disintegrate, releasing immunogenic intracellular molecules, which can trigger autoimmune inflammation and barrier disruption [174]. For example, cell-free DNA (cfDNA), an emerging SCZ marker, was documented in IBD, an SCZ comorbid autoimmune disorder [175,176]. Interestingly, gut microbiota releases microbial cell-free DNA (cfmDNA) that can be detected in the peripheral blood, indicating a potential measurable marker of intestinal barrier integrity [177]. For example, elevated Bacteroidetes and Firmicutes cfmDNA, documented in IBD, may also be a marker of SCZ with a potential role in screening individuals at high risk [178,179]. To our knowledge, there are no studies of cfmDNA in SCZ; however, elevated cfDNA was demonstrated in patients with a first episode of SCZ, linking this pathology once more to gut barrier disruption [176,180].

### *4.2. Autoantibodies as Markers of Microbial Translocation*

Over the past two decades, numerous "autoantibodies", including anti-N-methyl-Daspartate (NMDA) receptor antibodies, have been documented in SCZ, comprising phenomena difficult to reconcile with the DH. For example, the translocation of Corynebacterium glutamicum, a major glutamate producer, may account for NMDA receptor "autoantibodies", documented in SCZ [181,182] (Table 2). However, instead of reflecting autoreactivity, these "autoantibodies" may be conventional immunoglobulins directed at translocated microbial antigens.

**Table 2. Exogenous and endogenous AhR agonists and antagonists.**

| Exogenous Agonists | Endogenous Agonists | Dietary Antagonists | Pharmacological Antagonists |
|---|---|---|---|
| Benzotriazole UV stabilizer | Tryptophan photo metabolites and FICZ | quercetin | CH-223191 |
| Plasticizers (Bisphenol) | Indoles | apigenin | Alpha-naphtoflavone 3-methroxy-4-itriflavone |
| Clozapine | D3 hydroxyderivatives | luteolin | BAY2416964 |
| Carbidopa | DA | kaempferol | HBU651 |

Moreover, rather than "autoantibodies", immunoglobulins against Escherichia coli (E. coli) proteins yjjU, livG and ftsE, found in many SCZ patients, may reflect E. coli translocation through the dysfunctional intestinal barrier associated with this disorder [40]. Furthermore, γ-Aminobutyric acid (GABA)-generating Pseudomonas fluorescens may, upon migration into host systemic circulation, elicit anti-GABA antibodies, immunoglobulins documented in patients with SCZ [41,42]. As this topic was discussed elsewhere, it will not be explored in more detail here [183].

### *4.3 AhR, and Antipsychotic Drugs*

Discovered in 1976, AhR is a ligand-activated transcription factor and dioxin receptor, which regulates numerous cellular processes in response to exogenous and endogenous signals [184–186]. Currently, AhR is believed to be activated in a "tissue-specific" and "context-specific" manner which is not entirely clear, and more studies are needed to elucidate the ligands at this important receptor [187].

Under physiological circumstances, HSP90 retains AhR in the cytoplasm, preventing its ingress into the nucleus. HSP90 disassociation from AhR reveals a specific motif (adjacent to valine 647) that when exposed, promotes AhR nuclear entry, followed by either silencing or expression of several genes, possibly including the SCZ risk genes [188–190]. Indeed, the AhR/HSP90 complex has been implicated in psychosis and may exhibit opposite effects when residing in the cytoplasm vs. the nucleus. In general, high-affinity AhR ligands, primarily dioxin and plasticizers, induce neuronal apoptosis and cognitive deficit, while low-affinity AhR ligands and partial agonists or antagonists, such as quercetin, apigenin, or campherol, elicit neuroprotective effects [26,191,192]. Interestingly, aripiprazole-activated HSP90 has been associated with neurite outgrowth, suggesting involvement in neuroplasticity and cognition [193,194] (Figure 2). Moreover, both DA and clozapine are AhR ligands, while HSP90 has been involved in PD by inducing damage in midbrain DA neurons, suggesting that this complex plays a major role in neuropathology, probably accounting for the higher prevalence of SCZ in urban areas [53,195]. On the other hand, HSP90 inhibitors have emerged as therapies for neurodegenerative diseases and cancer [196]. Since DA is an AhR agonist, DA inhibition by antipsychotic drugs may have an antagonistic effect on the downstream AhR. This effect may strengthen the stability of AhR/HSP90 binding, maintaining this complex in the cytoplasm, thus preventing the transcription of SCZ risk genes [197].

In the gut, AhR is activated by tryptophan-derived microbial metabolites and participates in numerous physiological and pathological processes. Dietary AhR ligands promote STAT3 phosphorylation (pSTAT3), inducing the IL-22, the "guardian" of the gut barrier [198]. AhR ligands, including

DA, serotonin, and melatonin, may play a major role in interoceptive awareness [63–65].

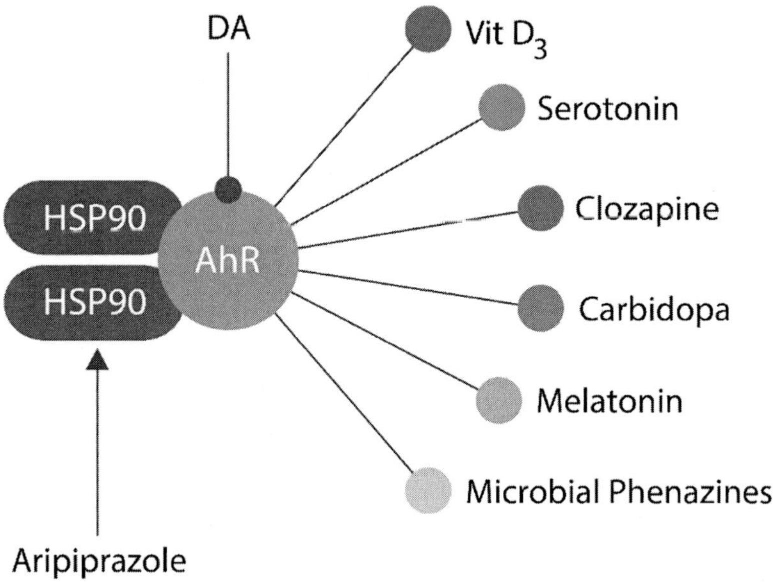


**Figure 2. AhR ligands associated with SCZ. DA is an AhR ligand, while aripiprazole binds HSP90. AhR agonists, vitamin D3, melatonin, and serotonin likely account for the increasing prevalence of SCZ with latitude, while pollutants, including dioxin, correlate with the increased prevalence of SCZ in urban environments. Microbial phenazines are natural phenothiazines, suggesting that these drugs are likely AhR. ligands.**

### *4.4. AhR and Environmental Pollutants*

Exposure to various environmental pollutants during development has been associated with SCZ, likely accounting for the higher prevalence of this disorder in individuals born or raised in urban areas [27,28]. Environmental pollutants, including dioxin, bind with high affinity to AhR, inducing neuronal apoptosis and cognitive dysfunction. For example, prenatal exposure to diethylhexyl phthalate (DEHP), a widely used plasticizer, has been shown to disrupt the thymus, inducing premature involution of this gland, a pathology encountered in SCZ [29,30,199,200]. In addition, this pollutant triggers gut barrier disruption and was linked to autism spectrum disorder (ASD), suggesting likely involvement in SCZ [31,32]. Moreover, DEHP has been implicated in ferroptosis, a nonapoptotic cell death, triggered by lipid peroxidation in the context of elevated intracellular iron levels and impaired redox systems [201]. Indeed, lipid peroxidation is accelerated by pollutants, including the atmospheric fine particulate matter (FPM), previously linked to neuropathology, including SCZ [33,34]. Ferroptosis and lipid peroxidation in biological barriers promote translocation-related pathology, including SCZ.

### *4.5. AhR and Latitude Variance*

The increasing prevalence rate of SCZ with distance from the equator indicates that daylight duration and light-activated AhR ligands play a major role in the pathogenesis of this disorder. The most studied sunlight-dependent AhR ligands include vitamin D3, and tryptophan photo-metabolites, such as 6-formylindolo [3,2-b]carbazole (FICZ), play a key role in latitude-dependent SCZ prevalence [35,202,203]. Upon vitamin D3/AhR binding, the receptor/ligand complex is shuttled into the nucleus where the transcription of multiple genes is initiated or suppressed [36–38]. In addition, FICZ upregulates IL22, protecting the gut barrier and BBB, likely explaining the lower prevalence of SCZ in warm climates [35,37]. Moreover, since latitude drives the diversity of gut microbiota, industrialized countries, found primarily at higher latitudes, exhibit less diverse microbes compared to equatorial areas of the globe [39].

Taken together, gut barrier disruption and microbial translocation, a common feature of SCZ, likely explain the association of this illness with being born and raised in urban environments as well as latitude variance, placing AhR at the very center of this pathology.

## 5. Non-Dopaminergic Antipsychotic Mechanisms of Neuroleptic Drugs

Several properties of antipsychotic agents appear difficult to reconcile with the DH, even when taking into consideration environmental and genetic factors [109]. For example, the antimicrobial properties of these drugs could alleviate psychosis by eliminating translocated microbes and subsequent inflammation [204]. The non-dopaminergic, therapeutic properties of antipsychotic drugs are likely driven by AhR, a protein involved in the regulation of antimicrobial, antiviral, and antiproliferative host defenses as well as pathogen clearance via reactive oxygen species (ROS), or autophagy [205–207]. For example, AhR-induced ROS can ameliorate psychotic symptoms by clearing intracellular pathogens, including Toxoplasma gondii, a SCZ-associated parasite [208]. In addition, neuroleptic drug-activated autophagy and clearance of molecular debris and damaged cells lower the organismal inflammatory burden, likely generating antipsychotic effects [209,210]. Conversely, dysfunctional autophagy and accumulation of cellular remains at the gut barrier and BBB may promote inflammation and microbial translocation into the host systemic circulation [66]. This may explain elevated translocation markers and the more diverse blood microbiome documented in SCZ patients [66,70,211].

Gut commensals enjoy immunological tolerance in the GI tract; however, this protection ceases upon migration outside the intestinal barrier, where they can be vehemently attacked by the host immune defenses [212]. Bactericidal antipsychotic drugs likely facilitate the clearance of both translocated microbes and damaged cells (by autophagy activation), lowering the odds of neuroinflammation and psychosis [213,214]. Other nondopaminergic beneficial effects of antipsychotic drugs, such as telomere elongation, microglial de-escalation, and inhibition of ferroptosis, may likely be explained by the agonist/antagonist AhR binding [6,200,215,216]. For example, AhR antagonists and some partial agonists, including resveratrol, quercetin, or the synthetic compound HBU651, were demonstrated to elongate telomeres, reverse microglial activation, and avert ferroptosis, placing AhR at the epicenter of SCZ pathology [217–220] (Table 2).

Taken together, the clinical efficacy of antipsychotic drugs may be mediated by both dopaminergic and non-dopaminergic pathways, the latter including lowering neuroinflammation, ferroptosis inhibition, telomere lengthening, and deactivation of microglia [215,221–223].

### *5.1. Antipsychotics as Antibacterials*

Firstand second-generation antipsychotic drugs possess antibacterial properties, suggesting that the elimination of translocated microbes may drive symptomatic relief in psychosis [224]. This is further substantiated by the current efforts to repurpose several antipsychotic drugs as antibiotics [225]. Conversely, antibiotics such as doxycycline and minocycline exert antipsychotic properties, indicating that postsynaptic DA blockade may not be the only mechanism for alleviating psychotic symptoms [226,227].

Other antipsychotic drugs with antimicrobial properties include phenothiazines, compounds capable of eliminating E. coli, a bacterium previously associated with SCZ [228,229]. Moreover, haloperidol exerts fungicidal action against Candida albicans (C. albicans), a BBB-crossing fungus, linked by previous studies to SCZ [230–232]. Furthermore, both antipsychotic drugs and IL-22, including the recombinant form, inhibit IFN-γ, a cytokine with established antifungal properties [233,234]. Interestingly, IL-22 exhibits fungicidal action against C. albicans as well as antipsychotic-like properties [231,235–238] (Table 3).

**Table 3. Antipsychotic-like properties of IL22 (or recombinant IL22).**

| Antipsychotic Drugs | Recombinant IL-22 | References |
|---|---|---|
| JAK-STAT activation | JAK-STAT activation | [239,240] |
| Neuroprotective | Neuroprotective | [241,242] |
| IFN-γ inhibitor | IFN-γ inhibitor | [243,244] |
| Activate autophagy | Activate autophagy | [245–247] |
| Antibacterial/antiviral | Antibacterial/antiviral | [230,248–250] |

### *5.2. Antipsychotics as Antivirals*

Many antipsychotic drugs possess antiviral properties inherited from their parent compound and phenothiazine dye, methylene blue (MB) [251]. For example, chlorpromazine exerts antiviral properties against SARS-CoV-2, the etiologic agent of the COVID-19 pandemic, and is currently in clinical trials (NCT04366739) for this viral infection [252]. Other viruses enter host cells via clathrin-dependent endocytosis (CDE) and are inhibited by several neuroleptics, including chlorpromazine, fluphenazine, perphenazine, prochlorperazine, and thioridazine, emphasizing an alternative, DA-independent mechanisms of action, likely mediated by AhR (functioning as an E3 ubiquitin ligase) [253–255].

Several antipsychotic drugs alter the biophysical properties of cell membranes by intercalating themselves into the lipid bilayer, blocking viral fusion with host cells. At the same time, this process may comprise an antipsychotic mechanism by depolarizing neuronal membranes, lowering pathological connectivity and likely calcium entry [256,257]. Moreover, several antipsychotics, including haloperidol, are cationic, amphiphilic compounds that accumulate in lysosomes, likely sabotaging viral replication as well as SCZ-associated lysosomal dysfunction [258,259].

### *5.3. Antipsychotics as Anticancer Drugs*

Several firstand second-generation antipsychotic drugs can arrest the cell cycle at the G2/M point, explaining their beneficial effects against some cancers [260,261]. In patients with SCZ, antipsychotic drugs were found to block the paradoxical attempt of mature neurons to re-enter the cell cycle, emphasizing another possible DA-independent mechanism of alleviating psychosis [262–266].

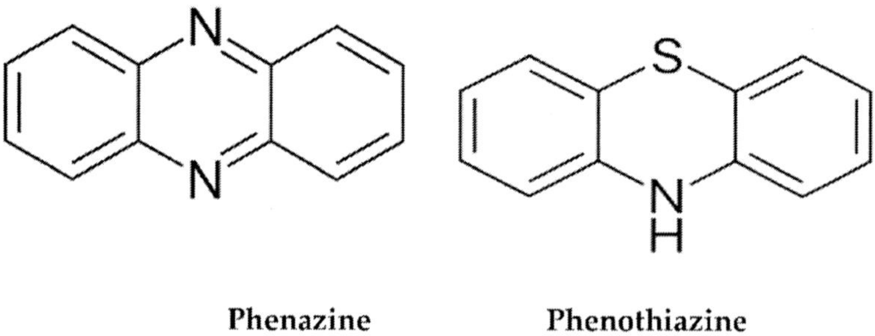


**Figure 3. Structural similarity between microbial phenazines and phenothiazines. In the gut, Pseudomonas aeruginosa is the main producer of phenazines. Phenazines upregulate ACh by inhibiting its degrading enzymes, acetylcholinesterase (AChE) and butyryl acetylcholinesterase (BChE), enhancing cholinergic transmission.**

### *5.4. Microbial Phenazines vs. Antipsychotic Phenothiazines*

Phenazines are ubiquitous nitrogen-based AhR ligands, released by a wide variety of bacteria, including gut commensals Pseudomonas spp. [267,268]. Like phenothiazine antipsychotics, phenazines exhibit anti-inflammatory, anticancer, antimicrobial, and neuroprotective properties, suggesting that they likely bind AhR [269]. Microbial phenazines are natural phenothiazines, generated by the gut commensals to eliminate pathogenic bacteria and malignant cells by ROS production [270–272] (Figure 3).

Phenothiazines are MB derivatives which led to the development of the first marketed antipsychotic drug, chlorpromazine, which in 1954 ushered in the era of psychopharmacology [273,274]. Since microbial phenazines are AhR ligands, phenothiazines very likely attach to AhR, suggesting an alternative antipsychotic mechanism [275,276].

## 6. Potential Applications

In this section, we take a closer look at several therapeutic modalities for optimizing intestinal permeability and increasing neurogenesis in both the CNS and the enteric nervous system (ENS). We discuss CAP enhancement, recombinant IL-22, and AhR ligands.

### *6.1. Cholinergic Anti-Inflammatory Pathway Augmentation*

In 2005, the Food and Drug Administration (FDA) approved VNS for the treatment of refractory major depressive disorder (MDD). More recent studies have shown that this treatment modality reduces paracellular intestinal permeability, suggesting beneficial effects in both IBD and SCZ [277–279]. For example, noninvasive transcutaneous VNS (tVNS), including trans-auricular (taVNS), currently utilized in clinical practice for the treatment of seizure disorder and migraine headaches, has been demonstrated to protect the intestinal barrier by parasympathetic nicotinic action on occludin and zonulin-1 (ZO-1) [280–283]. In addition, tVNS increases the abundance of beneficial gut microbes, Bifidobacterium and Lactobacillus, enhancing the gut barrier [284–286]. As inflammation negatively affects interoceptive awareness, tVMS may augment insight by increasing CAP function [287–289].

A variant of tVNS, ultrasound neuromodulation of the spleen, is based on the recent finding that memory T cells generate ACh in the gut and spleen, influencing microbial diversity [290–292]. Moreover, AChE and BuChE inhibitors may accomplish similar results to tVNS by increasing ACh levels [293,294]. A growing body of evidence has connected CAP and α7nAChR with increased neurogenesis in both the adult brain and ENS, emphasizing further central control of the gut barrier [295,296].

Taken together, ACh upregulation via therapeutics or vagal stimulation may have beneficial effects in SCZ by enhancing adult neurogenesis in both the CNS and ENS, lowering microbial translocation.

### *6.2. Recombinant IL-22 for IBD and SCZ*

The 2007 conclusion of the Human Microbiome Project and the subsequent finding that the brain and gut AhR/STAT3/IL-22 axis promotes neurogenesis in various niches shedding more light on the gut–brain interaction, suggesting that activating this molecular axis may be beneficial in SCZ [297–301].

IL-22, currently in clinical trials for IBD, exhibits antipsychotic-like properties and promotes thymus gland rejuvenation, suggesting beneficial effects in SCZ (NCT02847052) [302–305]. To our knowledge, at the time of this writing, there are no studies on IL-22 in SCZ. We have previously hypothesized that F-652, a recombinant human IL-22, can alleviate psychotic symptoms by blocking microbial translocation. Table 2 summarizes the overlapping action mechanisms of IL-22 (F-652) and antipsychotic drugs.

A member of the IL-10 cytokine family, IL-22, interacts with a heterodimeric protein comprising IL-22 and IL-10 receptors, which has been previously implicated in SCZ [305–307]. Moreover, IL-22 is an active participant in iron metabolism by inducing transcription of hepcidin and lowering ferroportin, sequestrating intracellular iron in ferritin [308,309]. This is significant as novel studies have shown that iron accumulates in SCZ brains, emphasizing that ferroptosis may be a key player in this pathology

[310–312]. Recombinant IL-22/F-652 may be beneficial in SCZ as it lowers the risk of ferroptosis by promoting iron storage in ferritin [313].

### *6.3. Dietary and Pharmacological AhR Ligands*

Excessive AhR activation was found to disrupt neurogenesis during the development, inducing growth arrest and apoptosis, a pathology encountered in ASD and SCZ [314,315]. Moreover, weight gain, one of the most common adverse effects of clozapine, is likely mediated by AhR and could be averted by this receptor's antagonist, CH-223191, a likely future metabolic syndrome treatment [316]. However, AhR antagonists also lower IL-22; therefore, studies of partial agonists/antagonists at this receptor are needed as these agents have the ability to selectively target AhR, avoiding adverse effects such as metabolic syndrome or IL-22 downregulation [317,318]. Moreover, selective AhR modulators (SAhRMs), such as flavonoids, may increase IL-22 without excessive AhR activation [318]. For example, quercetin apigenin, luteolin, kaempferol (KPF), and several common spices, including cloves, dill, thyme, nutmeg, and oregano, exert SAhRM properties, indicating selective induction of IL-22 without AhR overactivation [319,320]. Furthermore, synthetic flavonoids alpha-naphtoflavone, 3-methroxy-4-itriflavone, and their derivatives also possess SAhRM properties, suggesting potential benefits in SCZ [321]. AhR was discovered by Alan Poland et al., in 1976 and was characterized as a dioxin receptor [322]. A ligand-activated transcription factor, AhR responds to internal and external stimuli and the research focus has recently shifted from environmental toxins to ligands originating from the intracellular and extracellular body compartments. The discovery that AhR regulates transposable elements (including retrotransposons), DNA segments implicated in SCZ and ASD, has brought this transcription factor closer to the neuropsychiatric arena [323].

AhR has been known to induce cytochrome P450 1A1 (CYP1A1), an enzyme abundantly represented in the kidney, liver, and intestine, involved in phase one metabolism [324]. Approximately 70–80% of all drugs and exogenous molecules are metabolized by CYP1, 2, and 3 enzyme families [325]. CYP1A1 is responsible for the metabolism of fatty acids, steroid hormones, and heavy metals [326]. CYP1A1 was demonstrated to impair the phagocytosis of microorganisms, indicating interference with microbial translocation form the GI tract into the systemic circulation [327].

## 7. Wider Disparate Data and Future Directions

The investigation of how the above links to wider bodies of data should better clarify processes relevant to the pathophysiology and treatment of schizophrenia. As with many neuropsychiatric conditions, suboptimal mitochondrial function is often evident in diverse brain and systemic cells of people with schizophrenia [328]. Notably, AhR and α7nAChR are present on the mitochondrial membrane [329], indicating that direct effects on mitochondria, and therefore on core aspects of cellular function, are likely to be important aspects of pathophysiological alterations in schizophrenia. It is also important to note that AhR, via CYP1A2 and CYP1B1, O-demethylates melatonin to N-acetylserotonin (NAS). Variations in the NAS/melatonin ratio may be important given that NAS is a BDNF mimic via TrkB activation [330] and therefore drives more proliferative responses, whilst melatonin optimizes mitochondrial function and oxidant status, thereby impacting how mitochondrial oxidant production drives ROS-dependent microRNAs, and therefore modulating patterned gene expression. TrkB, like AhR and α7nAChR, is expressed on the mitochondrial membrane [330], indicating that variations in the AhR-driven NAS/melatonin ratio may have significant direct effects on mitochondrial function and thereby on patterned gene expression. It will be important for future research to determine how the mitochondrial presence of AhR, TrkB, and α7nAChR modulate core mitochondrial function and patterned gene expression, and thereby the changes in intercellular fluxes evident in schizophrenia.

This links to wider bodies of data showing increases in pro-inflammatory cytokines and dysregulated HPA axis, leading to increased indoleamine 2,3-dioxygenase (IDO) and tryptophan 2,3-dioxygenase (TDO), driving the raised levels of kynurenine and especially kynurenic acid evident in schizophrenia [331,332]. Both kynurenine and kynurenic acid activate AhR, whilst kynurenic acid may also antagonize the α7nAChR and N-methyl-daspartate (NMDA) receptor [332]. Wider immune dysregulation in schizophrenia may therefore be intimately linked to AhR and α7nAChR regulation, with consequences for mitochondrial function and intercellular interactions. Raised levels of systemic pro-inflammatory cytokines increase gut permeability, typically concurrent to gut dysbiosis, indicating how systemic inflammatory processes modulate the gut and the gut's influence on wider systemic processes, including its interaction with the vagal nerve. Variations in the levels of gut microbiome-derived butyrate may be especially important given the powerful influence of butyrate on mitochondrial function across body cells [333].

## 8. Conclusions

Several SCZ characteristics seem incongruent with DH, while some antipsychotic drugs appear to lower the positive symptoms of SCZ by DA-independent mechanisms. These discrepancies suggest that the third revision of DH may require further adjustment, as the dopaminergic transmission, receiving genetic and epigenetic input, may not be the final step in SCZ pathogenesis. DA is an AhR ligand; therefore, DA-lowering drugs may attenuate psychotic symptoms by indirectly modulating AhR. This seems to indicate that DA may play the role of an upstream effector which alters the function of AhR, the master regulator of exogenous and endogenous input. This may also explain the "delayed onset" of antipsychotic action, despite the fact that DA receptors are blocked very shortly after the dose.

Under physiological circumstances, the gut AhR/STAT3/IL22 axis optimizes microbiota composition and relays the status of "luminal milieu" to IC, directly regulating interoceptive awareness. Recombinant human IL-22/F-652 is an antimicrobial and antiviral molecule that promotes tissue repair, autophagy, and thymic regeneration, reversing SCZ-associated premature cellular and thymic senescence.

Stimulation of VN branches is a noninvasive procedure that promotes beneficial microbiota, lowering local and systemic inflammation. These procedures could correct SCZ-associated anosognosia as well as avert metabolic adverse effects. More AhR studies are needed to clarify this transcription factor's ligands and their selective actions in a tissueand context-dependent manner.

**Funding:** This research received no external funding. Institutional Review **Board Statement: Not applicable. Informed Consent Statement:** Not applicable.

**Data Availability Statement:** Not applicable.

**Conflicts of Interest:** The authors declare no conflict of interest.

## References

1. Berman JD, Burkhardt J, Bayham J, Carter E, Wilson A. Acute Air Pollution Exposure and the Risk of Violent Behavior in the United States. Epidemiology. 2019 Nov;30(6):799-806. doi: 10.1097/EDE.0000000000001085. PMID: 31430264.
2. Wei Q, Ji Y, Gao H, Yi W, Pan R, Cheng J, He Y, Tang C, Liu X, Song S, Song J, Su H. Oxidative stress-mediated particulate matter affects the risk of relapse in schizophrenia patients: Air purification intervention-based panel study. Environ Pollut. 2022 Jan 1;292(Pt B):118348. doi: 10.1016/j.envpol.2021.118348.
3. Khan A, Plana-Ripoll O, Antonsen S, et al. Environmental pollution is associated with an increased risk of psychiatric disorders in the US and Denmark. PLoS Biol. 2019;17(8):e3000353
4. Fu P, Yung KKL. Air Pollution and Alzheimer's Disease: A Systematic Review and Meta-Analysis. J Alzheimers Dis. 2020;77(2):701-714. doi: 10.3233/JAD-200483. PMID: 32741830.
5. Burkhardt, J., Bayham, J., Wilson, A., Carter, E., Berman, J.D., O'Dell, K., Ford, B., Fischer, E.V., & Pierce, J.R. (2019). The effect of pollution on crime: Evidence from data on particulate matter and ozone. Journal of Environmental Economics and Management.
6. Calderón-Garcidueñas L, Stommel EW, Rajkumar RP, Mukherjee PS, Ayala A. Particulate Air Pollution and Risk of Neuropsychiatric Outcomes. What We Breathe, Swallow, and Put on Our Skin Matters. Int J Environ Res Public Health. 2021 Nov 3;18(21):11568. Doi: 10.3390/ijerph182111568.
7. Ji Y, Liu B, Song J, Pan R, Cheng J, Su H, Wang H. Particulate matter pollution associated with schizophrenia hospital re-admissions: a time-series study in a coastal Chinese city. Environ Sci

Pollut Res Int. 2021 Nov;28(41):58355-58363. doi: 10.1007/s11356-021-14816-3.

8. Gao J, Wei Q, Pan R, Yi W, Xu Z, Duan J, Tang C, He Y, Liu X, Song S, Su H. Elevated environmental PM2.5 increases risk of schizophrenia relapse: Mediation of inflammatory cytokines. Sci Total Environ. 2021 Jan 20;753:142008. doi: 10.1016/j.scitotenv.2020.142008.
9. Parra KL, Alexander GE, Raichlen DA, Klimentidis YC, Furlong MA. Exposure to air pollution and risk of incident dementia in the UK Biobank. Environ Res. 2022 Jun;209:112895. doi: 10.1016/j.envres.2022.112895.
10. Brown JS Jr. Effects of bisphenol-A and other endocrine disruptors compared with abnormalities of schizophrenia: an endocrine-disruption theory of schizophrenia. Schizophr Bull. 2009 Jan;35(1): 256-78. doi: 10.1093/schbul/sbm147.
11. Moreno-Gómez-Toledano R, Sánchez-Esteban S, Cook A, Mínguez-Moratinos M, Ramírez-Carracedo R, Reventún P, Delgado-Marín M, Bosch RJ, Saura M. Bisphenol A Induces Accelerated Cell Aging in Murine Endothelium. Biomolecules. 2021 Sep 29;11(10):1429. doi: 10.3390/biom11101429.
12. Gale SD, Erickson LD, Anderson JE, Brown BL, Hedges DW. Association between exposure to air pollution and prefrontal cortical volume in adults: A cross-sectional study from the UK biobank. Environ Res. 2020 Jun;185:109365. doi: 10.1016/j.envres.2020.109365.
13. Martínez-Lazcano JC, González-Guevara E, del Carmen Rubio M, Franco-Pérez J, Custodio V, Hernández-Cerón M, Livera C, Paz C. The effects of ozone exposure and associated injury mechanisms on the central nervous system. Rev Neurosci. 2013;24(3):337-52. doi: 10.1515/revneuro-2012-0084.
14. Younan D, Wang X, Casanova R, Barnard R, Gaussoin SA, Saldana S, Petkus AJ, Beavers DP, Resnick SM, Manson JE, Serre ML, Vizuete W, Henderson VW, Sachs BC, Salinas J, Gatz M, Espeland MA, Chui HC, Shumaker SA, Rapp SR, Chen JC; Women's Health Initiative. PM2.5 Associated With Gray Matter Atrophy Reflecting

Increased Alzheimer Risk in Older Women. Neurology. 2021 Feb 22;96(8):e1190-e1201. doi: 10.1212/WNL.0000000000011149.
15. Rahman MM, Lorenzo M, Ban-Weiss G, Hasan Z, Azzouz M, Eckel SP, Conti DV, Lurmann F, Schlaerth H, Johnston J, Ko J, Palinkas L, Hurlburt M, Silva S, Gauderman WJ, McConnell R, Garcia E. Ambient temperature and air pollution associations with suicide and homicide mortality in California: A statewide case-crossover study. Sci Total Environ. 2023 May 20;874:162462. doi: 10.1016/j.scitotenv.2023.162462
16. McGarr GW, Fujii N, Schmidt MD, Muia CM, Kenny GP. Heat shock protein 90 modulates cutaneous vasodilation during exercise-heat stress but not during passive whole-body heating in young women. Physiol Rep. 2020 Aug;8(16):e14552. doi: 10.14814/phy2.14552.
17. Streicher JM. The role of heat shock protein 90 in regulating pain, opioid signaling, and opioid antinociception. Vitam Horm. 2019;111:91-103. doi: 10.1016/bs.vh.2019.05.010.
18. Hung HC, Kay SA, Weber F. HSP90, a capacitor of behavioral variation. J Biol Rhythms. 2009 Jun;24(3):183-92. doi: 10.1177/0748730409333171. PMID: 19465695.
19. Golomb BA, Stattin H, Mednick S. Low cholesterol and violent crime. J Psychiatr Res. 2000 Jul-Oct;34(4-5):301-9. doi: 10.1016/s0022-3956(00)00024-8. PMID: 11104842.
20. Tanos R, Patel RD, Murray IA, Smith PB, Patterson AD, Perdew GH. Aryl hydrocarbon receptor regulates the cholesterol biosynthetic pathway in a dioxin response element-independent manner. Hepatology. 2012 Jun;55(6):1994-2004. doi: 10.1002/hep.25571. PMID: 22234961; PMCID: PMC3340481.
21. Virkkunen M. Serum cholesterol levels in homicidal offenders. A low cholesterol level is connected with a habitually violent tendency under the influence of alcohol. Neuropsychobiology. 1983;10(2-3):65-9. doi: 10.1159/000117987. PMID: 6674827.
22. Sen P, Adewusi D, Blakemore AI, Kumari V. How do lipids influence the risk of violence, self-harm, and suicidality in people with psychosis? A systematic review. Aust N Z J Psychiatry. 2022 May;56(5):451-488. doi: 10.1177/00048674211025608

23. Herceg D, Mimica N, Herceg M, Puljić K. Aggression in Women with Schizophrenia Is Associated with Lower HDL Cholesterol Levels. Int J Mol Sci. 2022 Oct 6;23(19):11858. doi: 10.3390/ijms231911858. PMID: 36233163; PMCID: PMC9570159.
24. Sharma R. Emerging Interrelationship Between the Gut Microbiome and Cellular Senescence in the Context of Aging and Disease: Perspectives and Therapeutic Opportunities. Probiotics Antimicrob Proteins. 2022 Aug;14(4):648-663. doi: 10.1007/s12602-021-09903-3.
25. Kim, H.s., Kim, S., Shin, S.J. et al. Gram-negative bacteria and their lipopolysaccharides in Alzheimer's disease: pathologic roles and therapeutic implications. Transl Neurodegener 10, 49 (2021). https://doi.org/10.1186/s40035-021-00273-y
26. Severance EG, Yolken RH. From Infection to the Microbiome: An Evolving Role of Microbes in Schizophrenia. Curr Top Behav Neurosci. 2020;44:67-84. doi: 10.1007/7854_2018_84.
27. Mostafa S, Miller BJ. Antibiotic-associated psychosis during treatment of urinary tract infections: a systematic review. J Clin Psychopharmacol. 2014 Aug;34(4):483-90. doi: 10.1097/JCP.0000000000000150.
28. Page CE, Coutellier L. Reducing inhibition: A promising new strategy for treating schizophrenia. EBioMedicine. 2018 Sep;35:25-26. doi: 10.1016/j.ebiom.2018.07.043.
29. Schwartz DL. Quercetin as an Augmentation Agent in Schizophrenia. J Clin Psychopharmacol. 2016 Jun;36(3):282-3. doi: 10.1097/JCP.0000000000000498. PMID: 27035495.
30. Fan HR, Du WF, Zhu T, Wu YJ, Liu YM, Wang Q, Wang Q, Gu X, Shan X, Deng S, Zhu T, Xu TL, Ge WH, Li WG, Li F. Quercetin Reduces Cortical GABAergic Transmission and Alleviates MK-801-Induced Hyperactivity. EBioMedicine. 2018 Aug;34:201-213. doi: 10.1016/j.ebiom.2018.07.031.
31. Cleide S. Souza, Bruna S. Paulsen, Sylvie Devalle, Silvia Lima Costa, Helena L. Borges, Stevens K. Rehen. The pro-estrogenic flavonoid apigenin induces the commitment of human pluripotent stem cells to a neural lineage. Advances in Regenerative Biology, 2015; 2 (0) DOI: 10.3402/arb.v2.29244

32. Elisabetsky E, Costa-Campos L. The alkaloid alstonine: a review of its pharmacological properties. Evid Based Complement Alternat Med. 2006 Mar;3(1):39-48. doi: 10.1093/ecam/nek011.
33. Yan T, Li L, Sun B, Liu F, Yang P, Chen T, Li T, Liu X. Luteolin inhibits behavioral sensitization by blocking methamphetamine-induced MAPK pathway activation in the caudate putamen in mice. PLoS One. 2014 Jun 5;9(6):e98981.
doi: 10.1371/journal.pone.0098981. PMID: 24901319; PMCID: PMC4047057.
34. Wei KL, Gao GL, Chou YT, Lin CY, Chen SC, Chen YL, Choi HQ, Cheng CC, Su JJ. Sorafenib is an antagonist of the aryl hydrocarbon receptor. Toxicology. 2022 Mar 30;470:153118.
doi: 10.1016/j.tox.2022.153118.
35. Jeong J, Kim KH, Kim DY, Chandrasekaran G, Kim M, Pagire SH, Dighe M, Choi EY, Bak SM, Kim EY, Shin MG, Choi SY, Ahn JH. Identifying new aryl hydrocarbon receptor (AhR) antagonists using a zebrafish model. Bioorg Med Chem. 2019 Oct 1;27(19):115014. doi: 10.1016/j.bmc.2019.07.030.
36. McGovern K, Castro AC, Cavanaugh J, Coma S, Walsh M, Tchaicha J, Syed S, Natarajan P, Manfredi M, Zhang XM, Ecsedy J. Discovery and Characterization of a Novel Aryl Hydrocarbon Receptor Inhibitor, IK-175, and Its Inhibitory Activity on Tumor Immune Suppression. Mol Cancer Ther. 2022 Aug 2;21(8):1261-1272. doi: 10.1158/1535-7163.MCT-21-0984. PMID: 35666806.
37. Kang S, Lee AG, Im S, Oh SJ, Yoon HJ, Park JH, Pak YK. A Novel Aryl Hydrocarbon Receptor Antagonist HBU651 Ameliorates Peripheral and Hypothalamic Inflammation in High-Fat Diet-Induced Obese Mice. Int J Mol Sci. 2022 Nov 28;23(23):14871. doi: 10.3390/ijms232314871. PMID: 36499198; PMCID: PMC9736602.

# CHAPTER 4

# PTSD TRAUMATIC MEMORIES-DRIVEN AGGRESSION

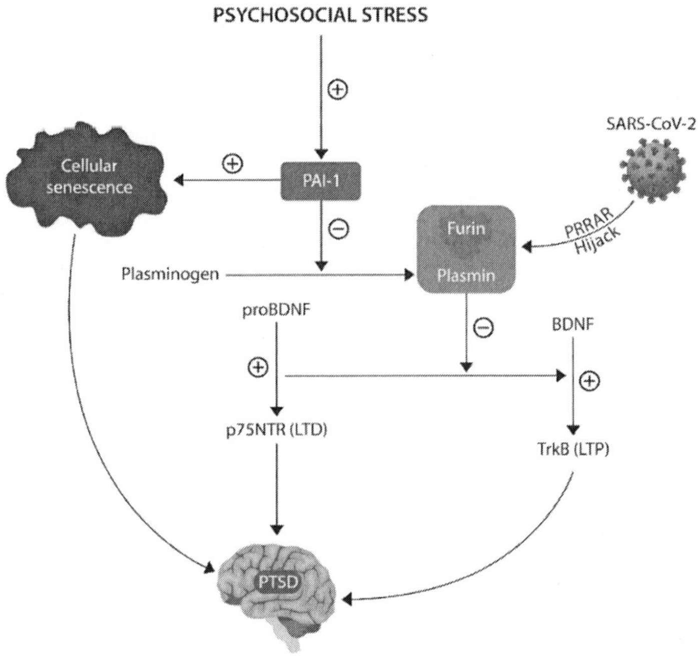


## Visual Abstract

**Psychosocial stress upregulates PAI-1, inducing endothelial and neuronal senescence. PAI-1 inhibits plasmin formation from plasminogen. Low plasmin (necessary for furin activation) disrupts the maturation of pro-BDNF to BDNF. The SARS-CoV-2 virus hijacks furin via the PRRAR motif, disrupting the generation of BDNF from pro-BDN, likely contributing to PTSD. This model explains premature cellular senescence and increased BDNF in PTSD.**

Posttraumatic stress disorder (PTSD) is a severe neuropsychiatric illness triggered by psychological stressors, which, like schizophrenia (SCZ), is marked by premature cellular senescence. Direct molecular aging due to psychosocial stress was documented recently by the detection of senescent markers, including p16INK4a, in PTSD patients (1)(2). Endothelial cells (ECs), due to their vascular architecture and turnover rate, are the first to be affected by normal aging, generating the body's most significant burden of senescent cells (3)(4)(5)(6). Moreover, high comorbidity with cardiovascular disease (CVD) further links PTSD to senescent endothelial (7).

The FURIN gene, a new player in neuropsychiatric illness, is highly expressed in ECs and maintains cellular senescence via brain-derived neurotrophic factor (BDNF) (8)(9)(10)(11). Furin is a proprotein convertase that turns precursor proteins into biologically active forms, including the pro-BDNF into BDNF. BDNF is elevated in PTSD, implicating overactive furin in this pathology (12). The ability to activate toxins or pathogens, such as anthrax, by proteolytic cleavage brought FURIN to the forefront of bioweapon manufacturing programs, where it remained up to the present day (13)(14).

## Traumatic memories are decentralized

As opposed to conventional memories, traumatic imprinting is believed to take place in the right amygdala and posterior cingulate cortex (PCC) (15)(16). Here, emotionally charged memories are processed without the involvement of the hippocampus and are experienced as if occurring in the present moment (17). Recent studies have shown that dysfunctional peripheral blood mononuclear cells could cause or exacerbate PTSD, suggesting that extracerebral cells and tissues are detrimental to traumatic recall (18)(19). This raises the question: can cognition generally “dwell” in the peripheral tissues? Indeed, early studies have found that single cells or unicellular life forms can process and recall information (20)(21). Moreover, furin contributes to protein folding and cognition via dendritic morphogenesis. This brings the question of where traumatic memories are stored.

## What is decentralized cognition?

Cognition and memory are precious human assets, making us unique and distinct from other species. For this reason, cognitive functions are likely distributed throughout the body to lower the odds of memory loss due to brain injuries or pathology. They are probably encoded in the molecular networks of all cells. For example, the cellular cytoskeleton communicates with the proteins of the extracellular matrix via integrins and lipid rafts (membrane windows that unite intra and extracellular molecular networks), generating global assemblies (22).

The proteins in molecular networks are believed to encode memory in a quantum manner by altering the conformational dynamics of various molecules. Indeed, proteins have unique properties that facilitate information processing and storage. Proteins fold along specific lines like origami, connect instantly with each other in a Lego-like fashion, and, like Transformers, build new structures from the old components. Moreover, proteins can exist as two-state systems, engendering logic gates, the building blocks of quantum circuits (23).

The molecular network-mediated memory allows information to be stored in neurons and most body cells, engendering a decentralized "blockchain" cognition. Indeed, phantom limb, pseudocyesis, psychogenic blindness, or cardiac transplant recipients adopting the donor's personality traits show that cells and molecules can harbor memories and behavioral patterns (24)(25).

In severe mental illness (SMI), including PTSD, cells throughout the body undergo premature cellular senescence, a phenotype triggered by dysfunctional tight junctions (TJs) (26)(27). At the level of the gut barrier and blood-brain barrier (BBB), senescent cells increase permeability further, enabling microbial migration into the host circulation and eventually reaching the brain. Senescent glial cells and multipotent stem cells stop replicating or replicate sporadically. In contrast, the opposite takes place in cancer, where there is uncontrolled proliferation, suggesting that senescence and tumorigenesis may act like the two faces of Janus.

Ancient viruses inherited from our predecessors, human endogenous retroviruses (HERVs), dwell in our DNA, comprising approximately 8% of the genome (28).

HERVs are activated by different pathologies, including cancer, SMI, or contemporary viruses, including SARS-CoV-2, the etiologic agent of the COVID-19 pandemic (29). Some HERVs have become "domesticated" and "work" for the human host. For example, HERV-W ENV. Encodes for a placental protein that, under pathological circumstances, may cause infertility (30). Another example, the activity-regulated cytoskeleton-associated (Arc) protein derived from an ancestral virus, is expressed primarily in the brain, promoting synaptic plasticity, learning, and long-term potentiation (31)(32).

A patient with cysticercosis, whom I treated years ago, comes to mind. He behaved, walked, and talked usually. The only complaint was mild forgetfulness and word-finding difficulties. The resident physician did a dementia work-up, including an MRI of the brain. When the results arrived, we were all surprised and wondered how this patient could be alive. He had very little brain parenchyma left. Numerous cysts were throughout his CNS, yet the patient seemed minimally impaired. This individual and others like him are proof that information and memories are stored not only in the brain but also in cells throughout the body. This may explain the patient's normal functioning despite losing cerebral volume. Indeed, consider the amount of information in the DNA, which is present in every single cell of the body, ensuring that the genetic information is not lost or altered. Furthermore, our muscles and tendons "remember" old postures we have long abandoned. Immune cells recall previous infections, while 36% of patients with heart transplants inherit bits and pieces of the donor's personality (33).

# Article for Chapter 4: Of Soldiers and Their Ghosts: Are We Ready for a Review of PTSD Evidence?


## Adonis Sfera[1], Jonathan J. Anton[2], Hassan Imran[1], Zisis Kozlakidis[3], Carolina Klein[4] and Carolina Osorio[1]

*1. California Department of State Hospitals, Patton, CA 92369, USA*
*2. Department of Biology, California Baptist University, Riverside, CA 92504, USA*
*3. International Agency for Research on Cancer, World Health Organization, 69366 Lyon, France*
*4. California Department of State Hospitals, Sacramento, CA 95814, USA*



## Abstract

Psychosocial trauma has accompanied mankind since time immemorial and has been sufficiently portrayed in art and literature to suggest that posttraumatic stress disorder may be as old as combat itself. Since war is more frequent in human history than peace, public health measures are confined to mitigating the detrimental impact of battlefield experiences on combat participants. At present, PTSD outcome studies show mixed results, marked by high nonresponse rates, therapy dropout, and completed suicide, suggesting that novel strategies are urgently needed. Those of us who work routinely with combat veterans have noted an increasing trend of patients preferring mindfulness-based therapies as opposed to trauma-centered treatments, such as prolonged exposure or trauma-focused cognitive behavioral therapy. Preference for mindfulness over trauma-based therapies appears to coincide with the shift in research focus from the amygdala and fear to the insular cortex and interoceptive awareness. Therefore, rethinking PTSD as insular pathology is driven by the recent findings that neurons in this cortical area not only regulate cardiac rhythm but also record past intestinal inflammations. These discoveries likely explain the high comorbidity of stress-related disorders with premature endothelial senescence and a dysfunctional intestinal barrier. Moreover, the identification of the cholinergic anti-inflammatory pathway and the revelation that endothelial cells express alpha-7 nicotinic receptors has brought PTSD prevention and early detection within reach. In this narrative review, we discuss the relationship between early vascular aging, gut barrier disruption, and PTSD. We also examine the link between this pathology and faulty interoceptive awareness, surmising that hypertension and decreased heart rate variability are PTSD risk factors, while lipopolysaccharide, lipopolysaccharide binding protein, soluble CD14, microbial cell-free DNA, acyloxyacyl hydrolase, and IL22 comprise early detection markers of this disorder.

**Keywords:** post traumatic stress disorder; hypertension; heart rate; microbial translocation; endothelial cells.

## 1. Introduction

Although the term "shell shock" was coined during World War I, battle trauma had likely entered human history long before modern warfare [1]. Ancient civilizations, unacquainted with the inner dimensions of the human mind, likely experienced war trauma as a mythical destiny based on the "rule of blood", traced in Ancient Greece to the House of Atreus, a primitive jurisprudence predating the "rule of law" [2,3].

"Nothing Matters to Me Now, But killing and blood and men in agony", exclaimed Trojan hero Achilles, suggesting that experiencing combat can beget new and often random acts of violence (Iliad 19.226). Indeed, combat scenarios, relived over and over by many contemporary veterans, appear to hijack selective neuronal assemblies implicated in emotional recall, keeping the traumatic event vividly alive. Although posttraumatic stress disorder (PTSD) patients maintain awareness of the subjective nature of their adversity-induced experiences, frequent misinterpretation of innocuous cues as danger signals likely reflects subtle defects of insight. In the section "PTSD and interoceptive awareness", we discuss "dysgnosia", a trauma-mediated partial agnosia, also known as "cognitive bias", a less accurate term unreflective of insight.

In the US, the lifetime prevalence of PTSD in the general population is in the range of 7–8%; however, it can surge to 14–16% in combat veterans and military personnel [4]. These data suggest that stress alone, without individual vulnerability, is insufficient to engender this pathology [4]. On the other hand, in susceptible individuals, the exposure to real or threatened death, severe injury, or sexual assault may be followed by pathology, manifested by nightmares, dissociative phenomena, hypervigilance, avoidance of situations reminiscent of the traumatic experience, and, in a subset of veterans, aggressive behavior directed at the self or others [5,6]. The question we ask here is what constitutes susceptibility, and can the high-risk phenotypes be identified early?

The common psychotherapeutic interventions for PTSD (VA/DoD Clinical Practice Guidelines revised in 2017) are primarily "amygdala-centered" and aim at correcting the cognitive bias, reducing fear associated with the traumatic scenario [7,8]. These approaches include prolonged exposure (PE), cognitive processing therapy (CPT), and trauma-focused cognitive behavioral therapy (CBT) with or without psychopharmacological interventions [9–11]. Although for many patients, these approaches are beneficial, nonresponse and treatment dropout rates are high, while the rate of suicide, the most concerning PTSD manifestation, is around 14%, compared to the lifetime risk of 3.7% in patients with major depressive disorder (MDD) [12]. Some clinicians have noticed that interventions incorporating exposure may sometimes trigger flashbacks, possibly accounting for the high therapy dropout rates [13]. In addition, vivid dreams, common adverse effects of antidepressant drugs, exacerbate nightmares in many patients, contributing to medication non-adherence [14].

Mindfulness-based therapies have emerged as alternative interventions for PTSD, aimed at enhancing interoceptive awareness by promoting conscious living in the "present moment" [15]. Preferred by many patients, mindfulness-based approaches have shown significantly lower dropout rates and have demonstrated statistically significant improvement on self-report [16,17]. This may be significant as the insular cortex (IC) houses a cardiac motor area, linking this neuroanatomical site to the autonomic features of PTSD [18]. For example, stress-induced tachycardia is likely mediated by the IC, while flashbacks and panic attacks may reflect a dysfunction in this neural hub. Moreover, aside from heart rate (HR), the IC has been associated with awareness of error, position of the body and limbs, linking cardiovascular system to insight [19–22].

The communication between the IC and vagus nerve (VN) was defined more than three decades ago, while recent studies have not only confirmed the existence of these pathways, but also found that transcutaneous auricular VN stimulation (taVNS) can enhance interoceptive awareness, suggesting a potential therapeutic strategy for PTSD [23,24]. In addition, the IC is tightly connected to the GI tract and was recently shown to store the memory of prior gut inflammations, likely explaining the high comorbidity between PTSD and inflammatory bowel disease (IBD), estimated at 19.5% [25,26]. Indeed, these findings were validated in neuroimaging studies, revealing impaired insular connectivity in patients with Chron's disease [27,28]. Interestingly, in one study, electrical stimulation of the IC was shown to increase the abundance of gut Prevotella and Bacteroides species, suggesting that insular neurons control microbiota composition [29].

## 2. PTSD and Interoceptive Awareness

Most PTSD models and therapies assume that excessive activation of amygdala triggers fearful memories, contributing to the pathogenesis of this disorder [30–32]. However, novel studies have shown that the inner perception of trauma may be more significant for the development of posttraumatic symptoms than the activation of fear-imbued memories [32]. For example, when processing traumatic experiences, the IC permeates the interoceptive and exteroceptive stimuli with autonomic coloring, generating a unique, individualized, inner perception of the catastrophic event [33,34]. In addition, the IC regulates empathy, compassion, and social cues, including the ability to interpret the feelings of others and adjust one's behavior accordingly [35]. This special form of insight is often impaired in PTSD patients, who frequently misinterpret neutral social signals as hostility, leading to hypervigilance, anxiety, and, occasionally, aggression [36]. Furthermore, dissociative phenomena, such as flashbacks and intrusive memories, may reflect disruption of insulamediated emotional intelligence as opposed to the amygdala and fear [37–39]. Indeed, neuroimaging

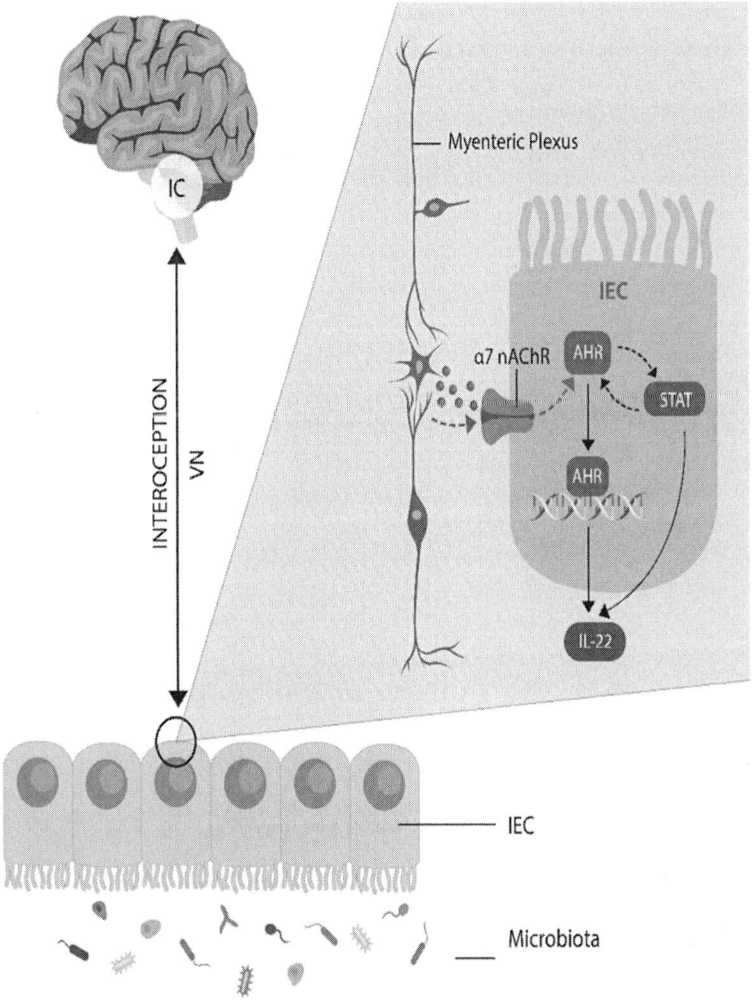


**Figure 1. The IC-IEC dialog is part of the gut–brain axis as well as the CAP. These systems enable interoceptive awareness, a two-way communication between insular neuronal networks and intestinal epithelial/endothelial cells. At the molecular level, myenteric-plexus-secreted acetylcholine (ACh) (via α7nAChR) activates the AhR/STAT3/IL22 system (which requires AhR entry into the nucleus, where it acts as a transcription factor). IL22, the "guardian of intestinal barrier", prevents MT into host tissues.**

studies of PTSD patients, experiencing active flashbacks, have revealed both dysconnectivity and impaired insular activation [40,41] (Figure 1).

Under normal circumstances, the IC receives input from the autonomic nervous system, comprising sympathetic, parasympathetic, and enteric divisions, as well as innate and adaptive immune data, maintaining a detailed inflammatory map [42–44]. In the gut, intestinal epithelial cells (IECs) express alpha 7 nicotinic acetylcholine receptor (α7nAChR), a major component of the cholinergic anti-inflammatory pathway (CAP) discovered in 2000 by Borovikova LV and colleagues. This system likely explains the beneficial effect of transcutaneous auricular vagal nerve stimulation (taVNS) on the intestinal barrier, where dopamine (DA)-activated aryl hydrocarbon receptor (AhR) upregulates interleukin 22 (IL22), maintaining physiological permeability [45–48] (Figure 1).

Under pathological circumstances, the IC has been implicated in a wide variety of syndromes marked by deficient insight, ranging from anosognosia to psychopathy, and frontotemporal dementia (FTD), linking insular neurons to disease awareness [19,49,50]. This is significant as several viral infections highly comorbid with PTSD, including SARS-CoV-2 and human immunodeficiency virus 1 (HIV-1), disrupt IC, inducing anosognosia for cognitive deficits. This suggests that insula is the likely the "dwelling place of insight" [51–53]. Moreover, as these viral infections induce intestinal inflammation, the GI tract likely plays a role in interoceptive awareness, justifying the vernacular expression "gut feeling", as a synonym for insight [26,27,54]. This is significant as patients with PTSD likely exhibit dysgnosia, a subtle insight deficit, interfering with the appreciation of situational reality [55,56]. For example, interpreting innocuous stimuli as danger signals may represent errors of insight, rather than amygdala-generated fearful stimuli [57]. In addition, like in frontotemporal dementia, PTSD patients may engage in aggressive acts while maintaining some degree of insight into the negative impact of this behavior [58]. Moreover, the fact that some patients with PTSD prefer mindfulness, instead of trauma-oriented therapies, may be the proof of concept that a dysfunctional IC may drive the pathogenesis of PTSD [13,59,60]. In the following subsections, we will discuss in more detail the role of the IC in emotional intelligence, cardiac, and gut connection, as well as PTSD risk factors, early detection markers, and public health approaches for preventing microbial translocation (MT) into the host circulation.

### *2.1. Heart Rate Variability as a PTSD Risk Factor*

In colloquial expression, the brain is the epitome of rational thinking and intelligence, while the heart is generally associated with feelings and emotion. Over the past two decades, the term "emotional intelligence" has been circulated widely, although the neuroanatomic "home" of this social skill has yet to be defined. Here, we suggest that social or emotional intelligence dwells in the IC and may be a function of von Economo neurons (VENs), which populate the anterior insula and the cingulate cortex [61–63]. Indeed, dysfunctional VENs have been associated with suicidal behavior and psychosis, while FTD is characterized by the selective loss of these cells [64]. Aside from neuropathology, VENs have been implicated in cardiac physiology as they regulate HR and blood pressure (BP), parameters associated with both emotional expression and environmental demands [65,66]. Indeed, VENs may comprise the heart motor center, which was recently identified in the IC, and plays a major role in the autonomic accompaniment of emotional experiences [67]. The IC communicates with the heart via VN and postganglionic cardiac neurons, likely explaining heart rate variability (HRV) in response to inner or outer stimuli, such as emotions or the environment [67]. Moreover, GI tract inflammation has been associated with decreased HRV, suggesting IC regulation of the autonomic nervous system [68]. Interestingly, dysfunctional resting HR as well as decreased HRV have been documented in psychopathy, a pathology associated with insular damage [69–71]. This may explain the evolutionary preservation of psychopathy, a phenotype likely conserved for its battlefield advantages.

Since under normal circumstances, VENs drive both empathy and HRV, in pathological conditions, these cells may trigger anxiety attacks, hypervigilance, avoidant behavior, or aggression [63,72,73]. HRV was previously identified as a PTSD risk factor, emphasizing the key role of the cardiovascular system in this pathology [74–76].

### 2.2. PTSD-Associated Hypertension (HTN)

Under physiological circumstances, the IC gathers real-time interoceptive and exteroceptive input, permeating it with autonomic hues, memories of past experiences, and personal values. These data are subsequently communicated to the cardiovascular system via insular–cardiac circuits, generating individualized homeostatic responses [77]. The IC-heart dialog regulates the HR and BP, parameters driven by both emotional experiences and environmental demands [78]. Indeed, the right IC has been associated with HTN, while the left induces vasodilation [79]. BP fluctuations accompany many human experiences, including emotion, physical pain, psychosocial stressors, infections, and pro-survival risk taking [80–82]. For example, the major HTN driver, angiotensin II (ANG II), has been associated with PTSD as renin-angiotensin (RAS) is a well-established component of the human stress response [83,84]. Indeed, ANG II has been associated with the neural expression of fear, while alamandine, a less-studied RAS member, lowers fear by acting on the rostral insula, likely averting the development of PTSD [78,85]. The role of RAS in neuropathology was emphasized during the COVID-19 pandemic, as SARS-CoV-2, the etiologic agent of this viral infection, employs angiotensin-converting enzyme 2 (ACE-2) as the entry portal into host cells.

RAS comprises two arms, the proinflammatory/prooxidative and anti-inflammatory/ antioxidative branch, which maintain the homeostasis of both BP and the human stress response. ACE-2 bridges the two RAS branches, indicating that a defect of this enzyme, including viral hijacking, can disable the entire protective RAS branch (Figure 2). This, in return, leads to endothelial barrier disruption and spill-over of neurotoxic molecules, including ANG II or endothelin-1 (ET-1), into the CNS, triggering pathology, including PTSD [86]. Indeed, this mechanism may explain the high comorbidity of some viral infections with both HTN and PTSD [87,88] (Figure 2). In addition, viruses have been known for disrupting both epithelial cells and ECs, increasing the permeability of biological barriers, including the intestinal and blood–brain barrier (BBB), enabling MT into the host systemic circulation [89]. As we have discussed this issue in another article, will not go into more detail here [90].

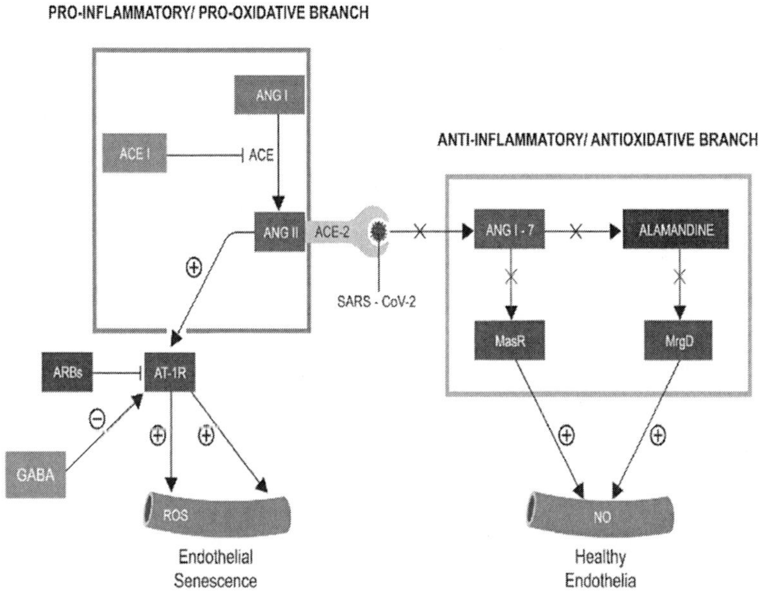


**Figure 2. The two RAS branches: pro-inflammatory/pro-oxidant and anti-inflammatory/antioxidant, are connected via ACE-2. When ACE-2 is disabled by various pathologies, including the SARS-CoV-2 virus attachment, the entire protective RAS branch is inhibited, disrupting the ECs (comprising the endothelial gut barrier) and enabling MT. ARBs and GABA oppose the effects of ANG II, averting EC senescence, barrier disruption, and MT.**

The COVID-19 pandemic emphasized the RAS-aryl hydrocarbon receptor (AhR) link, which plays a key role in orchestrating virus-induced senescence (VIS) in ECs [91–94]. Conversely, angiotensin receptor blockers (ARBs) and γ-aminobutyric acid (GABA) counteract EC senescence, indicating potential therapeutic effects in PTSD. Indeed, both GABA and ARBs have shown protective effects against psychosocial stress in both human and animal studies [95–97].

In summary, several lines of evidence implicate dysfunctional IC in PTSD pathogenesis, suggesting that impaired HRV and BP comprise risk factors for this disorder. At the molecular level, defective RAS and AhR contribute to PTSD by inducing premature epithelial and endothelial senescence, causing gut barrier disruption and MT. In the following sections, after a brief reminder of AhR physiology and pathology, we discuss PTSD resilience systems, HIF-1α and CAP, that not only counteract MT but also ameliorate IC homeostasis.

## 3. Aryl Hydrocarbon Receptor and Enteric Nervous System: Quick Reminder

The enteric nervous system (ENS), comprising the myenteric and submucosal plexus, is a semi-independent "gut brain" situated within the wall of the GI tract [98]. The ENS contains glial cells and three times as many neurons as the spinal cord. The ENS neurons exhibit unusual plasticity and a high level of neurogenesis as they are replaced every few weeks with newly born neuronal cells [99]. Moreover, the ENS neurons are regulated by AhR, which, depending on the attached ligand, may play a proor anti-apoptotic role [100]. Initially, AhR was believed to interact only with the environmental toxin dioxin (2,3,7,8tetrachlorodibenzo-p-dioxin). However, the discovery that the major neurotransmitters DA, serotonin (5HT), and melatonin, as well as several psychotropic drugs, including clozapine, are AhR ligands, brought this receptor into the neuropsychiatric arena [46,101–104]. Furthermore, when AhR binds to gut indole, it promotes adult neurogenesis in various brain niches, suggesting novel targets for major depressive disorder (MDD) and PTSD [105–108]. It has been well established that AhR regulates corticotropin releasing hormone (CRH), a major PTSD driver, involved in interoceptive awareness and the IC [109,110].

### *3.1. AhR and Cellular Senescence*

During development, AhR plays a key role in organogenesis; however, excessive activation of this transcription factor later in life has been associated with premature cellular senescence and neurodegeneration [111,112]. AhR is a transcription factor, stabilized in the cytosol by the heat shock protein 90 (Hsp90), a chaperone implicated in PTSD [113,114]. When AhR detaches from HSP90, it enters the nucleus, where it binds to AhR nuclear translocator (ARNT). This biochemical reaction is opposed by the aryl hydrocarbon receptor repressor (AhRR), an inhibitor of AhR signaling [115]. If not inhibited by AhRR, the AhR/ARNT heterodimer enters the genome, where it activates the DNA replication-related element (DRE), initiating the transcription of many genes, including IL22 [116–118].

The effects of AhR are dependent on the attached ligands and are tissueand contextspecific; thus, it may exert opposite effects in one cell type vs. another. For example, activated AhR blocks cellular senescence in hepatocytes and fibroblasts, while in renal cells, it precipitates this phenotype [119,120]. Another transcription factor, HIF-1α, averts premature EC senescence by opposing the effects of AhR on microvascular endothelia [121].

Moreover, HIF-1α also protects enteric neurons as hypoxia caused by IEC oxygen consumption exhibits neuroprotective properties [122]. In another article, we have discussed HIF-1α lactylation and dysfunction in PTSD pathogenesis so we will not dwell on this topic here [123].

### *3.2. PTSD, Premature EC Senescence, and Barrier Function*

It is well established that psychosocial stress activates the hypothalamic–pituitary– adrenal axis (HPA), and when the activation is chronic, it may precipitate PTSD. The initial step in HPA activation, is CRH synthesis in the paraventricular nucleus of the hypothalamus, a process mediated by AhR via acyloxyacyl hydrolase (AOAH). AOAH is an LPSinactivating enzyme capable of neutralizing the translocated endotoxin, thus preventing tissue damage. We surmise that low AOAH levels reflect PTSD severity and can serve as an early detection marker [109,124,125]. Another mechanism capable of neutralizing translocated bacteria or their components involves α7nAChRs and the CAP (see below) [126–128] (Figure 1). The CAP prevents premature vascular aging by enhancing the biosynthesis of nitric oxide (NO) in ECs, lowering the effects of psychosocial stress [129,130].

The question of why, under a similar level of trauma exposure, an individual develops PTSD while another does not, remains to be answered. However, as mentioned above, external (i.e., microbiome alterations) and internal (i.e., epigenetic changes) factors are likely involved. For example, psychosocial stressors have been associated with altered DNA methylation in epithelial and ECs, inducing senescence and increased gut barrier permeability [131–135]. Moreover, in ECs, impaired methylation of nuclear receptor subfamily 3 group C member 1 (NR3C1), a glucocorticoid receptor encoding gene, was demonstrated in both PTSD and cardiovascular disease (CVD), linking these conditions to premature endothelial aging [136–138]. In addition, AhRR methylation can promote PTSD and CVD via AhR/ARNT-induced EC senescence [139,140].

Recent studies have documented that AhR and HIF-1α exhibit opposing actions on ECs, as the former promotes while the latter opposes cellular senescence [111,126] (Figure 3).

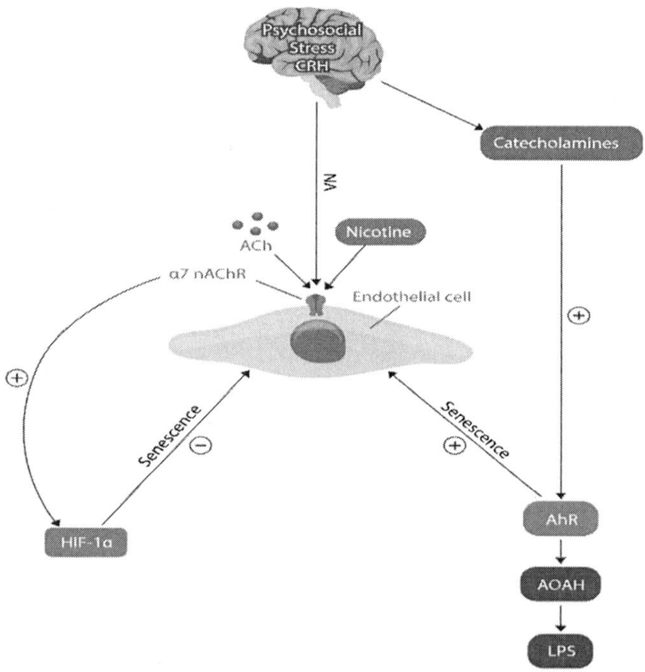


**Figure 3. Psychosocial stress (via HPA and CRH) induces EC senescence by upregulating catecholamines. This action is opposed by VN via ACh or nicotine signaling with α7nAChR, upregulating HIF-1α and counteracting EC senescence. Psychosocial-stress-induced catecholamines upregulate AhR, inhibiting AOAH and facilitating LPS accumulation. Both AhR and LPS promote EC senescence.**

For example, AhR facilitates DNA methylation, contributing to EC senescence, a phenotype that can also be induced by disabling HIF-1α [5,141,142].

## 4. PTSD Resilience Systems

Besides epigenetic mechanisms, psychosocial stress promotes EC senescence via four pathways: 1. AhR activation, 2. HIF-1α inhibition, 3. IL22 downregulation, and 4. disrupting tight junction molecules. These pathways enhance MT and the susceptibility for PTSD, as evidenced by previous findings:

1. MT markers are elevated in other disorders characterized by dysfunctional gut barrier, including HIV, IBD, and schizophrenia, conditions highly comorbid with PTSD [143–145].
2. Microbial cell-free DNA (mcfDNA) has been identified as a novel marker of MT and, to our knowledge, has not been evaluated for PTSD; however, it is utilized as a marker of sepsis, another condition characterized by MT [46,146,147].
3. Lowered AOAH allows unopposed translocation of LPS into the host circulation and may serve as a PTSD susceptibility marker [108].
4. Psychological stress downregulates intestinal IL22, increasing barrier permeability, suggesting that low levels of this cytokine may reflect PTSD susceptibility [148].
5. Preclinical studies have implicated dysfunctional tight junction proteins, claudins and occludins, in PTSD, suggesting that these biomolecules can serve as markers of this pathology [149–151].

MT drew the attention of researchers and clinicians in the 1980s, during the HIV epidemic, as this virus, known for depleting IL22, has been associated with the disruption of the intestinal barrier [152]. This is significant as recent studies have found increased prevalence of mental illness in the offspring of mothers suffering from MDD during pregnancy. Since these pregnancies were associated with elevated levels of MT markers, these molecules may reflect psychopathology risk before birth [153–156]. Therefore, testing for MT biomarkers should be part of prenatal screening for mental illness in offspring.

### *4.1. Resilience Mechanism #1: The Cholinergic Anti-Inflammatory Pathway (CAP)*

Intestinal macrophages are innate immune cells that recognize gut pathogens and clear both acute and chronic inflammation. These cells also regulate mucus secretion and intestinal motility, participating actively in the barrier function [157]. Macrophages express α7nAChRs and are directly innervated by the VN, averting premature epithelial and EC senescence [158] (Figure 4).

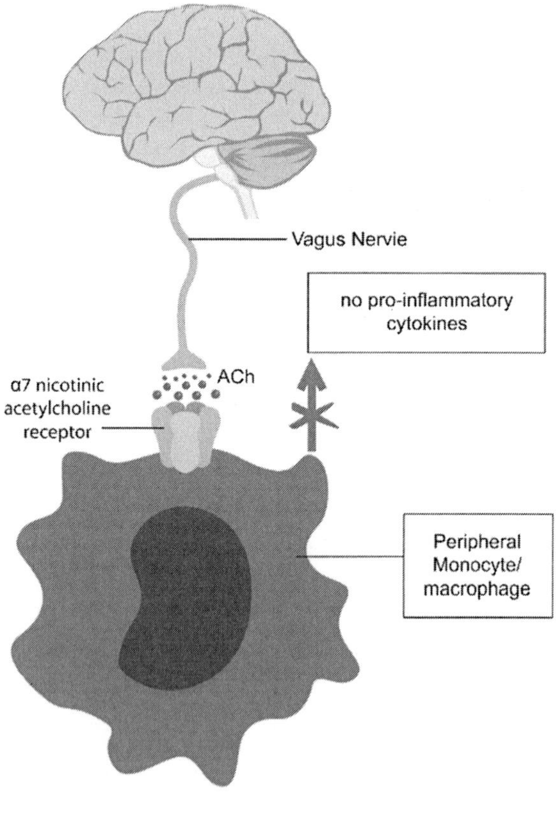


**Figure 4. The VN communicates with the IC and comprises the CAP. Macrophages/monocytes, like ECs and IECs, express α7nAChR and are innervated by the VN, inhibiting the release of proinflammatory cytokines. The CAP is part of the interoceptive system as well as the gut–brain axis.**

Due to the rapid turnover of enteric neurons and accelerated efferocytosis, intestinal macrophages are much more active compared to those in other tissues [159,160]. For this reason, dysfunctional elimination of dead cells and accumulation of molecular debris can trigger gut barrier disruption and inflammation. Conversely, taVNS may restore the integrity of the gut barrier, lowering the odds of PTSD [161–164] (Figure 4). Moreover, as mentioned above, IECs express α7nAChRs and are subject to the CAP, which protects the barrier function [165,166]. This is significant as it likely explains the high comorbidity of PTSD with IBD and HIV, disorders characterized by gut barrier dysfunction [25,88]. In addition, AOAH and IL22 protect the intestinal barrier against microbial and LPS translocation, indicating that these proteins could be used to identify PTSD early [124,167].

Dysfunctional CAP and macrophage-mediated efferocytosis can cause accumulation of cellular and molecular debris and gut barrier disruption [168].

### *4.2. Resilience Mechanism #2: HIF-1α and PTSD Resilience*

HIF-1α is a transcription factor activated by local hypoxia that plays a key role in averting premature cellular senescence, including that of ECs. Senescence is a cellular program of averting malignant transformation by inducing cell entry into a state of permanent proliferation arrest, while maintaining an active metabolism. Although protective against cancer, the senescent phenotype releases a detrimental secretome, known as senescenceassociated secretory phenotype (SASAP), which can disseminate senescence to the healthy neighboring cells [169]. Replicative cellular senescence was discovered by Leonard Hayflick in 1965, who demonstrated that cells do not replicate indefinitely, but after 40–60 divisions, they undergo telomere erosion and permanently exit the cell cycle [170,171].

Many neuropsychiatric disorders, including PTSD, have been associated with accelerated aging and shorter telomeres, indicating that psychosocial stress can induce premature cellular senescence [172,173]. Early endothelial aging in PTSD has been documented in many studies, suggesting that psychosocial stress primarily affects the endothelia and epithelia, contributing to increased intestinal permeability [174–176]. For example, MT has been documented in several PTSD studies, linking this pathology to an impaired gut barrier [177]. HIF-1α opposes MT via telomere elongation, reversing the effects of premature vascular aging, thus lowering the odds of PTSD [178,179].

As opposed to peripheral arteries in which HIF-1α rejuvenates endothelia, in the lungs, hypoxia causes pulmonary arterioles to constrict, leading to pulmonary artery resistance, which, under chronic conditions, may lead to right ventricular failure [180–182]. This may explain the high prevalence of obstructive sleep apnea (OSA) in PTSD patients, linking chronic hypoxia to this pathology [183,184]. Indeed, chronic HIF-1α elevation is detrimental, while intermittent hypoxemia is physiological and protects the endothelial barrier, suggesting that hyperbaric oxygen may comprise an effective treatment strategy for both PTSD and OSA. Indeed, several recent studies have reported amelioration of PTSD symptoms with hyperbaric oxygen, suggesting that more studies are needed to clarify this issue [185,186].

Aside from the endothelial barrier, HIF-1α also protects the intestinal epithelial barrier [187,188]. The mechanism of hypoxia-induced gut barrier repair is complex, but it comes down to IL22 upregulation. Microbiota-derived short-chain fatty acids (SCFAs) induce a degree of GI tract hypoxia due to increased oxygen consumption by the IECs. This, in turn, upregulates HIF-1α in mucosal ILC3, increasing the production of IL22 [189,190]. Although HIF-1α expression can be easily measured in blood serum, due to its fluctuating levels, it may not be an ideal PTSD marker; therefore, IL22, which indirectly reflects

HIF-1α status, is likely a more reliable indicator of gut barrier integrity.

Taken together, PTSD association with gut barrier dysfunction is driven by the pre-mature senescence of endothelial and epithelial cells. MT markers can be used to identify PTSD susceptibility prior to the development of clinical symptoms and should be included in prenatal care to screen for offspring mental health.

# 5. Early Detection Markers

In this section, we take a closer look at individual markers that could be used to identify PTSD in the premorbid phase, allowing prevention. Many markers of intestinal permeability have been utilized; however, at present, there is no gold standard test for MT [191]. Aside from the existing peripheral blood bacteria-detecting assays, including LPS, LBP, CD14, or AOAH, we propose two new tests, mcfDNA (measured via Karius Test®), and IL22 (measured via Singulex-Erenna®), which, when combined, may have higher specificity for MT. Indeed, we chose this battery of microbial tests as they measure both LPS translocation (LBP, CD14, and AOAH) and barrier integrity. LPS was chosen because of its predictive value for neuropathology. For example, human and animal studies show that maternal exposure to LPS during pregnancy contributes to high susceptibility for anxiety disorders, including PTSD, in offspring [192–196] (Table 1).

## *5.1. LPS*

LPS is a component of the outer membrane of Gram-negative bacteria that consists of lipid A, the O antigen, and the core oligosaccharide [197]. Circulatory LPS originates in the GI tract, although lower amounts can be derived from the oral microbiome, and even food [198,199]. LPS is an inducer of host inflammatory responses and induces the release of IL1 alpha, IL1 beta, IL6, IL10, tumor necrosis factor alpha (TNF-alpha), and cyclooxygenase-2 as well as nitric oxide synthase (NOS), an enzyme that metabolizes arginine into nitric oxide (NO) and citrulline [200]. Interestingly, citrulline is an established marker of gut barrier integrity as well as an enhancer of athletic performance, suggesting anti-inflammatory properties [201,202]. In contrast, as a posttranslational modification, citrullination (due to excess citrulline) is detrimental as it promotes inflammation and autoimmunity [203,204].

Upon crossing into the host tissues, LPS is detected by Toll-like receptor 4 (TLR4), a protein that activates nuclear factor kappa B (NF-κB) and interferon regulatory factor 3 (IRF3), promoting the release of proinflammatory cytokines [205]. Minute amounts of LPS can lead to PTSD as this toxin (the lethal dose for humans is 1 to 2 μg) stimulates host immunity, inducing premature cellular senescence [206–209].

Psychosocial trauma can also activate TLR4, a process known as sterile inflammation, suggesting that the body does not discern very well between biological and psychosocial stress [210,211]. This may be significant as various disorders of unclear etiology, usually labeled as "psychogenic" or "functional", such as fibromyalgia or psychogenic fever, may be explained by the concept of sterile inflammation [212]. Conversely, psychotherapy, antidepressant drugs, and exercise have been demonstrated to lower TLR4 [213–215].

Sterile inflammation engenders pathology via TLR4-induced assembly of inflammasome (NOD)-like receptor protein 3 (NLRP3), which can be activated by LPS, psychosocial stress, a high-fat diet, and other environmental factors, including air pollution [216–218]. Excessive NLRP3 activation has been documented in PTSD, while inhibition of this inflammasome can ameliorate the symptoms, likely through AhR [219–221] (Figure 5). In addition, LPS has been reported to directly induce EC senescence in biological barriers, promoting MT [209,222].

Dysfunctional NLRP3 was demonstrated to aberrantly activate microglia, triggering the elimination of healthy neurons, a pathology manifested in PTSD as gray matter loss [223–225]. Indeed, neuroimaging studies have revealed decreased gray matter in PTSD, suggesting abnormal microglial activation [226–228].

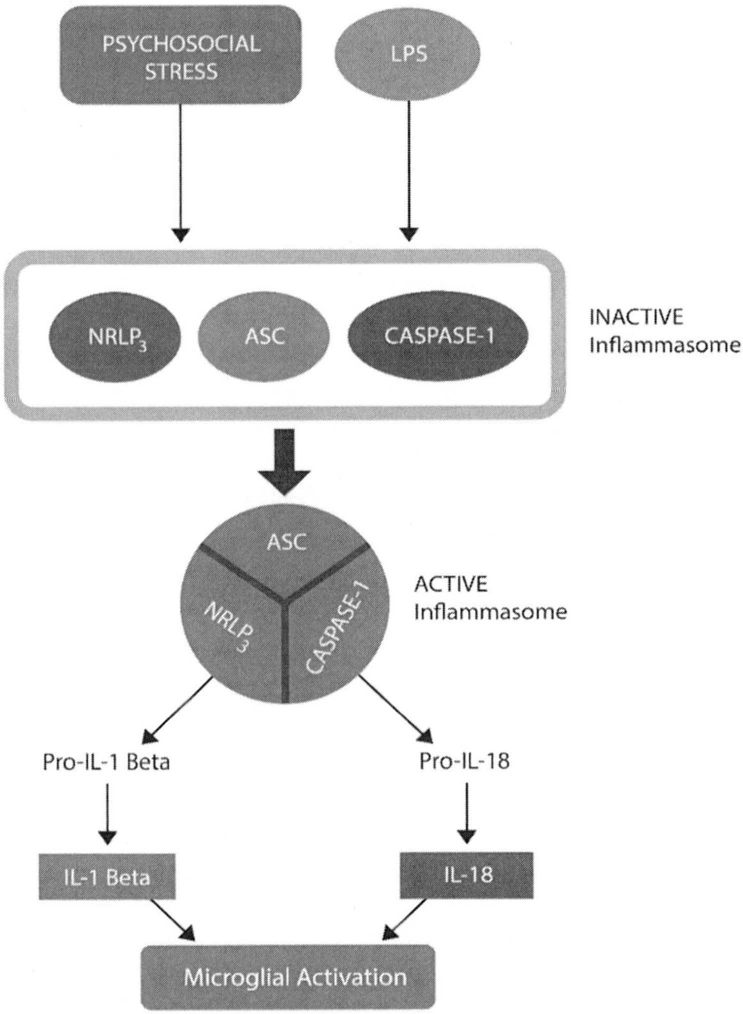


**Figure 5. NLRP3 inflammasome activation: psychosocial stress and LPS trigger inflammation by inducing inflammasome assembly. Inflammasomes comprise a sensor, the nucleotide-binding oligomerization domain (NOD), in this case the (NOD)-like receptor protein 3 (NLRP3), apoptosisassociated speck-like protein containing a caspase recruitment domain (ASC), and caspase-1. In the presence of proinflammatory endogenous or exogenous stimuli, these molecules assemble and the inflammasome becomes biologically active, transforming premature IL-1 beta and IL-18 into their biologically active forms, which, in turn, activates microglia.**

### 5.2. LBP and CD14

Upon LPS migration from the gut into the host systemic circulation, it binds LBP, a secretory phase-one molecule, as well as CD14, the receptor of the LPS-LPB complex [229]. Together, LBP/LPS/CD14 initiate cellular secretory responses that are much stronger than those of LPS alone, suggesting that these translocation markers enhance the pathological effects of translocated microbes or their components [230]. LBP serum levels are upregulated (normal range 5 to 10 μg/mL) and elevated LPB binds LPS with higher affinity, exacerbating PTSD [226,231]. Conversely, low LBP attenuates host inflammation, lowering the susceptibility for PTSD. In this regard, psychosocial stress has been demonstrated to upregulate LBP, inducing depressive symptoms and PTSD exacerbations, thus validating the role of the LBP/LPS/CD14 complex in these pathologies [232]. Conversely, the soluble form of CD14 (sCD14) is a reliable microbial translocation marker upregulated in sepsis, schizophrenia, and cancer, indicating that it likely comprises a valid signature of PTSD susceptibility [143,233,234].

### 5.3. Microbial Cell-Free DNA (mcfDNA)

Microbial cell-free DNA (mcfDNA) is a novel plasma marker utilized in infectious diseases that may also have potential to be used to detect translocated bacteria in PTSD [235]. The mcfDNA test was developed by Karius Inc. (Redwood City, CA 94065, USA) in 2017 (Karius Test®) and may accurately detect microbial translocation in PTSD [236]. To our knowledge, Karius Test® has never been used in PTSD; however, mcfDNA could serve as an early detection marker for this pathology. Further studies are needed to assess the validity of this marker in PTSD.

### 5.4. Acyloxyacyl Hydrolase (AOAH)

AOAH is a leukocyte-secreted lipase that hydrolyzes LPS by breaking the acyloxyacyl bonds [124]. For example, mice with higher AOAH levels were found to recover more rapidly from Gram-negative infections, while AOAH-deficient rodents exhibited not only more severe infection but also chronic pain, anxiety, and depression-like behaviors [109]. Interestingly, it was recently reported that AOAH regulates CRH via AhR, implicating this enzyme in PTSD pathogenesis [109]. In this regard, as AOAH eliminates LPS, low levels of this protein likely reflect PTSD vulnerability. Indeed, preclinical studies have shown that genetic treatment with the AOAH gene lowers LPS, suggesting a potential therapeutic strategy for Gram-negative sepsis and likely PTSD [237].

### *5.5. IL22*

IL22 is a member of the IL-10 family of cytokines that is synthesized by several lymphocyte types, including T helper (Th) 17 cells, γδ T cells, NKCs, and ILCs3 [238]. IL22 functions as a master regulator of gut barrier permeability as it modulates gut microbiota as well as the function of intestinal mucosa ILCs [239]. Luminal IL22 is generated by ILC3 and functions to enhance the beneficial gut microbes Bifidobacterium and Lactobacillus spp., increasing PTSD resilience. Along this line, we have suggested recombinant human IL22 as a treatment for schizophrenia and believe that this cytokine can also be beneficial in PTSD [240,241]. Indeed, psychological stress was demonstrated to disrupt IL22 as well as the gut barrier function, indicating that exogenous IL22 could restore the integrity of the intestinal barrier [148]. IL22 serum levels can be measured via Singulex-Erenna®, an ultrasensitive assay, indicating that detection of this cytokine is currently possible [242].

Taken together, based on several clinical and preclinical studies, PTSD susceptibility may be measured using MT markers, including elevated LPS, LBP, CD14, and lowered AOAH. Downregulated IL22, a marker of gut barrier integrity, likely reflects PTSD vulnerability. If validated, these biomarkers could be useful for discerning individuals at high risk of PTSD and adjusting or developing deployment policies accordingly.

**Table 1. Microbial markers, sources, and physiological role.**

| Markers | Origin or Function | References |
|---|---|---|
| HRV | GI tract inflammation lowers HRV | [68] |
| BP | Right vs. left IC = vasopressor vs. vasodilation | [79] |
| LPS (elevated) | Gut, oral microbiome, food origin | [198–200] |
| sCD14 (elevated) | Receptor for LPS/LBP heterodimer | [229] |
| LBP (elevated) | Enhances the action of LPS | [230] |
| AOAH (low) | Neutralizes translocated LPS | [124] |
| IL22 (low) | Impaired barrier function | [239] |

## 6. Conclusions

PTSD has accompanied human history for millennia. However, under a similar level of trauma exposure, who develops and who does not develop this condition remains poorly defined.

Shifting the research focus from the amygdala and fear to the IC and interoceptive awareness has brought forth new potential treatments as well as diagnostic opportunities, suggesting that dysgnosia may be corrected by interventions at the body periphery, such as taVNS. Since the IC is in close communication with both the heart and the GI tract, cardiac and gut biomarkers can be utilized for identifying PTSD susceptibility. For example, high-risk phenotypes, offspring of mothers with a history of MDD and bacterial (or viral) infections during pregnancy, may be identified early through postnatal screening.

This article emphasizes the prevalence of PTSD after war trauma, an aspect that may appear relevant only to military personnel, the police force, and their families. However, since a significant number of people from all walks of life are exposed daily to overwhelming stressors, including assaults, motor vehicle accidents, shootings, and hold-ups, this report may have significance for PTSD in general.

The battery of markers proposed here reflect intestinal barrier permeability (IL22) and translocation of microbial components (LPS, LBP, CD14, and

AOAH). As they also mirror the BBB integrity, these biomarkers likely reveal the presence of bacteria or LPS in the CNS, including the IC.

**Author Contributions:** Conceptualization: A.S. and C.O.; writing and original draft preparation: Z.K.; Data curation and writing: C.K.; writing review: H.I.; Project administration J.J.A. All authors have read and agreed to the published version of the manuscript.

**Funding:** This research received no external funding.

**Conflicts of Interest:** The authors declare no conflict of interest. Where authors are identified as personnel of the International Agency for Research on Cancer/WHO, the authors alone are responsible for the views expressed in this article and they do not necessarily represent the decisions, policy or views of the International Agency for Research on Cancer/WHO.

## References

1. Rentscher KE, Carroll JE, Repetti RL, Cole SW, Reynolds BM, Robles TF. Chronic stress exposure and daily stress appraisals relate to biological aging marker p16 INK4a. Psychoneuroendocrinology. 2019;102:139–148. doi: 10.1016/j.psyneuen.2018.12.006
2. Razzoli M, Nyuyki-Dufe K, Gurney A, et al. Social stress shortens lifespan in mice. Aging Cell. 2018;17(4):e12778. doi: 10.1111/acel.12778
3. Yousefzadeh MJ et al. Tissue specificity of senescent cell accumulation during physiologic and accelerated aging of mice. Aging Cell 19, e13094 (2020). 10.1111/acel.13094
4. Grosse L et al. Defined p16(High) Senescent Cell Types Are Indispensable for Mouse Healthspan. Cell Metab 32, 87–99.e86 (2020). 10.1016/j.cmet.2020.05.002
5. Piao L, Zhao G, Zhu E, Inoue A, Shibata R, Lei Y, Hu L, Yu C, Yang G, Wu H, Xu W, Okumura K, Ouchi N, Murohara T, Kuzuya M, Cheng XW. Chronic Psychological Stress Accelerates Vascular Senescence and Impairs Ischemia-Induced Neovascularization: The Role of Dipeptidyl Peptidase-4/Glucagon-Like Peptide-1-Adiponectin

Axis. J Am Heart Assoc. 2017 Sep 28;6(10):e006421. doi: 10.1161/JAHA.117.006421.

6. Lehmann ML, Poffenberger CN, Elkahloun AG, Herkenham M. Analysis of cerebrovascular dysfunction caused by chronic social defeat in mice. Brain Behav Immun. 2020 Aug;88:735-747. doi: 10.1016/j.bbi.2020.05.030.
7. Beristianos MH, Yaffe K, Cohen B, Byers AL. PTSD and Risk of Incident Cardiovascular Disease in Aging Veterans. Am J Geriatr Psychiatry. 2016 Mar;24(3):192-200. doi: 10.1016/j.jagp.2014.12.003. Epub 2014 Dec 9. PMID: 25555625.
8. Zhang Y, Gao X, Bai X, Yao S, Chang YZ, Gao G. The emerging role of furin in neurodegenerative and neuropsychiatric diseases. Transl Neurodegener. 2022 Aug 23;11(1):39. doi: 10.1186/s40035-022-00313-1.
9. Yang X, Yang W, McVey DG, Zhao G, Hu J, Poston RN, Ren M, Willeit K, Coassin S, Willeit J, Webb TR, Samani NJ, Mayr M, Kiechl S, Ye S. FURIN Expression in Vascular Endothelial Cells Is Modulated by a Coronary Artery Disease-Associated Genetic Variant and Influences Monocyte Transendothelial Migration. J Am Heart Assoc. 2020 Feb 18;9(4):e014333. doi: 10.1161/JAHA.119.014333.
10. AbdelMassih AF, Ye J, Kamel A, Mishriky F, Ismail HA, Ragab HA, El-Qadi L, Malak L, Abdu M, El-Husseiny M, Ashraf M, Hafez N, AlShehry N, El-Husseiny N, AbdelRaouf N, Shebl N, Hafez N, Youssef N, Afdal P, Hozaien R, Menshawey R, Saeed R, Fouda R. A multicenter consensus: A role of furin in the endothelial tropism in obese patients with COVID-19 infection. Obes Med. 2020 Sep;19:100281. doi: 10.1016/j.obmed.2020.100281.
11. Anerillas C, Herman AB, Munk R, Garrido A, Lam KG, Payea MJ, Rossi M, Tsitsipatis D, Martindale JL, Piao Y, Mazan-Mamczarz K, Fan J, Cui CY, De S, Abdelmohsen K, de Cabo R, Gorospe M. A BDNF-TrkB autocrine loop enhances senescent cell viability. Nat Commun. 2022 Oct 20;13(1):6228. doi: 10.1038/s41467-022-33709-8. Erratum in: Nat Commun. 2022 Dec 7;13(1):7540. PMID: 36266274; PMCID: PMC9585019.

12. Wu GWY, Wolkowitz OM, Reus VI, Kang JI, Elnar M, Sarwal R, Flory JD, Abu-Amara D, Hammamieh R, Gautam A, Doyle FJ 3rd, Yehuda R, Marmar CR, Jett M, Mellon SH; SBPBC. Serum brain-derived neurotrophic factor remains elevated after long-term follow-up of combat veterans with chronic post-traumatic stress disorder. Psychoneuroendocrinology. 2021 Jul 22;134:105360. doi: 10.1016/j.psyneuen.2021.105360. Epub ahead of print. PMID: 34757255.
13. Farkas CB, Dudás G, Babinszky GC, Földi L. Analysis of the Virus SARS-CoV-2 as a Potential Bioweapon in Light of International Literature. Mil Med. 2023 Mar 20;188(3-4):531-540. doi: 10.1093/milmed/usac123. PMID: 35569934; PMCID: PMC9384074
14. Molloy SS, Bresnahan PA, Leppla SH, Klimpel KR, Thomas G. Human furin is a calcium-dependent serine endoprotease that recognizes the sequence Arg-X-X-Arg and efficiently cleaves anthrax toxin protective antigen. J Biol Chem. 1992 Aug 15;267(23): 16396-402. PMID: 1644824.
15. Perl O, Duek O, Kulkarni KR, Gordon C, Krystal JH, Levy I, Harpaz-Rotem I, Schiller D. Neural patterns differentiate traumatic from sad autobiographical memories in PTSD. Nat Neurosci. 2023 Dec;26(12):2226-2236. doi: 10.1038/s41593-023-01483-5.
16. Iyadurai L, Visser RM, Lau-Zhu A, Porcheret K, Horsch A, Holmes EA, James EL. Intrusive memories of trauma: A target for research bridging cognitive science and its clinical application. Clin Psychol Rev. 2019 Apr;69:67-82. doi: 10.1016/j.cpr.2018.08.005. Epub 2018 Aug 23. PMID: 30293686
17. van der Kolk BA. The body keeps the score: memory and the evolving psychobiology of posttraumatic stress. Harv Rev Psychiatry. 1994 Jan-Feb;1(5):253-65. doi: 10.3109/10673229409017088. PMID: 9384857.
18. Andrews JA, Neises KD. Cells, biomarkers, and post-traumatic stress disorder: evidence for peripheral involvement in a central disease. J Neurochem. 2012 Jan;120(1):26-36. doi: 10.1111/j.1471-4159.2011.07545.x.
19. Benedict TM, Keenan PG, Nitz AJ, Moeller-Bertram T. Post-Traumatic Stress Disorder Symptoms Contribute to Worse Pain and

Health Outcomes in Veterans With PTSD Compared to Those Without: A Systematic Review With Meta-Analysis. Mil Med. 2020 Sep 18;185(9-10):e1481-e1491. doi: 10.1093/milmed/usaa052.
20. Dussutour A. Learning in single cell organisms. Biochem Biophys Res Commun. 2021 Jul 30;564:92-102. doi: 10.1016/j.bbrc.2021.02.018
21. Cheikhi A, Wallace C, St Croix C, Cohen C, Tang WY, Wipf P, Benos PV, Ambrosio F, Barchowsky A. Mitochondria are a substrate of cellular memory. Free Radic Biol Med. 2019 Jan;130:528-541. doi: 10.1016/j.freeradbiomed.2018.11.028.
22. Agnati LF, Zunarelli E, Genedani S, Fuxe K. On the existence of a global molecular network enmeshing the whole central nervous system: physiological and pathological implications. Curr Protein Pept Sci. 2006 Feb;7(1):3-15. doi: 10.2174/138920306775474086.
23. Miyamoto T, Razavi S, DeRose R, Inoue T. Synthesizing biomolecule-based Boolean logic gates. ACS Synth Biol. 2013 Feb 15;2(2):72-82. doi: 10.1021/sb3001112. PMID: 23526588; PMCID: PMC3603578.
24. Al-Juhani A, Imran M, Aljaili ZK, Alzhrani MM, Alsalman RA, Ahmed M, Ali DK, Fallatah MI, Yousuf HM, Dajani LM. Beyond the Pump: A Narrative Study Exploring Heart Memory. Cureus. 2024 Apr 30;16(4):e59385. doi: 10.7759/cureus.59385.
25. Carter, B.; Khoshnaw, L.; Simmons, M.; Hines, L.; Wolfe, B.; Liester, M. Personality Changes Associated with Organ Transplants. Transplantology 2024, 5, 12-26. https://doi.org/10.3390/transplantology5010002
26. Feng Y, Shen J, He J, Lu M. Schizophrenia and cell senescence candidate genes screening, machine learning, diagnostic models, and drug prediction. Front Psychiatry. 2023 Apr 11;14:1105987. doi: 10.3389/fpsyt.2023.1105987. PMID: 37113536; PMCID: PMC1012 6505.
27. Solana, C.; Pereira, D.; Tarazona, R. Early Senescence and Leukocyte Telomere Shortening in SCHIZOPHRENIA: A Role for Cytomegalovirus Infection? Brain Sci. 2018, 8, 188. https://doi.org/10.3390/brainsci8100188

28. Nelson PN, Carnegie PR, Martin J, et al. Demystified. Human endogenous retroviruses. Mol Pathol. 2003;56(1): 11-18. doi:10.1136/mp.56.1.11
29. Charvet B, Brunel J, Pierquin J, Iampietro M, Decimo D, Queruel N, Lucas A, Encabo-Berzosa MDM, Arenaz I, Marmolejo TP, Gonzalez AI, Maldonado AC, Mathieu C, Küry P, Flores-Rivera J, Torres-Ruiz F, Avila-Rios S, Salgado Montes de Oca G, Schoorlemmer J, Perron H, Horvat B. SARS-CoV-2 awakens ancient retroviral genes and the expression of proinflammatory HERV-W envelope protein in COVID-19 patients. iScience. 2023 May 19;26(5):106604. doi: 10.1016/j.isci.2023.106604
30. Gholami barzoki , M., Shatizadeh Malekshahi, S., Heydarifard, Z. et al. The important biological roles of Syncytin-1 of human endogenous retrovirus W (HERV-W) and Syncytin-2 of HERV-FRD in the human placenta development. Mol Biol Rep 50, 7901–7907 (2023). https://doi.org/10.1007/s11033-023-08658-0
31. Sibarov DA, Tsytsarev V, Volnova A, Vaganova AN, Alves J, Rojas L, Sanabria P, Ignashchenkova A, Savage ED, Inyushin M. Arc protein, a remnant of ancient retrovirus, forms virus-like particles, which are abundantly generated by neurons during epileptic seizures, and affects epileptic susceptibility in rodent models. Front Neurol. 2023 Jul 7;14:1201104. doi: 10.3389/fneur.2023.1201104. PMID: 37483450; PMCID: PMC10361770.
32. Shepherd JD. Arc An endogenous neuronal retrovirus? Semin Cell Dev Biol. 2018 May;77:73-78. doi: 10.1016/j.semcdb.2017.09.029. Epub 2017 Sep 24. PMID: 28941877; PMCID: PMC5862763.
33. Liester MB. Personality changes following heart transplantation: The role of cellular memory. Med Hypotheses. 2020 Feb;135: 109468. doi: 10.1016/j.mehy.2019.109468.

# CHAPTER 5

# SCHIZOPHRENIA, A DISORDER OF ABNORMAL AGING: LACTYLATION AND AGGRESSION

Compared to the population at large, patients with chronic schizophrenia (SCZ) or schizophrenia-like disorders (SLDs) exhibit elevated central lactate, a metabolic signature of premature brain aging (1). Early senescence, decreased life span, and short telomeres have been documented in patients with SCZ over the past two decades. However, this condition is rarely conceptualized as a disorder of abnormal aging (2)(3)(4). Increased brain age gap (BAG), the difference between predicted and chronological age, has been demonstrated by neuroimaging in SCZ, SLDs, and traumatic brain injury (TBI), emphasizing the role of accelerated aging in these pathologies (5)(6)(7).

Glycolysis, the preferred metabolic modality of schizophrenic brains, results in excessive intra and extracellular lactate as well as local acidic pH, a phenomenon associated not only with anxiety and panic attacks but also with violence and aggression (8)(9)(10)(11)(12). Lactate utilization as the primary energy source is likely the result of dysfunctional mitochondria and abnormal oxidative phosphorylation (OXPHOS), limiting the metabolic options of neuronal cells to glycolysis (13)(14)(15)(16). Indeed, lactate is considered a biological marker of both chronic mental illness and aging, highlighting psychiatric metabolomics as an emerging area of research (17)(18).

## SCZ as a "segmental progeria"

SCZ is characterized by premature cellular senescence, low-grade inflammation (inflammation), and metabolic rewiring to glycolysis as the primary brain energy source (4)(19)(20). Like senescence in general, premature brain aging in SCZ and SLDs is accompanied by inflammation triggered by the activation of nucleotide-binding oligomerization domain (NOD)-like receptor protein 3 (NLRP3) inflammasome. NLRP3 activation promotes metabolic rewiring with upregulated lactate, linking inflammation to cellular energetics (Fig, 1) (21)(22)(23). Conversely, lactate deactivates NLRP3, lowering inflammation. This engenders a vicious circle in which NLRP3 increases lactate levels while lactate lowers NLRP3.

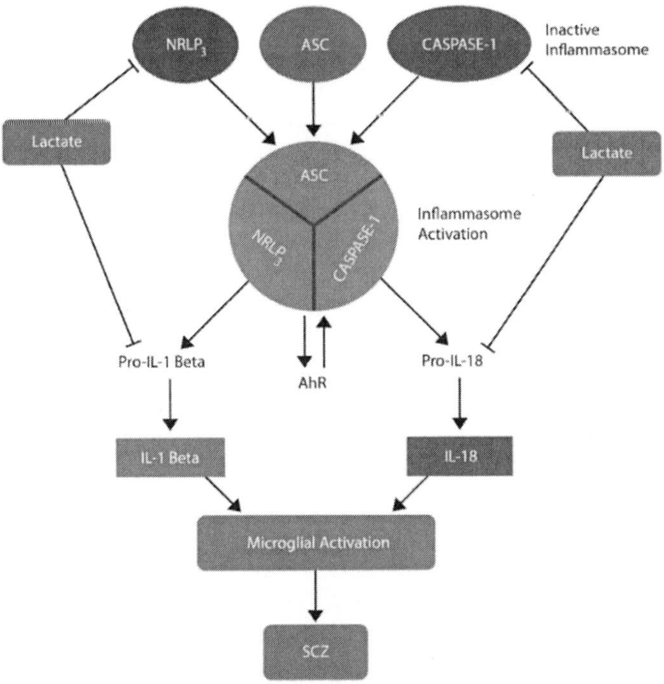


**When disassembled, NLRP3, ASC, and Caspase-1 inflammasome components are biologically inactive. Inflammatory signaling requires inflammasome assembly, which generates pro-interleukin -1β (IL-1β) and pro-IL-18, which become activated into IL-1β and IL-18. In the CNS, IL-1β and IL-18 may aberrantly activate microglia, contributing to neurotoxicity and neuronal loss, a characteristic of SCZ and neurodegenerative disorders. Lactate inhibits inflammasomes at several steps, including NLRP3, Caspase-1, pro-IL1β, and pro-IL-18.**

NLRP3 inflammasome comprises several proteins that must assemble to initiate an inflammatory response. For example, inflammasome components, NLRP3, adaptor molecule apoptosis-associated speck-like protein (ASC), and caspase-1 (CASP-1) are biologically inactive when disconnected; however, upon assembly, they generate pro-interleukin-1 β and pro-interleukin-18, which promote inflammation by becoming active interleukins, IL-1β and IL-18 (Fig. 1).

Cellular senescence refers to a permanent proliferation arrest with an active metabolism, extensive cellular remodeling, and a detrimental secretome, known as senescence-associated secretory phenotype (SASP), which can spread senescence to the neighboring healthy cells in an exocrine/paracrine manner.

Senescence was first described by Hayflick 1961, who showed that cells do not replicate indefinitely but undergo telomere shortening and exit the cell cycle after 40-60 divisions (24). Although lactate can inhibit inflammasome activation, it paradoxically drives SASP, promoting brain aging and related pathology (25)(26)(27). Indeed, SASP-induced senescent microglia may, under pathological circumstances, eliminate viable neurons, a pathology documented in neurodegenerative disorders, SCZ, and SLDs (28)(29)(30)(31)(32). Under physiological circumstances, microglia are neuroprotective as they prevent inflammation caused by the accumulation of molecular debris and damaged and infected cells (33). Novel studies have connected senescent microglia and brain aging with histone H3K18 lactylation, linking neuropathology to the epigenome (34)(35).

## Psychiatric metabolomics in SCZ and SLDs

Lactatylation, a newly discovered post-translational modification (PTM), is directly correlated with lactate levels, the end-product of glycolysis. Activation consists of adding lactate to the lysine residues of histone proteins, a phenomenon known as KLA. KLA promotes the open chromatin conformation, facilitating the transcription of many genes, including those that are usually silenced . Like other PTMs, lactylation requires "writer" and "eraser" proteins to add and remove histone lactate. In this regard, acetylation is highly intertwined with acetylation and utilizes identical reading and writing enzymes, histone acetyltransferase (HAT), and histone deacetylases 1-3 (HDACs 1-3). For example, HAT p300 is a "writer" (adds lactate to histone lysine residues), while HDACs, including sirtuin-2 (SIRT-2), are "erasers" (remove lactate from histone proteins) (36). The molecular underpinnings of the lactylation-acetylation connection are poorly defined, but the consensus is that both "relax" chromatin conformation, enabling gene transcription (37)(38)(39). Physiologically, lactylation promotes neurogenesis and angiogenesis, processes disrupted in SCZ with aggressive behaviors (40)(41)(42). This suggests that impaired lactylation may facilitate the expression of genes that should be silenced, such as SCZ vulnerability genes, while commonly expressed genes may be pathologically silenced. For example, decreased expression of monoaminoxidase A (MAOA) and oxytocin receptor (OXTR) genes, previously associated with aggression, highlights the link between lactylation and disruptive behavior in SCZ or SLDs.

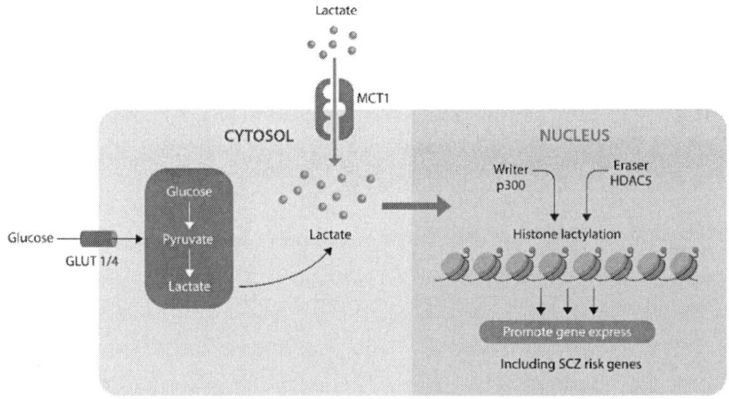


**Lactate, derived from glucose, enters cells via glucose transporters (GLUTs). Glycolysis transforms glucose into lactate (via pyruvate). Lactate can also enter cells directly via monocarboxylate transporter 1 (MTC1). Lactylation can add or remove lactate to and from histone lysine residues (KLA) in the nucleus. Lactylation relaxes chromatin conformation, enabling gene transcription. Impaired lactylation may lead to the expression of customarily silenced genes, such as SCZ vulnerability genes, activating pathology.**

## Warburg effect and aggression

Aerobic glycolysis, also known as the Warburg effect, refers to the generation of lactate in the presence of oxygen, a phenomenon observed in senescent, malignant, and activated immune cells, including microglia (26)(43)(44). Senescent cells undergo a metabolic shift from OXPHOS to glycolysis and generate adenosine triphosphate (ATP) from lactate (26). Both cancer and SCZ brains utilize lactate as the primary energy source, and recent clinical and preclinical studies have linked aggressive behavior to glycolysis (45)(46). Indeed, novel studies have found that aggression is triggered by the activation of NLRP3 inflammasome, which upregulates glycolysis (47).

Under physiological circumstances, lactate and lactylation decrease macrophage/microglia inflammation, reducing the injury of peripheral organs by suppressing the assembly of NLRP3 and caspase-1 (CASP-1) as well as the activation of Pro-IL-1β, Pro-IL-18 (48)(49)(50) (Fig. 1). Moreover, normal lactate levels promote synaptic plasticity and exhibit antipsychotic and antidepressant properties, probably by optimizing autophagy (51). Furthermore, adequate lactate and lactylation were reported to inhibit inflammasome assembly, deactivating microglia, highlighting a novel target for SCZ and SLDs (52) (Fig. 1).

Inflammaging in SCZ and SLDs promotes glycolysis. However, excessive lactate may be detrimental as it may induce further senescence by upregulating SASP (53). Indeed, lactate is a two-edged sword; on the one hand, it lowers inflammation via NLRP3, while on the other, it promotes senescence by upregulating SASP. Therefore, lactylationn may not only activate neurotoxic microglia but can also epigenetically contribute to SCZ by facilitating the expression of risk genes, such as disrupted in schizophrenia 1 (DISC-1) (54)(55)(Fig.1).

There is a close cooperation between the aryl hydrocarbon receptor (AhR), which binds both dioxin, and the NLRP3 promoter xenobiotic response element (XRE), highlighting potential AhR dysfunction in chronic mental illness (56)(57)(58). Along this line, previous studies have linked AhR/NLRP3 dialog with aggressive behavior and SCZ (23)(59)(60). In addition, AhR was demonstrated to induces cellular senescence, suggesting involvement in SCZ-associated inflammaging (61)(62). The AhR/SCZ link is further substantiated by the fact that dopamine (DA), serotonin (5-HT), and several antipsychotic drugs are AhR ligands, further implicating this receptor in neuropathology (8)(63).

## Conclusion

Psychiatric metabolomics is a new field that connects cellular energetics with the pathogenesis of psychotic disorders. Conceptualized as accelerated aging conditions, the outcome of SCZ and SLDs could be facilitated via metabolic strategies.

Lactate is the primary source of ATP in cancer, chronic mental illness, and senescent cells. Malignancies prefer glycolysis because excessive lactate lowers host immunity, facilitating tumorigenesis. SCZ and SLDs are characterized by shorter telomeres and premature brain aging, a phenotype marked by higher glycolytic flux and elevated lactate levels. Impaired lactate signaling and dysfunctional lactylation may disrupt neuroplasticity and adult neurogenesis, promoting neuroinflammation, microglial activation, and neuronal loss.

Psychiatric metabolomics opens new avenues for treating chronic SCZ and SLDs by targeting NLRP3 inhibitors, lactylation "writer," and "eraser" proteins. In addition, conceptualizing chronic mental illness as a disorder of accelerated aging is likely to bring senolytic and senomorphic drugs into the psychiatric arena.

# Article for Chapter 5: The Role of Lactylation in Mental Illness: Emphasis on Microglia

## Adonis Sfera[1], Carolina Klein[2], Johnathan J. Anton[3], Zisis Kozlakidis[4] and Christina V. Andronescu[5]

*1. Patton State Hospital, Riverside, CA 92369, USA*
*2. Napa State Hospital, 2100 Napa Vallejo Hwy, Napa, CA 94558, USA*
*3. Department of Biomedical Sciences, California Baptist University, 8432 Magnolia Ave., Riverside, CA 92504, USA*
*4. International Agency for Research on Cancer, World Health Organization, 69000 Lyon, France*
*5. Department of Cell Biology, Stanford University, 450 Serra Mall, Stanford, CA 94305, USA*

### Abstract

A paradigm shift is currently taking place in the etiopathogenesis of neuropsychiatric disorders as immunometabolism is replacing the earlier neurotransmitter model. According to the new concept, cellular bioenergetics drives information processing in the central nervous system; therefore, neuropathology is conceptualized as a direct consequence of impaired metabolism. Along the same lines, endoplasmic reticulum stress and gut barrier dysfunction are emerging as novel targets in schizophrenia and affective disorders, linking immune responses to cellular distress. Furthermore, microglia, the brain's innate immune cells, acquire energy through oxidative phosphorylation, while in the resting state, and glycolysis upon activation, contributing to lactate accumulation and reduced brain pH. The same metabolic signature characterizes neuropsychiatric disorders as the central nervous system derives adenosine triphosphate from aerobic glycolysis, upregulating lactate and generating an acidic environment.

Although known for over three decades, the link between dysmetabolism and neuropathology was poorly defined until the discovery of brain-resident innate lymphoid cells, including natural killer cells, and lactylation of histone and nonhistone proteins. In this perspective article, we examine three anti-inflammatory microglial systems relevant for neuropsychiatry: lactate, oxytocin, and the aryl hydrocarbon receptor. We also discuss potential interventions for restoring microglial homeostasis.

**Keywords:** microglia; neuropathology; lactylation; oxytocin; aryl hydrocarbon receptor.

## Introduction

Severe neuropsychiatric illnesses, including schizophrenia and affective disorders, have been associated with brain metabolic disturbances, including excessive aerobic glycolysis and upregulated lactate, emphasizing that in the central nervous system (CNS) bioenergetics and information processing are highly intertwined [1–4]. Aerobic glycolysis and upregulated lactate, known as the Warburg effect, are the preferred energy sources of cancer cells and likely drive the pathogenesis of neuropsychiatric disorders [5,6]. Although low levels of lactate are neuroprotective, in excess it was demonstrated to induce neuronal apoptosis and decreased glutamatergic and GABAergic neurotransmission, hallmarks of neuropathology [7,8]. Along this line, a novel schizophrenia (SCZ) study has found that oral flora-derived lactate crosses the blood–brain barrier (BBB), generating CNS acidity [9,10].

Microglia are the CNS-resident macrophages known for vigilantly scanning the brain parenchyma, searching for tissue damage, molecular debris, and invading pathogens [10,11]. When changes are detected, microglia become activated and bioenergetically dependent on lactate [10]. Inflamed microglia, a characteristic of several neuropsychiatric disorders, release proinflammatory cytokines and adopt a neurotoxic phenotype [12]. Hence, targeting microglial lactate is an emerging immunometabolic strategy in neuropsychiatric disorders [13–15] (see the section on Potential Therapeutic Strategies).

Recent studies have revealed that lactate is an essential CNS metabolite which promotes synaptic plasticity and exerts anti-inflammatory, antipsychotic, and antidepressant properties [16–20]. These are mediated by suppression of nuclear factor kappa B (NF-κB) via lactate signaling with its receptor hydroxycarboxylic acid receptor 1 (HCAR1) (also known as G-protein-coupled receptor 81 (GPR81)) [18]. In addition, lactate promotes axonal myelination as well as the rehabilitation of injured oligodendrocytes (OLs), highlighting a potential treatment modality for multiple sclerosis (MS) [21–23].

Lactylation is a post-translational modification (PTM) which utilizes lactate as a substrate; therefore, excessive availability of this metabolite promotes lactylation-mediated pathologies, including malignant transformation, Alzheimer's disease (AD), and neuropsychiatric disorders [24–27]. Lysine lactylation (Kla), discovered in 2019 by Yingming Zhao, can be a physiological or pathological process, depending on the lactylation levels, which regulates gene transcription by metabolically reprograming the neurons and glia [28,29] (Figure 1). In addition, the lactylation of nonhistone proteins, such as the high-mobility group box 1 (HMGB1), hypoxia-inducible factor 1 alpha (HIF-1α), and the membrane-organizing extension spike protein (moesin), was associated with tumorigenesis and schizophrenia, further linking dysfunctional lactylation to various pathologies [30–32].

Another major discovery took place in 2022, when a subpopulation of oxytocin (OXT)producing microglia was discovered, revealing a novel anti-inflammatory phenotype of these cells, likely distinct from the resting state [33,34]. Indeed, OXT signaling with OXT receptors (OXTRs), expressed on microglia, astrocytes, and oligodendrocytes, was reported to lower not only neuroinflammation but also depression, suicidal behavior, and psychosis, highlighting new potential pharmacological targets [35–44]. In addition, OXT promotes myelination and supports the nervous system white matter, likely explaining the reason this hormone was patented as an MS treatment (US patent 3274060A) [38,45,46].

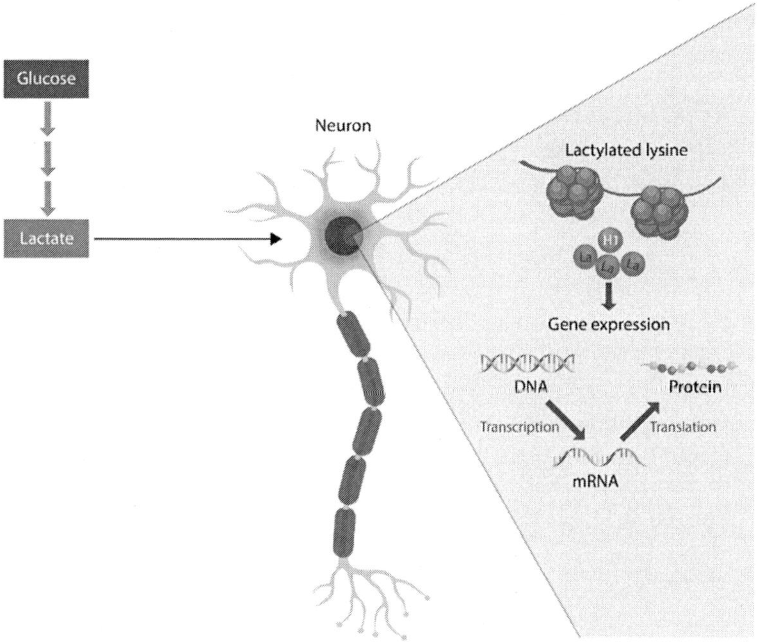


**Figure 1. Excessive lactate derived from glucose metabolism can lead to excessive histone lysine lactylation (Kla), promoting pathologies, such as cancer, AD, schizophrenia, and related neuropsychiatric illnesses. Histone lactylation alters gene expression that in return affects translation and protein synthesis.**

The aryl hydrocarbon receptor (AhR), a cytosolic ligand-activated transcription factor, regulates the expression of numerous genes, including those involved in the response to environmental pollutants, polarization of microglia, myelination, and inflammation [47–49]. In the CNS, AhR exerts anti-inflammatory properties on microglia and astrocytes, promoting restorative neurogenesis and post-insult tissue regeneration [50]. However, in ischemic strokes, AhR may activate microglia, triggering inflammation, suggesting that this receptor is not only tissue-specific but also dependent on the pathology type [51]. In addition, AhR modulates meningeal innate lymphoid cells (ILCs), especially the protective CD56bright natural killer cells (NKCs), promoting a tolerant, IL-10-generating phenotype [52,53]. Conversely, dysfunctional NKCs promote neuroinflammation by aberrantly eliminating the anti-inflammatory resting microglia, disrupting immune homeostasis by selectively sparing the activated, inflamed cells [54].

In this perspective article, we take a closer look at three anti-inflammatory microglial systems relevant for neuropsychiatry, lactate, OXT, and AhR, as well as potential interventions for restoring microglial homeostasis.

## Lactate and Mental Illness4

Major neuropsychiatric illnesses, including schizophrenia and affective disorders, have been associated with decreased brain pH, lactic acid accumulation and upregulated glycolysis [1,2,8]. From a bioenergetic perspective, the brain cells of mentally ill individuals resemble cancer cells, as adenosine triphosphate (ATP) is acquired through aerobic glycolysis, or the Warburg effect, decreasing the brain pH, while oxidative phosphorylation (OXPHOS) is downregulated.

Lactate plays a key role in the CNS where it functions as a metabolite as well as a neurotransmitter. Lactate is endowed with anti-inflammatory properties as it inhibits NK-kB, promotes myelination, and regulates microglial function [22,55]. Indeed, microglia possess the molecular machinery to shift metabolism according to phenotype; resting microglia rely on OXPHOS, while activated microglia utilize aerobic glycolysis [23].

Innate lymphoid cells (ILCs) signaling with microglia and the discovery of histone and nonhistone proteins lactylation have contributed to a better understanding of the role of aerobic glycolysis in neuropsychiatric disorders. Although lactate is neuroprotective and mediates synaptic plasticity, excessive lactylation can alter neuronal function, shifting them to an energy state akin to malignant cells [56–58] (see section Microglia, lactylation and mental illness). For example, aberrant neuronal cell cycle reentry and aneuploidy have been observed in patients with SCZ, suggesting that lactate triggers "reprimitivization" of brain cells or the acquisition of stem cell properties [30,59–63]. This is further substantiated by the neuronal progenitor cells' dependency on aerobic glycolysis, suggesting that local acidity promotes undifferentiated cellular phenotypes [64,65]. Indeed, in an acidic environment, somatic mammalian cells could be epigenetically reprogrammed into pluripotent stem cells, while L-lactate has been shown to induce neurogenesis in adult hippocampal neurons [66–68]. Moreover, exposed to lactate, cardiomyocytes were demonstrated to reenter the cell cycle in a manner reminiscent of neurons, emphasizing the link between low pH and postmitotic cells' replication attempts [69].

Moesin is a member of the ezrin-radixin-moesin (ERM) family of proteins which are constituent parts of the cellular cytoskeleton, and thus implicated in mitosis [70]. In AD, moesin activates neuronal cell cycle reentry, indicating that lactylation of this protein may promote neuropsychiatric pathology [71–73]. Indeed, moesin was implicated in schizophrenia and plays a major role in the aberrant NKCs activation [74–76] (Figure 2).

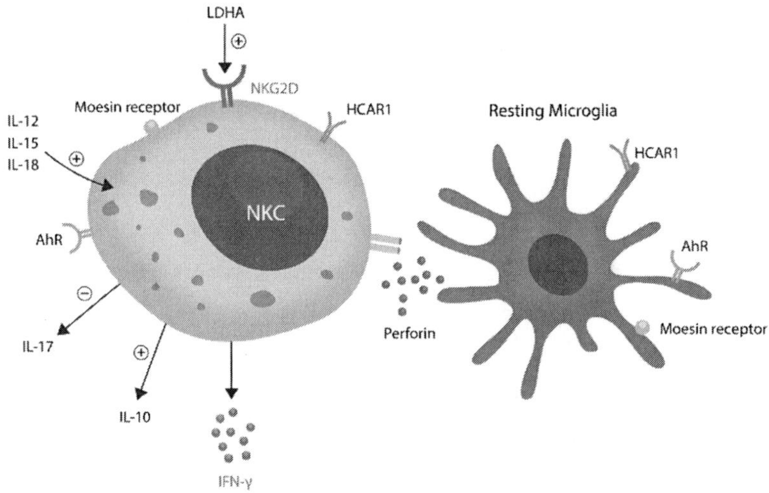


**Figure 2. Aberrant elimination of resting microglia by lactate-activated NKCs. LDHA or LDH-5 can activate NKC via NKG2D receptors. IL-12, IL-15, and IL-18 activate NKCs, facilitating the release of IL-10, IL17, and IFN-γ. NKCs express HCAR1, AhR, and moesin receptors, proteins previously implicated in neuropathology. Activated NKCs release perforin, a toxic molecule known for eliminating resting microglia. Because activated microglia are not killed, this is a likely mechanism of tilting the balance toward inflammation**

Histone Kla, a reversible PTM, is regulated by EP300 and class I histone deacetylases (HDAC1–3), enzymes which add and remove lactate to and from the histone proteins [77–79]. Both HDAC1–3 and EP300 have been implicated in SCZ and/or the adverse effects of antipsychotic drugs via the brain-derived neurotrophic factor (BDNF) [80–82]. As BDNF gene histone modifications contribute to fear extinction, this system's malfunction likely triggers Kla-mediated neuropsychiatric symptoms, such as excitation, social defeat, anxiety, and stress [83,84]. Interestingly, the neuroprotective properties of BDNF consist of preventing neuronal cell cycle reentry, further linking attempted mitosis to psychopathology [85].

NKCs are members of ILCs which are activated by lactate and sense pathological changes, migrating to the affected sites, including the brain parenchyma [86]. Lactateactivated NKCs were found to eliminate resting microglia but not the activated phenotype, suggesting that the pathological loss of anti-inflammatory microglia triggers neuroinflammation and the related pathology [54] (Figure 2). Moreover, as activated microglia have been linked to neurotoxicity and demyelination, pathological NKCs may predispose to autoimmune inflammation, including multiple sclerosis (MS) [12,87,88]. This is significant as impaired NKCs were found in the first episode of SCZ in antipsychotic-naïve individuals, suggesting that manipulation of these cells could ameliorate psychotic symptoms [89].

Recent studies have revealed an alternative source of brain lactate, the microbial community residing in various body compartments, including the oral cavity and the GI tract [1,9]. Indeed, the high lactate producers Bifidobacterium and Lactobacillus spp. have been shown to maintain the integrity of intestinal epithelial cells (IECs) and the survival of other commensals [90,91]. However, excessive lactate accumulation in the GI tract can trigger pathology by lowering the production of short-chain fatty acids (SCFA), biomolecules in charge of numerous CNS and peripheral physiological functions [92]. Indeed, the lactateinduced anti-inflammatory and immunosuppressive milieu can predispose to cancer as well as microbial and viral infections [93–95]. For example, lactate signaling with microglial HCAR1 promotes tissue regeneration and healing; however, it may also induce pathology by suppressing the phagocytosis of malignant or pathogen-infected cells [94–96].

## Mental Illness, Lactylation, and Microbes

Histone Kla is not limited to mammals as it was also demonstrated in prokaryotes, linking microbial lactate to host neuropathology [97]. For example, Escherichia coli (E. coli) proteins YiaC and CobB induce histone lactylation, likely explaining the association of this bacterium with schizophrenia [98]. This was exemplified in the 2011 outbreak of E. coli in Germany which was accompanied by psychosis, linking this pathogen to mental illness [99,100]. In another example, urinary tract infection (UTI), caused primarily by

E. coli, is known for the potential to trigger new-onset psychosis or the exacerbation of psychotic symptoms in stable patients with schizophrenia, further illustrating the link between this pathogen and mental illness [101,102].

Lactylation of nonhistone proteins, HMGB1, HIF-1α, and moesin, was associated with both schizophrenia and E. coli infection, linking this microbe once more to neuropathology [30,31,103–106]. Moreover, Toxoplasma gondii, an intracellular protozoan, previously associated with SCZ, is another example of pathogen-mediated lactylation, causing host neuropathology [107]. Indeed, a recent study found that Toxoplasma gondii, containing 523 lactylated proteins, eliminates host inhibitory synapses by aberrantly activating microglia [108,109]. Moreover, Toxoplasma gondii was demonstrated to induce endoplasmic reticulum (ER) stress as well as intestinal barrier disruption, pathologies associated with mental illness [110,111].

Taken together, lactate is a CNS protective metabolite that not only contributes to energy metabolism and signaling but also serves as a substrate for lactylation. Excessive lactate accumulation from local metabolism or the microbiome may trigger lactylationassociated pathology, such as cancer, AD, or neuropsychiatric illness.

## Oxytocin and Microglia in Mental Illness

Oxytocin (OXT)-oxytocin receptor (OXTR) signaling comprises a microglial antiinflammatory pathway. OXT is a neuropeptide synthesized in the hypothalamus and stored in the posterior pituitary prior to being released into the systemic circulation. OXT is both a hormone and a neurotransmitter, the former mediating parturition and lactation, while the latter affects social behavior, affiliation, intimacy, and mother–infant bonding [112]. A recent study found that the OXT concentration in the brain can reach levels 1000 times higher than in the systemic circulation, highlighting the importance of this biomolecule for CNS function [113].

Low blood OXT levels were reported in patients with SCZ marked by negative symptoms, while intranasal administration of OXT was shown to ameliorate this condition [114,115]. Indeed, like lactate, OXT modulates synaptic plasticity and upregulates adult hippocampal neurogenesis, enhancing long-term potentiation and memory, properties that likely mediate this hormone's antipsychotic and antidepressant properties [116–118].

OXT decreases microglial inflammation by lowering ER stress via translation initiation factor 2 alpha/transcription factor ATF4 (eIF-2α–ATF4), a common autophagic pathway disrupted in SCZ and major depressive disorder (MDD) [119–121]. For example, eIF-2α– ATF4 lowers ER stress by upregulating Sigma-1 receptors (Sig-1Rs), proteins involved in several neuropsychiatric disorders. Indeed, several antidepressant and antipsychotic drugs, including fluvoxamine, sertraline, and haloperidol, lower ER stress, suggesting that the therapeutic properties of these agents could be mediated by eIF-2α–ATF4 [122,123]. Aside from lowering ER stress, Sig-1Rs protect the intestinal barrier and BBB, linking eIF-2α–ATF4 to microbial translocation [124,125]. It stands to reason, therefore, that strengthening the gut barrier and lowering ER stress in intestinal epithelial cells (IECs) are emerging strategies for neuropsychiatric disorders (Table 1) (clinical trials identifier NCT03183609) [126–131]).

**Table 1. The action mechanisms of Lactate, OXT, and AhR.**

| Lactate | OXT | AhR | References |
|---|---|---|---|
| Deactivates microglia by NF-kB inhibition | Deactivates microglia via eIF-2α–ATF4 pathway | Deactivates microglia via NF-kB | [4,15,50] |
| Excess lactate promotes Kla | No known effect on lactylation | Increases LDHA and lactate | [24,132] |
| Lowers ER stress | Lowers ER stress | Lowers ER stress | [16,33,133] |
| Augments gut barrier function | Augments gut barrier | Augments gut barrier | [90,124,134] |
| Upregulated in schizophrenia | Downregulated in schizophrenia | Implicated in schizophrenia | [1,135,136] |

Several studies have connected OXT with the selective serotonin reuptake inhibitors (SSRIs), emphasizing that this hormone may contribute, at least in part, to the action mechanism of antidepressant drugs [137,138]. Moreover, sexual dysfunction, a common SSRI adverse effect, was associated with decreased OXT blood levels, linking this hormone further to the serotonergic system [139,140]. This is significant as OXT exerts antidepressant properties of its own and may be indicated in situations when other antidepressants are to be avoided, such as during pregnancy and the postpartum period as well as in patients with sexual dysfunction.

Aside from the antidepressant action, OXT exerts antipsychotic properties, documented as early as the 1970s and 1980s, followed by clinical trials of intranasal OXT in 2010, studies which have produced encouraging results for schizophrenia patients [35,135,141] (clinical trials identifier NCT0162 1737).

In 2022, it was discovered that a subpopulation of microglial cells is capable of generating OXT, drawing the attention of researchers and clinicians to the anti-inflammatory properties of these cells [33,34]. Indeed, OXT signaling with OXTR, expressed on microglia, astrocytes, and oligodendrocytes, lowers neuroinflammation, depression, suicidal behavior, and psychosis, indicating that OXT signaling is a significant neuropsychiatric target [35–44] (see section Microglia, lactylation and mental illness).

Taken together, OXT and lactate exert antipsychotic and antidepressant properties through different mechanisms. Impaired OXT signaling may trigger neuropathology by increasing ER stress in IECs, disrupting the GI tract barrier.

## Aryl Hydrocarbon Receptor and Mental Illness

ILCs are mucosa-anchored lymphocytes which express transcription factors instead of Tor B-cell receptors; they are activated by specific cytokines and generate their own cytokine output. ILCs, comprised of NKCs, ILCs types 1, 2, 3, and regulatory ILCs (ILCreg), are situated at the biological barriers, including the gut and meninges [142,143]. Human ILCs express AhR which is abundantly represented on CD56bright NKC, emphasizing further the protective role of these lymphocytes [53,144]. Glycolytic enzymes, lactate dehydrogenase A (LDHA) or lactate dehydrogenase-5 (LDH-5), activate NKG2D receptors, regulating CD56bright NKC responses, suggesting that excessive lactate likely disrupts the function of these lymphocytes [144,145].

Aside from AhR and lactate, NKCs, including CD56bright, are activated by IL-12, IL-15, and IL-18, releasing interferon γ (IFN-γ) and IL-10 (Figure 2) [1–4]. In addition, AhR lowers the proinflammatory IL-17 previously implicated in both SCZ and MS [146–148].

Moreover, dysfunctional IL-12, IL-15, IL-18, IFN-γ, and IL-10 have been associated with schizophrenia, highlighting further the key role NKCs in this pathology [149,150]. AhR also suppresses microglial and astrocytic inflammation, switching these cells from inflammatory to the restorative phenotype [51,151,152].

Aberrant elimination of resting microglia by NKCs is likely the root cause of neuroinflammation, documented in many neuropsychiatric disorders; therefore, rescuing these cells should be explored as a therapeutic strategy

[53,54]. For example, the expansion of circulating CD56bright NKCs has been associated with improved MS symptoms, suggesting that these cells may also play a beneficial role in SCZ and affective disorders [153,154]. Indeed, a low CD56 lymphocyte count was demonstrated in antipsychotic-naïve patients with schizophrenia, and it was upregulated by treatment, emphasizing the beneficial properties of these cells [134] (for the role of AhR in microglial cells, see the section Microglia, lactylation and mental illness). As CD56bright NKCs express AhR, the clinical symptoms may respond to the pharmacological manipulation of this receptor [155] (discussed in the section on Potential Therapeutic Strategies).

In the gut, AhR protects the intestinal barrier by binding microbiota-derived metabolites as well as the SCFAs, linking dysfunctional AhR signaling to gut barrier disruption and microbial translocation [156,157].

Novel studies have shown that AhR functions in a tissue-specific manner, dependent on the ligand affinity, likely accounting for the variable, often opposite, responses elicited in one organ vs. another [158,159]. For example, endogenous AhR ligands, such as tryptophan and microbial metabolites, may exacerbate breast cancer while exerting salutary effects in colorectal carcinoma [132,160–163]. Moreover, in the gut, AhR enhances the barrier function while inducing liver toxicity, illustrating the difficulties encountered in trying to develop AhR therapeutics. Having said that, selective modulators, such as flavonoids and isoflavones, may offer a solution [164–167] (Table 2) (see the section on potential interventions).

AhR promotes myelination and lowers ER stress, suggesting that MS, MDD, schizophrenia, and bipolar disorder may be exacerbated by the dysfunction of this protein [133,186]. Interestingly, carbidopa and the unique antipsychotic drug clozapine are AhR agonists, linking this receptor to the dopaminergic system and probably explaining both the efficacy as well as the side effects of these agents [187,188]. Moreover, dopamine is an AhR ligand, further implicating this receptor in mental illness [136]. Indeed, AhR was implicated in schizophrenia by the earlier studies, emphasizing a novel psychopharmacological target [189]. In a rodent model, clozapine attenuates experimental autoimmune encephalomyelitis (EAE), suggesting that the unique anti-suicide properties of this drug (not shared with other antipsychotic agents) may be mediated by AhR [190]. Yet another study saw that agranulocytosis, an autoimmune-like adverse effect of clozapine, was associated with DRB1*15:01, a rare human leukocyte antigen (HLA), and a major MS risk factor, linking agranulocytosis to this genetic marker [191,192].

**Table 2. Potential interventions for restoring the homeostasis of anti-inflammatory microglia.**

| Lactate | OXT | AhR | References |
|---|---|---|---|
| L-lactate | Intranasal OXT | Flavonoids | [114,168,169] |
| Lactylation inhibitors | ARBs | Nattokinase | [169–171] |
| Demethylzeylasteral (DML) | ISRIB | Isoflavones | [172–174] |
| Sirtuins | PAK inhibitors | Laquinimod | [170,175,176] |
| Sodium oxamate | MIF-1 | CH 22391 | [177–179] |
| Gallnut extract CN102836354A | OT-1 (TC OT 39) | Triptans (Sumatriptan) | [180–182] |
| Galloflavin (NSC 107022) | WAY 267464 | CD56bright NKCs | [183–185] |

Taken together, AhR exerts antidepressant and antipsychotic properties by several mechanisms: 1. microglial deactivation, 2. lowering ER stress, 3. enhancing the gut barrier, 4. upregulating lactate, and 5. myelination. These protective effects may explain the unique clozapine properties (Table 1).

## Microbial Translocation Outside the GI Tract

In our previous work, we have discussed microbial translocation from the GI tract into the host systemic circulation, suggesting that the pathogenesis of several idiopathic diseases could be explained by the immune responses to extraintestinal microbial proteins [193]. As higher gut and BBB permeability markers, including the soluble form of CD14 (sCD14), were documented in neuropsychiatric illness, this pathology may, at least in part, result from microbial migration through the gut barrier [194–196].

Various antigens of GI tract microbes, including Bacteroides, Bifidobacterium, Acinetobacter, and Pseudomonas, have been shown to exhibit molecular mimicry with the host myelin basic protein (MBP), suggesting that autoantibodies against myelin, documented in MS, schizophrenia, and bipolar disorder, may be conventional immunoglobulins directed at the displaced microbes or their components [197–199]. In addition, as myelin contains a serotonin binding site, the autoantibodies against serotonin, found in MS and MDD, may be classical antibodies against serotonin-producing microbes, such as Clostridia or staphylococci [200,201]. Furthermore, bacterial N-acetylmuramyl dipeptide was reported to mimic myelin, likely triggering antibodies upon translocation into host tissues [202]. These findings are significant as they emphasize that strengthening the gut barrier to lower microbial

migration likely comprises a novel therapeutic strategy in neuropsychiatric disorders. In fact, inflammation in response to translocated microbial proteins was previously associated with suicidal behavior, suggesting that gut barrier restoration should be instituted as a therapy in mental illness [203–205]. Indeed, some antidepressant drugs currently utilized in clinical practice were demonstrated to optimize the gut barrier function, suggesting an alternative, noncanonical, mechanism of action [206]. Microbial translocation across the gut barrier has been documented in MDD, suicidal behavior, bipolar disorder, aggression in SCZ, and neurodegeneration, suggesting that the loss of anti-inflammatory microglia plays a crucial role in neuropathology [196,202–205,207,208].

## Potential Therapeutic Strategies

Lactate, OXT, and AhR are therapeutic targets rarely considered in the treatment of neuropsychiatric disorders; however, they play a major role in the CNS and immune metabolism.

## Lactate

Novel studies have shown that peripheral administration of L-lactate exerts antidepressant effects by increasing hippocampal lactic acid which upregulates neurogenesis and inhibits microglial activation [168,209] (Table 2).

1. Lactylation inhibitors are compounds belonging to several classes of therapeutics, such as LDHA inhibitors, demethylzeylasteral (DML), and phytotherapeutics, including polyphenols. Here, we review only the agents that can cross the BBB, lower ER stress, and strengthen the intestinal barrier [210,211]. These are as follows.
2. Sirtuins: Studies in oncology have reported that sirtuins (SIRT), especially SIRT2, can remove lactate from the histone lysine, showing that de-lactylation may comprise a novel strategy for microglial depolarization, an approach likely beneficial in MDD and SCZ [170]. The effect of SIRT in these disorders has been documented by earlier research [212–214].
   Demethylzeylasteral (DML) inhibits lactylation of histone H3, a protein associated with MDD, suggesting that it could exert antidepressant properties [172,215].
3. LDH inhibitors Lactate-HCAR1 signaling is regulated by LDHA or LDH-5, glycolytic enzymes upregulated by psychological stress, suggesting that inhibiting these enzymes could be therapeutic for neuropsychiatric illness [216]. LDH inhibitors, include the following:
   3.1 Sodium oxamate, a structural analog of pyruvate, is known for lowering ER stress by promoting protective autophagy, properties beneficial for neuropsychiatric disorders [177,217]. To the best of our knowledge this compound has not been evaluated for psychiatric conditions.
   3.2 Chinese Gallnut Extract from Galla chinensis is a traditional Chinese medicine and a potent LDHA inhibitor which was patented for the treatment of MDD and is currently in clinical trials (Chinese patent CN102836354A) (US patent 10098854B2) (clinical trials identifier NCT04080752) [180,218].

3.3 Galloflavin or NSC 107022 is a polyphenol found in berries which upregulates SIRT6, a key regulator of neuronal mitochondria [183,219]. Dysfunctional SIRT6 was associated with depression-like behavior in mice, suggesting potential benefits for humans with MDD [220]. Galloflavin has been patented as a modulator of protein kinases that can treat a variety of conditions, ranging from cancer to neuropsychiatric disorders (US patent 2003 0187007A1).

## OXT

OXT signaling with OXTRs has been shown to inhibit activated microglia and increase the number of NKCs, a phenomenon documented in schizophrenia [221]. Recently, an OXT-generating microglial population was identified, suggesting that anti-inflammatory microglia may regulate many physiological functions that could cause pathology when disrupted [222,223].

### *Angiotensin IV (ANG IV) as an OXT Agonist*

Several studies demonstrated that microglia express a functional renin-angiotensin system (RAS), including angiotensin II type 1 receptors (AT-1Rs) [224]. Conversely, AT-1R blockers (ARBs), especially the BBB-crossing candesartan, have been found therapeutic in schizophrenia and MDD, linking dysfunctional RAS to inflamed microglia [171]. This is significant as angiotensin II (ANG II) is a negative OXT regulator; thus, ARBs may not only depolarize these cells but also enhance OXT release [33,34,224,225]. Indeed, angiotensin IV was reported to upregulate OXT in vitro and in vivo, probably by inhibiting oxytocinase, the hydrolyzing enzyme of this hormone [226].

OXT inhibits eIF-2α–ATF4 signaling, a pathway implicated in ER stress, suggesting that the beneficial neuropsychiatric effects of OXT can likely be attributed to autophagy [44]. Indeed, the antiretroviral drug nelfinavir has been shown to promote ER stress by eIF2α phosphorylation; in contrast, the integrated stress response inhibitor (ISRIB), a protein with antidepressant and antipsychotic properties, inhibits nelfinavir-induced ER stress via eIF2α dephosphorylation [173]. The related drugs, p21-activated kinase (PAK) inhibitors, were found beneficial in SCZ, emphasizing new potential targets in this disorder [175]. IRIB was patented in Australia as a broad therapeutic agent that may be useful in pathologies involving learning, memory, immunity, intermediary metabolism, insulin production, and resistance to unfolded protein stress (Australian patent 2020229748A1).

## *OXT Fragments*

OXT, comprised of nine amino acids, was found to rctain biological properties even when cleaved in shorter segments. For example, melanocyte-inhibiting factor-1 (MIF-1), the N-terminal segment of oxytocin, possesses antidepressant and antipsychotic properties, suggesting that OXTR can be activated by related small ligands [178,227]. MIF-1 was patented for cancer, autoimmune diseases, fibrotic diseases, inflammation, and neurodegenerative diseases (international patent WO2009040045A2). Several OXT-like molecules have also been studied, including lipo-oxytocin-1 (LOT-1), a synthetic OXTR agonist (also known as TC OT 39), and WAY-267464, an OXTR agonist and vasopressin 1 receptor (V1AR) antagonist [181,184]. The efficacy of these ligands for neuropsychiatric disorders has not been evaluated in clinical trials; however, several patents were obtained for use in neurological and psychiatric disorders (international patent WO2018107216A1) (EP2326341B1).

## AhR

AhR binds diverse ligands derived from the environment, diet, microbes, and cellular metabolism, enabling cells to adapt to the changing exogenous or endogenous conditions. Drugs, chemicals, and plant-derived compounds, including isoflavones, attach with different affinities to AhR [228]. Nattokinase, a soybean fermented by Bacillus subtilis var. natto, contains AhR-binding flavonoids [169]. Indeed, several isoflavones, including, soybeans, genistein, daidzein, glycitein, formononetin, biochanin, and phytoestrogens, have been found to exert antidepressant and antipsychotic properties [174,229,230].

i. Laquinimod, a quinolone-3-carboxamide developed for the treatment of MS, is a selective AhR ligand that demonstrated encouraging results in animal models of MDD and anxiety [176].

ii. CH223191 is an antagonistic selective AhR ligand with a favorable profile for neuropsychiatric disorders [179]. This compound was patented in the US for cancer treatment but has still to enter clinical trials for neuropsychiatric disorders (US patent 20160175278A1).

iii. Sumatriptan, a selective 5-hydroxy-triptamine (5-HT1) receptor agonist, activates human AhR, exerting anti-inflammatory properties, suggesting beneficial effects on activated microglia [182,231].

iv. Dimethyl fumarate, indicated for MS, is not an AhR ligand; however, it upregulates the protective AhR-expressing CD56bright NKCs which eliminate the detrimental autoreactive immune cells to avert autoimmunity [232,233]. For this reason, CD56bright NKCs expansion via AhR or transplantation may comprise a potential therapeutic strategy for neuropsychiatric illness. For example, CD56bright NK cells allogeneic or stem cell transplantation, a treatment used for acute myeloid leukemia, could be therapeutic in both MS and schizophrenia [185,234].

## Microglia, Lactylation, and Mental Illness

Although microglia comprise less than 10% of the brain cells, it plays a major role in neuropsychiatric pathology [235]. Resting microglia are neuroprotective as evidenced by in vivo two-photon imaging of fluorescent-labeled neurons and microglia, demonstrating that these cells participate in the plasticity of neuronal circuits [236]. Resting microglia actively communicate with other brain cells, including astrocytes, neurons, and ILCs [237–239]. Recent studies have shown that microglia express monocarboxylate transporters (MCTs) and HCAR1, suggesting that lactate plays an important role in the reprograming of these cells [240,241]. Numerous studies have found that young and healthy brains rely on glycolysis and lactate, while aging brains lose glycolytic ability [242]. For example, dysfunctional glycolysis was associated with AD pathology as well as schizophrenia [243,244]. Excessive lactate generation contributes to lactylation of histone and nonhistone proteins, engendering pathology [245].

Microglia are brain resident macrophages that express OXT receptors, suggesting that these proteins contribute to anti-inflammatory microglia, a likely protection against mental illness [246,247].

Microglia express AhR, proteins involved in several pathologies, including glioblastoma [248]. AhR is a new receptor of interest in schizophrenia, not only because it binds dopamine but also because schizophrenia-associated exogenous toxins, such as plasticizers, are ligands at this receptor [249,250]. In addition, many protective metabolites synthesized by gut microbes, including indole and tryptophan, are AhR ligands, suggesting that the gut–brain axis likely operates through this receptor [251].

It has been reported that aberrantly activated microglia become neurotoxic and engage in the elimination of healthy neurons or synapses, a pathology involved in schizophrenia [252–254].

## Limitations

Many compounds described above are phytotherapeutics, primarily natural products, such as sirtuins, or traditional foods, including nattokinase and the Chinese Gallnut Extract, that have been used by humans for hundreds of years. The ability of these molecules to act as AhR ligands suggests beneficial effects in neuropsychiatric illness, and clinical trials should be initiated to assess their efficacy. Likewise, the ability of sirtuins to remove histone lysine lactate has reawakened the interest in these compounds, previously studied for neurodegenerative disorders, as potential medical foods or dietary interventions.

Furthermore, several compounds mentioned above have been patented in different countries and some are currently in clinical trials, while others have not reached that stage yet. However, the profile of these agents, estimated by their action mechanism described in the patent application, suggests that they should be evaluated as antidepressant or antipsychotic agents. For example, dimethyl fumarate was patented in Europe for the treatment of MS; however, as this drug exerts neuroprotective as well as anti-inflammatory effects on astrocytes and microglia, it likely possesses antidepressant and antipsychotic properties which should be evaluated in clinical trials.

Additionally, we need to state that most of the pathophysiological mechanisms described in this article are newly elucidated. As the details become increasingly available, it would be much easier to prioritize different potential therapeutic targets. Moreover, understanding these mechanisms will eventually allow for an in-depth stratification of neuropsychiatric patients, and a move toward an improved precision medicine approach.

## Conclusions

Increasing awareness of the shortcomings of the neurotransmitter paradigm contributed to the development of a new concept, metabolism-driven information processing. This model, illustrated by the previously known association of neuropsychiatric pathology with excessive aerobic glycolysis, was put in perspective by the discovery of ILCs and lactylation. The consequences of excessive brain lactate and increased local acidity include the following:

1. The aberrant elimination of anti-inflammatory resting microglia by pathologically activated NKCs.
2. The reactivation of the neuronal cell cycle with resultant aneuploidy or apoptosis as these cells lack the molecular machinery to complete mitosis.
3. Several interventions may restore the homeostasis of anti-inflammatory microglia, including 1. lowering lactylation, 2. enhancing OXT signaling, 3. modulating AhR, and 4. expanding CD56NKCs. These strategies lower the ER stress and strengthen the gut barrier, limiting microbial migration outside of the GI tract, thus decreasing the risk of microglial activation by translocated bacterial antigens.

More studies are needed to clarify the role of lactylation of histone and nonhistone proteins in mental illnesses and the interaction of lactylation with meningeal ILCs.

Where authors are identified as personnel of the International Agency for Research on Cancer/WHO, the authors alone are responsible for the views expressed in this article and they do not necessarily represent the decisions, policy, or views of the International Agency for Research on Cancer/WHO.

**Author Contributions:** Conceptualization, A.S., C.K. and Z.K.; methodology, C.V.A.; formal analysis,

J.J.A. and C.V.A.; data curation, J.J.A.; writing—original draft preparation, A.S.; writing—review and editing, C.K. and Z.K. All authors have read and agreed to the published version of the manuscript.

**Funding:** This research received no external funding.

**Institutional Review Board Statement:** Not applicable.

**Informed Consent Statement:** Not applicable.

**Data Availability Statement:** Not applicable.

**Conflicts of Interest: Where authors are identified as personnel of the** International Agency for Research on Cancer/WHO, the authors alone are responsible for the views expressed in this article and they do not necessarily represent the decisions, policy or views of the International Agency for Research on Cancer/WHO.

**Abbreviations**

NF-κB = nuclear factor kappa B; HCAR1 = hydroxycarboxylic acid receptor 1; GPR81 = Gprotein-coupled receptor 81; Kla = lysine lactylation; OXT = oxytocin; OXTRs = receptors; AhR = aryl hydrocarbon receptor; NKCs = natural killer cells; ERM = ezrin-radixin-moesin; HDAC1 = class I histone deacetylases; ILC = innate lymphoid cells; HMGB1 = high-mobility group box 1; HIF-1α = hypoxia-inducible factor 1α; BDNF = brain-derived neurotrophic factor; IEC = intestinal epithelial cells; SCFA = short-chain fatty acids; ISRIB = integrated stress response inhibitor; MIF-1 = melanocyte-inhibiting factor-1; OXPHOS = oxidative phosphorylation; V1AR = vasopressin 1 receptor; SCZ = schizophrenia.

## References


1. Ross JM, Öberg J, Brené S, Coppotelli G, Terzioglu M, Pernold K, Goiny M, Sitnikov R, Kehr J, Trifunovic A, Larsson NG, Hoffer BJ, Olson L. High brain lactate is a hallmark of aging and caused by a shift in the lactate dehydrogenase A/B ratio. Proc Natl Acad Sci U S A. 2010 Nov 16;107(46):20087-92. doi: 10.1073/pnas.1008189107.
2. Feng Y, Shen J, He J, Lu M. Schizophrenia and cell senescence candidate genes screening, machine learning, diagnostic models, and drug prediction. Front Psychiatry. 2023 Apr 11;14:1105987. doi: 10.3389/fpsyt.2023.1105987.
3. Okusaga OO. Accelerated aging in schizophrenia patients: the potential role of oxidative stress. Aging Dis. 2013 Dec 4;5(4):256-62. doi: 10.14336/AD.2014.0500256.
4. Papanastasiou E, Gaughran F, Smith S. Schizophrenia as segmental progeria. J R Soc Med. 2011 Nov;104(11):475-84. doi: 10.1258/jrsm.2011.110051. PMID: 22048679; PMCID: PMC3206717.
5. Tesli N, Bell C, Hjell G, Fischer-Vieler T, I Maximov I, Richard G, Tesli M, Melle I, Andreassen OA, Agartz I, Westlye LT, Friestad C, Haukvik UK, Rokicki J. The age of violence: Mapping brain age in psychosis and psychopathy. Neuroimage Clin. 2022;36:103181. doi: 10.1016/j.nicl.2022.103181.
6. Cole JH, et al. Brain age and other bodily 'ages': implications for neuropsychiatry. Mol Psychiatry. 2019;24(2):266–281. doi: 10.1038/s41380-018-0098-1.
7. Amgalan A, Maher AS, Ghosh S, Chui HC, Bogdan P, Irimia A. Brain age estimation reveals older adults' accelerated senescence after traumatic brain injury. Geroscience. 2022 Oct;44(5):2509-2525. doi: 10.1007/s11357-022-00597-1.
8. Park HJ, Choi I, Leem KH. Decreased Brain pH and Pathophysiology in Schizophrenia. Int J Mol Sci. 2021 Aug 4;22(16):8358. doi: 10.3390/ijms22168358. PMID: 34445065; PMCID: PMC8395078.
9. Hagihara H, Catts VS, Katayama Y, Shoji H, Takagi T, Huang FL, Nakao A, Mori Y, Huang KP, Ishii S, Graef IA, Nakayama KI,

Shannon Weickert C, Miyakawa T. Decreased Brain pH as a Shared Endophenotype of Psychiatric Disorders. Neuropsychopharmacology. 2018 Feb;43(3):459-468. doi: 10.1038/npp.2017.167.

10. Liu WP, Song YQ, Zheng W, Wang XP, Ding N, Zhu J. Aggressive behavior and elevated lactate dehydrogenase at baseline confer inferior prognosis in patients with primary cutaneous lymphoma. Clin Lymphoma Myeloma Leuk. 2013 Oct;13(5):534-40. doi: 10.1016/j.clml.2013.04.011.
11. Rowland LM, Pradhan S, Korenic S, Wijtenburg SA, Hong LE, Edden RA, Barker PB. Elevated brain lactate in schizophrenia: a 7 T magnetic resonance spectroscopy study. Transl Psychiatry. 2016 Nov 29;6(11):e967. Doi: 10.1038/tp.2016.239. PMID: 27898072; PMCID: PMC5290358.
12. George DT, Hibbeln JR, Ragan PW, Umhau JC, Phillips MJ, Doty L, Hommer D, Rawlings RR. Lactate-induced rage and panic in a select group of subjects who perpetrate acts of domestic violence. Biol Psychiatry. 2000 May 1;47(9):804-12. doi: 10.1016/s0006-3223(99)00300-5. PMID: 10812039.
13. Coco, M., Alagona, G., Rapisarda, G., Costanzo, E., Calogero, R. A., Perciaevalle, V., & Perciavalle, V. (2010). Elevated blood lactate is associated with increased motor cortex excitability. Somatosensory and Motor Research, 27(1), 1–8. https://doi.org/10.3109/08990220903471765
14. Dogan AE, Yuksel C, Du F, Chouinard VA, Öngür D. Brain lactate and pH in schizophrenia and bipolar disorder: a systematic review of findings from magnetic resonance studies. Neuropsychopharmacology. 2018 Jul;43(8):1681-1690. doi: 10.1038/s41386-018-0041-9.
15. Wiley CD, Campisi J. From Ancient Pathways to Aging Cells-Connecting Metabolism and Cellular Senescence. Cell Metab. 2016 Jun 14;23(6):1013-1021. doi: 10.1016/j.cmet.2016.05.010.
16. Sullivan, C.R., Mielnik, C.A., Funk, A. et al. Measurement of lactate levels in postmortem brain, iPSCs, and animal models of schizophrenia. Sci Rep 9, 5087 (2019). https://doi.org/10.1038/s41598-019-41572-9
17. Ross JM, Öberg J, Brené S, Coppotelli G, Terzioglu M, Pernold K, Goiny M, Sitnikov R, Kehr J, Trifunovic A, Larsson NG, Hoffer BJ,

Olson L. High brain lactate is a hallmark of aging and caused by a shift in the lactate dehydrogenase A/B ratio. Proc Natl Acad Sci USA. 2010;107(46):20087–20092.

18. Caddye E, Pineau J, Reyniers J, Ronen I, Colasanti A. Lactate: A Theranostic Biomarker for Metabolic Psychiatry? Antioxidants (Basel). 2023 Aug 22;12(9):1656. doi: 10.3390/antiox12091656.
19. Henkel ND, Wu X, O'Donovan SM, Devine EA, Jiron JM, Rowland LM, Sarnyai Z, Ramsey AJ, Wen Z, Hahn MK, McCullumsmith RE. Schizophrenia: a disorder of broken brain bioenergetics. Mol Psychiatry. 2022 May;27(5):2393-2404. doi: 10.1038/s41380-022-01494-x.
20. Nguyen TT, Eyler LT, Jeste DV. Systemic Biomarkers of Accelerated Aging in Schizophrenia: A Critical Review and Future Directions. Schizophr Bull. 2018 Feb 15;44(2):398-408. doi: 10.1093/schbul/sbx069. PMID: 29462455; PMCID: PMC5815075.
21. Finucane OM, Sugrue J, Rubio-Araiz A, Guillot-Sestier MV, Lynch MA. The NLRP3 inflammasome modulates glycolysis by increasing PFKFB3 in an IL-1β-dependent manner in macrophages. Sci Rep. 2019 Mar 11;9(1):4034. doi: 10.1038/s41598-019-40619-1.
22. Liu R, Tang W, Wang W, Xu F, Fan W, Zhang Y, Zhang C. NLRP3 Influences Cognitive Function in Schizophrenia in Han Chinese. Front Genet. 2021 Dec 10;12:781625.
doi: 10.3389/fgene.2021.781625
23. Ozdamar Unal G, Hekimler Ozturk K, Inci HE. Increased NLRP3 inflammasome expression in peripheral blood mononuclear cells of patients with schizophrenia: a case-control study. Int J Psychiatry Clin Pract. 2023 Jun;27(2):111-117.
doi: 10.1080/13651501.2022.21062
24. Hayflick L., Moorhead P. S. (1961). The serial cultivation of human diploid cell strains. Exp. Cell Res. 25, 585–621 10.1016/0014-4827(61)90192-6
25. Dou X, Fu Q, Long Q, Liu S, Zou Y, Fu D, Xu Q, Jiang Z, Ren X, Zhang G, Wei X, Li Q, Campisi J, Zhao Y, Sun Y. PDK4-dependent hypercatabolism and lactate production of senescent cells promotes cancer malignancy. Nat Metab. 2023 Nov;5(11):1887-1910. Doi: 10.1038/s42255-023-00912-w.

26. James EL, Michalek RD, Pitiyage GN, de Castro AM, Vignola KS, Jones J, Mohney RP, Karoly ED, Prime SS, Parkinson EK. Senescent human fibroblasts show increased glycolysis and redox homeostasis with extracellular metabolomes overlapping with irreparable DNA damage, aging, and disease. J Proteome Res. 2015 Apr 3;14(4):1854-71. doi: 10.1021/pr501221g.
27. Paluvai H, Di Giorgio E, Brancolini C. The Histone Code of Senescence. Cells. 2020 Feb 18;9(2):466. doi: 10.3390/cells9020466. PMID: 32085582; PMCID: PMC7072776.
28. Li J, Wang Y, Yuan X, Kang Y, Song X. New insight in the cross-talk between microglia and schizophrenia: From the perspective of neurodevelopment. Front Psychiatry. 2023 Feb 16;14:1126632. doi: 10.3389/fpsyt.2023.1126632.
29. Zhuo, C., Tian, H., Song, X. et al. Microglia and cognitive impairment in schizophrenia: translating scientific progress into novel therapeutic interventions. Schizophr 9, 42 (2023). https://doi.org/10.1038/s41537-023-00370-z
30. Yanuck SF. Microglial Phagocytosis of Neurons: Diminishing Neuronal Loss in Traumatic, Infectious, Inflammatory, and Autoimmune CNS Disorders. Front Psychiatry. 2019 Oct 3;10:712. doi: 10.3389/fpsyt.2019.00712.
31. Ng PY, McNeely TL, Baker DJ. Untangling senescent and damage-associated microglia in the aging and diseased brain. FEBS J. 2023 Mar;290(5):1326-1339. doi: 10.1111/febs.16315. Epub 2021 Dec 14. PMID: 34873840; PMCID: PMC9167891.
32. Corley, E. et al. Microglial-expressed genetic risk variants, cognitive function and brain volume in patients with schizophrenia and healthy controls. Transl. Psychiatry 11, 490 (2021).
33. Chen Z, Trapp BD. Microglia and neuroprotection. J Neurochem. 2016 Jan;136 Suppl 1:10-7. doi: 10.1111/jnc.13062. Epub 2015 Mar 10. PMID: 25693054.
34. Wei L, Yang X, Wang J, Wang Z, Wang Q, Ding Y, Yu A. H3K18 lactylation of senescent microglia potentiates brain aging and Alzheimer's disease through the NFκB signaling pathway. J

Neuroinflammation. 2023 Sep 11;20(1):208. doi: 10.1186/s12974-023-02879-7.

35. van der Kamp, M.W. (2013). Lactate Dehydrogenase – Computational Studies. In: Roberts, G.C.K. (eds) Encyclopedia of Biophysics. Springer, Berlin, Heidelberg. https://doi.org/10.1007/978-3-642-16712-6_236

36. Zu, H., Li, C., Dai, C. et al. SIRT2 functions as a histone deacetylase and inhibits the proliferation and migration of neuroblastoma cells. Cell Discov 8, 54 (2022). https://doi.org/10.1038/s41421-022-00398-y

37. Xie, Y.; Hu, H.; Liu, M.; Zhou, T.; Cheng, X.; Huang, W.; Cao, L. The role and mechanism of histone lactylation in health and diseases. Front. Genet. 2022, 13, 949252.

38. Bredy, T.W.; Wu, H.; Crego, C.; Zellhoefer, J.; Sun, Y.E.; Barad, M. Histone modifications around individual BDNF gene promoters in the prefrontal cortex are associated with extinction of conditioned fear. Learn. Mem. 2007, 14, 268–276.

39. Fan, H.; Yang, F.; Xiao, Z.; Luo, H.; Chen, H.; Chen, Z.; Liu, Q.; Xiao, Y. Lactylation: Novel epigenetic regulatory and therapeutic opportunities. Am J Physiol Endocrinol Metab. 2023, 324, E330–E338.

40. Smagin DA, Park JH, Michurina TV, Peunova N, Glass Z, Sayed K, Bondar NP, Kovalenko IN, Kudryavtseva NN, Enikolopov G. Altered Hippocampal Neurogenesis and Amygdalar Neuronal Activity in Adult Mice with Repeated Experience of Aggression. Front Neurosci. 2015 Dec 1;9:443. doi: 10.3389/fnins.2015.00443.

41. Rampino A, Annese T, Torretta S, Tamma R, Falcone RM, Ribatti D. Involvement of vascular endothelial growth factor in schizophrenia. Neurosci Lett. 2021 Aug 24;760:136093. doi: 10.1016/j.neulet.2021.136093. Epub 2021 Jun 30. PMID: 34216717.

42. Al-Onaizi M, Al-Khalifah A, Qasem D, ElAli A. Role of Microglia in Modulating Adult Neurogenesis in Health and Neurodegeneration. Int J Mol Sci. 2020 Sep 19;21(18):6875. doi: 10.3390/ijms21186875. PMID: 32961703; PMCID: PMC7555074.

43. Towriss, M.; MacVicar, B.; Ciernia, A.V. Modelling Microglial Innate Immune Memory In Vitro: Understanding the Role of Aerobic Glycolysis in Innate Immune Memory. Int. J. Mol. Sci. 2023, 24, 8967. https://doi.org/10.3390/ijms24108967
44. Koppenol WH, Bounds PL, Dang CV. Otto Warburg's contributions to current concepts of cancer metabolism. Nat Rev Cancer. 2011 May;11(5):325-37. doi: 10.1038/nrc3038. Epub 2011 Apr 14. Erratum in: Nat Rev Cancer. 2011 Aug;11(8):618. PMID: 21508971.
45. Chandrasekaran S, Rittschof CC, Djukovic D, Gu H, Raftery D, Price ND, Robinson GE. Aggression is associated with aerobic glycolysis in the honey bee brain(1). Genes Brain Behav. 2015 Feb;14(2):158-66. doi: 10.1111/gbb.12201.
46. Rittschof CC, Coombs CB, Frazier M, Grozinger CM, Robinson GE. Early-life experience affects honey bee aggression and resilience to immune challenges. Sci Rep. 2015 Oct 23;5:15572. doi: 10.1038/srep15572. PMID: 26493190; PMCID: PMC4616062.
47. Yang K, Xu J, Fan M, Tu F, Wang X, Ha T, Williams DL, Li C. Lactate Suppresses Macrophage Pro-Inflammatory Response to LPS Stimulation by Inhibition of YAP and NF-κB Activation via GPR81-Mediated Signaling. Front Immunol. 2020 Oct 6;11:587913. doi: 10.3389/fimmu.2020.587913.
48. Yu Q, Liu M, Dai W, Xiong Y, Mu X, Xia M, Li Y, Ma S, Su Y, Wu J, Liu C, Xie Y, Zhao T, Lu A, Weng N, Zheng F, Sun P. The NLRP3 inflammasome is involved in resident intruder paradigm-induced aggressive behaviors in mice. Front Pharmacol. 2023 Jan 25;14: 974905. Doi: 10.3389/fphar.2023.974905.
49. Wang J, Yang P, Yu T, Gao M, Liu D, Zhang J, Lu C, Chen X, Zhang X, Liu Y. Lactylation of PKM2 Suppresses Inflammatory Metabolic Adaptation in Pro-inflammatory Macrophages. Int J Biol Sci. 2022 Oct 24;18(16):6210-6225. doi: 10.7150/ijbs.75434.
50. Zhou Y, Yang L, Liu X, Wang H. Lactylation may be a Novel Posttranslational Modification in Inflammation in Neonatal Hypoxic-Ischemic Encephalopathy. Front Pharmacol. 2022 Jun 2;13:926802. Doi: 10.3389/fphar.2022.926802.
51. Sun W, Jia M, Feng Y, Cheng X. Lactate links glycolysis and autophagy through lactylation. Autophagy. 2023 Dec;19(12):3240-

3241. doi: 10.1080/15548627.2023.2246356. Epub 2023 Aug 18. PMID: 37565742; PMCID: PMC10621282.

52. Fang Yu, Yan Meng, Kehong Chen, Yani He, #4668 CITRATE SYNTHASE LACTYLATION PROMOTES THE TRANSITION FROM ACUTE KIDNEY INJURY TO CHRONIC KIDNEY DISEASE BY ACTIVATING NLRP3 INFLAMMASOME, Nephrology Dialysis Transplantation, Volume 38, Issue Supplement_1, June 2023, gfad063c_4668, https://doi.org/10.1093/ndt/gfad063c_4668
53. Sabbatinelli J, Prattichizzo F, Olivieri F, Procopio AD, Rippo MR, Giuliani A. Where Metabolism Meets Senescence: Focus on Endothelial Cells. Front Physiol. 2019 Dec 18;10:1523. Doi: 10.3389/fphys.2019.01523.
54. Hagihara H, Shoji H, Otabi H, Toyoda A, Katoh K, Namihira M, Miyakawa T. Protein lactylation induced by neural excitation. Cell Rep. 2021 Oct 12;37(2):109820. doi: 10.1016/j.celrep.2021.109820.
55. Jouroukhin Y, Kageyama Y, Misheneva V, Shevelkin A, Andrabi S, Prandovszky E, Yolken RH, Dawson VL, Dawson TM, Aja S, Sesaki H, Pletnikov MV. DISC1 regulates lactate metabolism in astrocytes: implications for psychiatric disorders. Transl Psychiatry. 2018 Apr 12;8(1):76. doi: 10.1038/s41398-018-0123-9. PMID: 29643356
56. Ojo ES, Tischkau SA. The Role of AhR in the Hallmarks of Brain Aging: Friend and Foe. Cells. 2021 Oct 13;10(10):2729. doi: 10.3390/cells10102729. PMID: 34685709; PMCID: PMC8534784.
57. Huai, W., Zhao, R., Song, H. et al. Aryl hydrocarbon receptor negatively regulates NLRP3 inflammasome activity by inhibiting NLRP3 transcription. Nat Commun 5, 4738 (2014). https://doi.org/10.1038/ncomms5738
58. Cheng Z, Huo X, Dai Y, Lu X, Hylkema MN, Xu X. Elevated expression of AhR and NLRP3 link polycyclic aromatic hydrocarbon exposure to cytokine storm in preschool children. Environ Int. 2020 Jun;139:105720. doi: 10.1016/j.envint.2020.105720.
59. Pham-The, T.; Nishijo, M.; Pham, T.N.; Vu, H.T.; Tran, N.N.; Tran, A.H.; Hoang, L.V.; Do, Q.; Nishino, Y.; Nishijo, H. Perinatal Dioxin

Exposure and Attention Deficit Hyperactivity Disorder (ADHD) Symptoms in Children Living in a Dioxin Contamination Hotspot in Vietnam. Toxics 2022, 10, 212. https://doi.org/10.3390/toxics10050212

60. Nishijo M, Pham TT, Pham NT, Duong HTT, Tran NN, Kondoh T, Nishino Y, Nishimaru H, Do QB, Nishijo H. Nutritional Intervention with Dried Bonito Broth for the Amelioration of Aggressive Behaviors in Children with Prenatal Exposure to Dioxins in Vietnam: A Pilot Study. Nutrients. 2021 Apr 25;13(5):1455. doi: 10.3390/nu13051455.

61. Salminen A. Mutual antagonism between aryl hydrocarbon receptor and hypoxia-inducible factor-1α (AhR/HIF-1α) signaling impacts aging. Cell Signal. 2022 Nov;99:110445. doi: 10.1016/j.cellsig.2022.110445

62. Jia Y, Zhang C, Hua M, Wang M, Chen P, Ma D. Aberrant NLRP3 inflammasome associated with aryl hydrocarbon receptor potentially contributes to the imbalance of T-helper cells in patients with acute myeloid leukemia. Oncol Lett. 2017 Dec;14(6):7031-7044. doi: 10.3892/ol.2017.7177.

63. Fehsel K, Schwanke K, Kappel BA, Fahimi E, Meisenzahl-Lechner E, Esser C, Hemmrich K, Haarmann-Stemmann T, Kojda G, Lange-Asschenfeldt C. Activation of the aryl hydrocarbon receptor by clozapine induces preadipocyte differentiation and contributes to endothelial dysfunction. J Psychopharmacol. 2022 Feb;36(2):191-201. doi: 10.1177/02698811211055811.

# CHAPTER 6

# BRAIN OSCILLATIONS AND VIOLENT CRIME

Oscillations or vibrations are fundamental properties of all matter, including biological systems (1)(2)(3). For example, simple organisms, including yeast, were shown to communicate with their counterparts via synchronized glycolytic oscillations, indicating that this is likely a highly conserved mechanism (4). Indeed, it is believed that specific frequencies may be ideal for encoding and transmitting information, suggesting that oscillations may play a role in neurotransmission, functioning in parallel with the synaptic and exocrine/paracrine systems (5)(6).

How brain oscillatory frequencies relate to information processing in neuronal networks is partially transparent. However, growing evidence has demonstrated that neurons can function as oscillators, making cognition possible by synchronizing with identical frequency oscillators in other brain regions (7)(8). Adaptive resonance theory (ART) and communication through coherence (CTC) are two neurophysiological models that utilize inter-region signaling to explain information processing (9)(10). For example, the auditory cortex generates spontaneous oscillations in response to the exogenous oscillatory input, synchronizing with the environment (11).

Synchronized oscillations may engender a body-wide communication platform, connecting structures inside and outside the CNS. For example, gastrointestinal (GI) tract microbes entrain "brain-like" oscillations, suggesting that the gut-brain axis may be driven by this modality (12)(13)(14)(15)(16)(17). This is in line with another novel discovery that oscillations drive the expression of microbial genes, division, cell cycle progression, and antibiotic resistance (17)(18)(19). Furthermore, the metabolism drives the GI tract microbiota oscillations, suggesting that the enteric nervous system (ENS) may function as an oscillatory sensor and direct this information to the CNS (2).

## Interoceptive awareness and oscillations

Synchronization of oscillatory activity is believed to drive human awareness, while desynchronization and inhibition of inter-regional signaling occur in general anesthesia and induce unconsciousness (20)(21)(22). For example, gamma (γ) oscillations (30-100 Hz) promote connectivity between different brain regions, which are essential for body movement, memory, and emotion (23)(24). Gamma waves drive interoceptive awareness and cognition, contributing to emotional intelligence and the ability to see things from another person's perspective (25)(26). Moreover, awareness of one's limbs, body parts, pain, or well-being constitutes insight or interoceptive awareness. In psychopathology, including SCZ, anosognosia (lack of understanding) is a marker of higher severity of symptoms and aggressive behaviors (27)(28).

## Insight, the role of local hormones and inhibitory neurons

It is believed that local γ -aminobutyric acid (GABA) neurons generating somatostatin (SST) produce γ oscillations associated with higher-order brain functions, including insight (29). In contrast, dysfunctional γ oscillations were associated with CNS pathology, including AD, PD, and SCZ, linking anosognosia with the loss of GABA interneurons (30)(31)(32)(33) (Fig. 1).

## The brain on death row

Several studies interrogating EEG frequencies in the perpetrators of violent crime on death row found diminished or absent γ frequencies in the inmates with SCZ, suggesting impaired cognition and insight (34). These electrophysiological changes, low activity in the right prefrontal cortex, and increased striatum reflect cortico-subcortical desynchronization (35)(36)(37). The altered prefrontal coherence, especially hypo-frontality, likely reflects impaired information processing of subcortical stimuli and the inability to distinguish them from imaginary content (38).

## Lowering criminal behaviors by enhancing gamma BAND

Since decreased or absent high-frequency γ oscillations were found in violent criminals, is it possible to lower crime by inducing gamma frequencies?

Along this line, noninvasive stimulatory techniques, such as low-level laser therapy (LLLT), transcranial alternating current stimulation (tACS), or transcranial magnetic stimulation (TMS), may enhance the gamma band synchronization, improving insight into criminal behavior (39)(40)(41)(42). Indeed, a 40 Hz auditory steady-state response (ASSR) stimulated the brain to generate gamma waves, opening novel therapeutic avenues for noninvasive treatments for anosognosia and negative symptoms of SCZ (43)(44)(45)(46). In addition, SST has been implicated in CNS synchronization and brain plasticity, suggesting that loss of this hormone may promote negative and cognitive symptoms in SCZ (47)(48). Aging downregulates SST and upregulates the non-pituitary growth hormone (npGH), inducing premature neuronal senescence, which lowers the γ band (49)(50)(51). Since SST-generating GABAergic interneurons are depleted in SCZ, stimulation at 40 Hz may be compensatory, inducing a similar frequency in the cortex (52).

# Article for Chapter 6: Local Hormones and Neurolipidomics in Schizophrenia

## Adonis Sfera[1], Sabine Hazan[2], Peter G. Bota[3], Jonathan J. Anton[4] and Garth L Nicolson[5]

*1 Patton State Hospital, Loma Linda University, University of California at Riverside.*
*2 Progenabiome.*
*3 California university of Science and Medicine.*
*4 California Baptist University, department of biology.*
*5 Institute for Molecular Medicine in Huntington Beach, California.*

**Received:** October 20, 2023; **Accepted:** November 22, 2023; **Published:** November 30, 2023



**Citation:** Adonis Sfera, Sabine Hazan, Peter G Bota, Jonathan J Anton, Garth L Nicolson. Local Hormones and Neurolipidomics in schizophrenia. American J Neurol Res. 2023; 2(1):1-4.

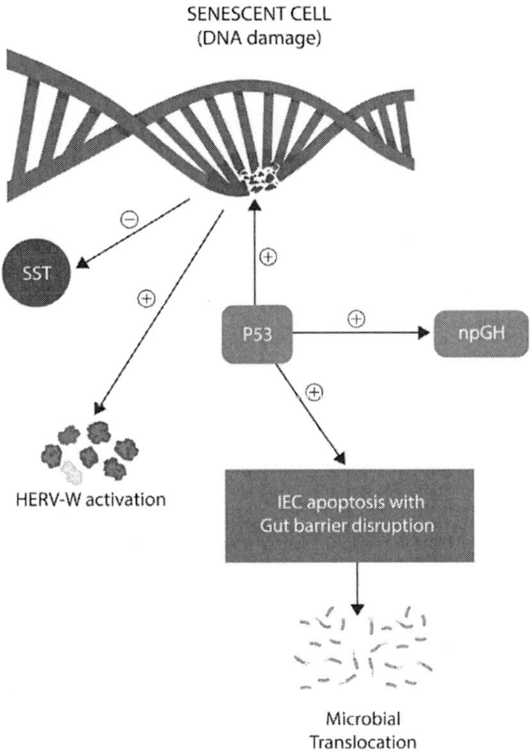


## Graphical Abstract

1. SCZ is associated with genomic damage and premature cellular senescence, affecting both somatic and postmitotic cells.
2. Premature neuronal senescence contributes to gray matter loss, involving the neurites and synapses of inhibitory interneurons.
3. Loss of somatostatin-expressing GABA interneurons may drive the gray matter loss in schizophrenia.
4. Deficient somatostatin upregulates non-pituitary growth hormone, inducing DNA damage and p53-mediated neuronal senescence.

## Abstract

Chronic mental illnesses, including schizophrenia, have been associated with premature brain aging manifested on neuroimaging as gray matter loss. This has been associated with impaired insight (anosognosia) and suboptimal treatment outcome. Novel strategies for addressing premature brain aging are urgently needed and somatostatin up regulation may avert gray matter loss. Recent studies, involving non-pituitary growth hormone and p53, have offered early glimpses into the molecular underpinnings of cellular senescence in SCZ. Moreover, age-downregulated somatostatin and activation of Human Endogenous Retroviruses likely drive the negative and cognitive symptoms of SCZ.

In this perspective article, we discuss the following: 1) neuropsychiatric implications of premature brain aging, 2) potential therapies for restoring the homeostasis of somatostatin and non-pituitary growth hormone.

**Keywords:** Schizophrenia, Neurodevelopmental diseases.

## Introduction

Schizophrenia (SCZ) and schizophrenia-like disorders (SLDs) are neurodevelopmental diseases with an average global prevalence of 1%. Antipsychotic drugs, extremely effective for acute psychosis, are much less helpful in the chronic phase, marked primarily by negative and cognitive symptoms [1]. In addition, SCZ outcome studies show that a dismal 13.5% of patients achieve sustained recovery at any time after the first psychotic episode, suggesting that the currently available antipsychotic drugs do not target the central pathology of this illness [2-4].

SCZ neuroimaging studies have consistently reported progressive brain shrinkage, while microscopy found gray matter loss at the expense of dendritic spines and synapses. These findings comprise the proof of concept that the available treatment strategies do not address gray matter loss [5]. Indeed, several studies have found accelerated brain atrophy with some antipsychotic drugs, indicating that maintenance treatment may require different approaches than acute episodes.

Novel studies have emphasized the role of p53, somatostatin (SST), and non-pituitary growth hormone (npGH) in SCZ-associated neuronal senescence [6,7]. In addition, p53 and senescence can activate human endogenous retroviruses (HERVs), ancestral pathogens, residing in the human genome, previously linked to SCZ with negative symptoms [8].

The role of hormones in the etiology of neuropsychiatric disorders is well-established as these conditions often become manifest at puberty or postpartum, life milestones marked by significant stress and "hormonal storms". In addition, endocrinopathies, including Cushing's syndrome, hypopituitarism, and primary hyperparathyroidism (PHPT) have been associated with SCZ, emphasizing the intertwinement of endocrinology and neuropathology [9-12]. Moreover, gut microbes, synthesize several hormones, including SST and npGH, likely implicating

the microbiome in SCZ [13-17]. Indeed, commensal flora can synthesize many SCZ-relevant neurotransmitters, including dopamine (DA), serotonin (5HT), norepinephrine (NE), acetylcholine (ACh), melatonin, somatostatin (SST), and oxytocin (OXT), further linking mental illness to various endocrinopathies [18-21].

Numerous studies have connected SCZ with the premature cellular (including neuronal) senescence, emphasizing that DNA damage or defective genomic repair is the likely cause of this pathology [22-24]. It is well-established that SCZ patients live on average 15 to 20 years shorter than their healthy counterparts and develop age-related diseases while still young, highlighting the role of premature aging in this disorder. Indeed, some scholars refer to SCZ as "segmental" progeria, to emphasize this correlation [25].

Gamma oscillations (30-100 Hz) on electroencephalogram (EEG) are altered in SCZ patients, probably reflecting the loss of SSTexpressing gamma-aminobutyric acid (GABA) neurons, known for promoting network oscillations [26-29]. Interestingly, both GABA and SST are synthesized by the gut microbes, which are also known for entraining "brain-like" oscillations, linking the microbiome to the EEG waves [30-35]. This is not surprising as in bacteria, oscillations control gene expression, division, cell cycle progression, and antibiotic resistance [35-37].

Do gut microbes communicate with the host via synchronized oscillations? Many believe that certain frequencies may be ideal for low-energy encoding and transmitting information to distant body tissues, suggesting that this platform may be functioning in parallel with the synaptic and exocrine/paracrine neurotransmission [38,39]. Indeed, synchronized oscillations were documented in many tissues, including the endocrine glands, which are known for releasing hormones in regular spurs [40-43]. At the molecular level, the DNA double helix as well as the p53 genomic repair system, generate spontaneous oscillations, suggesting that macromolecules may engender their own signaling platform a global molecular network [44]. For example, genome oscillations and gamma waves may generate a quantum code for almost instant information transfer to distant tissues and cells [45,46]. Along this line, desynchronization or uncoupling of a brain region from other areas was demonstrated in general anesthesia or ketamine-induced dissociation states, indicating that awareness requires network synchronization [47,48]. Conversely, noninvasive stimulatory techniques, such as photobiomodulation or transcranial magnetic stimulation (TMS), may avert gray matter loss by optimizing synchronization [49,50]. Indeed, a 40 Hz auditory steady-state response (ASSR) is believed to be an insight biomarker of SCZ, suggesting novel therapeutic avenues for addressing anosognosia and the negative symptoms [51-54]. In addition, SST has been implicated not only in central nervous system (CNS) synchronization but also in brain plasticity, suggests that loss of this hormone may account for the negative and cognitive symptoms of SCZ [55,56]. Indeed, aging downregulates SST and upregulates npGH, linking local hormones to premature neuronal senescence and decreased gamma band [57-59]. Since SST-generating GABAergic interneurons are depleted in SCZ, desynchronization may explain the information processing difficulties [60].

In the GI tract, accumulation of npGH induces intestinal epithelial cells (IECs) senescence via p53 and insulin growth factor-1 (IGF1), enabling microbes and/or their molecule to migrate into the systemic circulation, eventually reaching the brain [61,6]. Indeed, microbial translocation may be averted by novel approaches, such as lipid replacement therapy (LRT) and or 3-phosphoinositidedependent protein kinase-1 (PDK1) inhibitors [62].

In this article, we take a closer look at the role of SST and npGH in neuronal senescence, microbial translocation, gray matter loss, and HERV-W activation. We also discuss some potential strategies for restoring the homeostasis of npGH and somatostatin.

## Natural Progression of Schizophrenia

The gray matter loss in SCZ, demonstrated in both antipsychotic naïve patients and in those treated with these drugs, suggests that this disorder progresses despite the available therapeutics [63,64]. This is in line with the discouraging SCZ outcome studies, and the continuous need for long-term psychiatric hospitals [65,5].

SCZ starts with a premorbid phase with very few or no symptoms, followed by a prodrome with behavioral changes, but without overt psychosis, which gradually transitions into the psychotic phase marked by acute positive symptoms, multiple hospitalizations, and medication nonadherence. The last phase, beginning in the late 40s or early 50s, is characterized by negative and cognitive symptoms, significant disability and poor response to medications [66] (Figure 1).

## Antipsychotics: Electron Donors or Receivers?

Several studies have found that psychotropic drugs which give away electrons do not deplete the CNS gray matter, while electron accepting therapeutics do, suggesting that biophysical properties of these drugs may be more important for the treatment outcome than their receptor affinity or agonist/antagonist status [67,68]. This quantum conceptualization of antipsychotics opens a new research vista the development of electron donor drugs. For example, dopamine agonists and dopamine (DA) itself are electron donors, while most, but not all, antipsychotic drugs are electron acceptors, suggesting that partial DA antagonists may be preferable for SCZ maintenance treatment [69]. This is significant as electron donors, DA and DA agonists were shown to promote gamma oscillations, while antagonists had the opposite effect [70]. This raises the question of the "anionic brain": do externalized anionic phospholipids such as phosphatidylserine (PS), a marker of cellular senescence, contribute to the loss of gray matter? It has been established that PS on the cytoplasmic side of cell membranes binds several kinases, containing the pleckstrin homology (PH) domain. This molecular leitmotif regulates cell membranerecruited kinases, including PDK1, implicated in SCZ [71]. Since PS is externalized in senescent cells, bringing about the "anionic brain", downstream PDK1-mediated phosphorylation is disrupted, likely disinhibiting glycogen synthase kinase 3 beta (GSK3β), a SCZ-associated enzyme (see below in Natural and synthetic PDK1 inhibitors). For this reason, LRT may stabilize the function of cell membranes, restoring the homeostasis of these kinases.

We construe, that SST downregulation and the subsequent surge in npGH contribute to premature neuronal senescence and the negative and cognitive symptoms of SCZ. This model is supported by the postmortem mRNA studies, demonstrating low SST and NMDA in patients with negative symptoms [72]. In addition, preclinical studies, have shown that knockdown of parvalbumin (PV) or SST neurons, resembles negative symptoms of SCZ [73].

## Premature Senescence and Somatostatin Loss

The most consistent neuroimaging findings in SCZ, gray matter loss and enlargement of lateral ventricles, indicate that reversing this pathology could ameliorate the negative and cognitive symptoms, likely improving the outcome [74-76].

For example, in SCZ, reduced gamma oscillations due to the loss of gray matter volume may be a measurable marker of negative symptoms. At the molecular level, npGH-mediated DNA damage and p53-induced cellular senescence likely drive the gray matter loss [22]. In this regard, recent studies have shown that the interplay between npGH and p53 contributes to the accumulation of damaged DNA and premature senescence (77). Excessive genomic damage downregulates SST, increasing npGH, which in return, promotes brain aging and senescence-mediated pathology [72,78].

Moreover, p53 upregulation activates HERVs, viral fossils previously connected to SCZ [79].

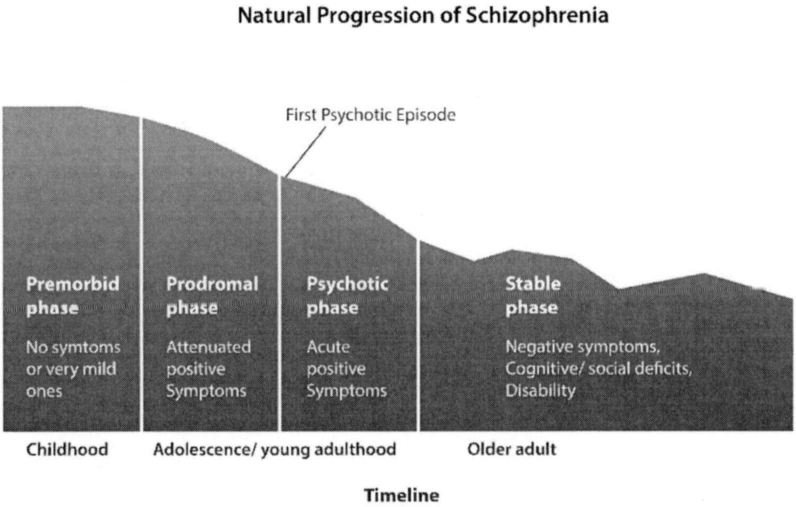


**Figure 1: SCZ is believed to be a neurodevelopmental disorder, which starts "in utero". There are usually no symptoms, or very few symptoms in the initial, premorbid phase. The following prodromal phase is marked by behavioral changes but no overt psychosis. The subsequent psychotic phase is characterized by acute positive symptoms, multiple hospitalizations, and medication nonadherence. The last SCZ phase, beginning around the age of 50, is characterized by negative and cognitive symptoms, significant disability, and poor response to medications. As patients get older, cognitive disorders usually begin during this phase.**

Under physiological circumstances, SST augments NMDA, while in SCZ, NMDA is hypofunctional, probably reflecting neuronal senescence and loss of this hormone [80]. Therefore, SST augmentation may comprise a strategy for developing etiopathogenetic treatments for the negative and cognitive symptoms of SCZ [72]. Indeed, in neuronal membranes, SST enhances protein kinase B (also called AKT), inhibiting GSK3β, an enzyme suppressed by lithium and several antipsychotic drugs. In addition, SST, activates phosphoinositide 3-kinases (PI3K)/AKT pathway, further suppressing GSK3β [81]. Moreover, AKT upregulation can be accomplished by lowering the neuronal membrane ceramide, highlighting the key role of membrane lipidome in SCZ (see below in Lipid rafts: hubs of cellular senescence).

In IECs, the complex interaction between IGF-1, p53, and npGH, induces premature cellular senescence, disrupting the gut barrier. This facilitates microbial translocation from the GI tract into the host circulation, ultimately reaching the CNS. For example, upon brain entry, microbial LPS was shown to induce neuroinflammation and premature aging, a pathology observed in AD. Indeed, gut microbiota LPS was found postmortem in the brains of AD patients, confirming translocation [82]. Others found, specific microbiota and immunoglobulins in patients with SCZ with negative symptoms, further linking this pathology to microbial migration outside the GI tract [83]. Interestingly, gut microbes, Bacillus subtilis and Escherichia coli can synthesize SST, demonstrating a possible feedback mechanism of counteracting excessive npGH [84,85].

It is believed that gray matter loss in SCZ occurs at the expense of neurites and synapses of the inhibitory parvalbumin (PV)expressing GABAergic interneurons, a subgroup of which release SST. It is noteworthy that neurons secreting vasoactive intestinal polypeptide (VIP) inhibit SST and GABA, disinhibiting the pyramidal cells [86,87] (Figure 3). For this reason, VIP inhibitors should be assessed for negative and cognitive symptoms of SCZ.

During the development and childhood, inhibitory GABAergic interneurons are underdeveloped and appear gradually during adolescence and early adulthood. In contrast, the number of excitatory synapses decreases during this time as the CNS undergoes adolescence-mediated recalibration [5,88]. The loss of gray matter volume and gamma oscillations in SCZ and AD is believed to be the result of excessive microglial "pruning" of neurites and synapses [73,89-91]. However, senescence-depleted SST may lead to the loss of dendritic arborizations, producing the same pathological effect as over-pruning [92].

Cellular senescence is an anticancer program marked by resistance to apoptosis, irreversible proliferation arrest, active metabolism, and a specific secretome, known as the senescence-associated secretory phenotype (SASP) which contains enzymes, cytokines, and npGH [6]. These molecules spread

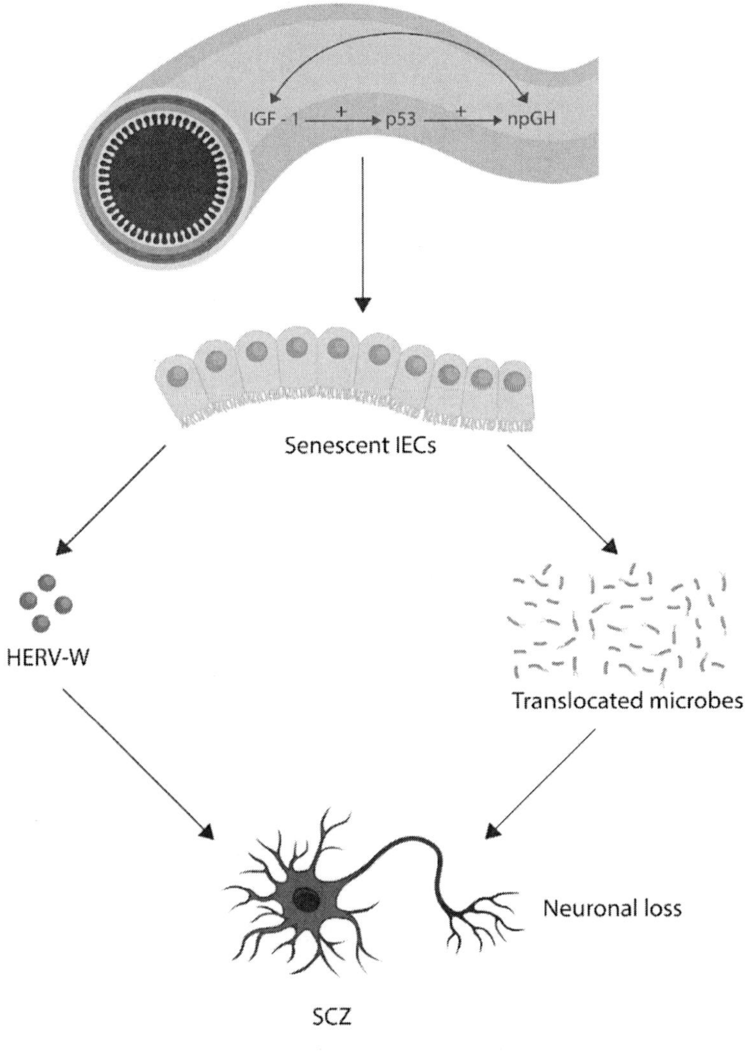


**Figure 2: Cellular senescence, an anticancer program, is activated by damaged DNA. The genome guardian, p53 initiates the senescence phenotype and repairs the genome. Senescence lowers SST and increases the levels of npGH which also upregulates IGF-1. In the GI tract, senescent intestinal epithelial cell (IECs) can disrupt the permeability of gut barrier, enabling microbial migration across the lamina propria. Premature neuronal senescence also activates HERVs, viral fossils comprising 8% of the human genome. Translocated bacteria and their molecules can reach the brain, causing neuronal damage by activating microglia.**

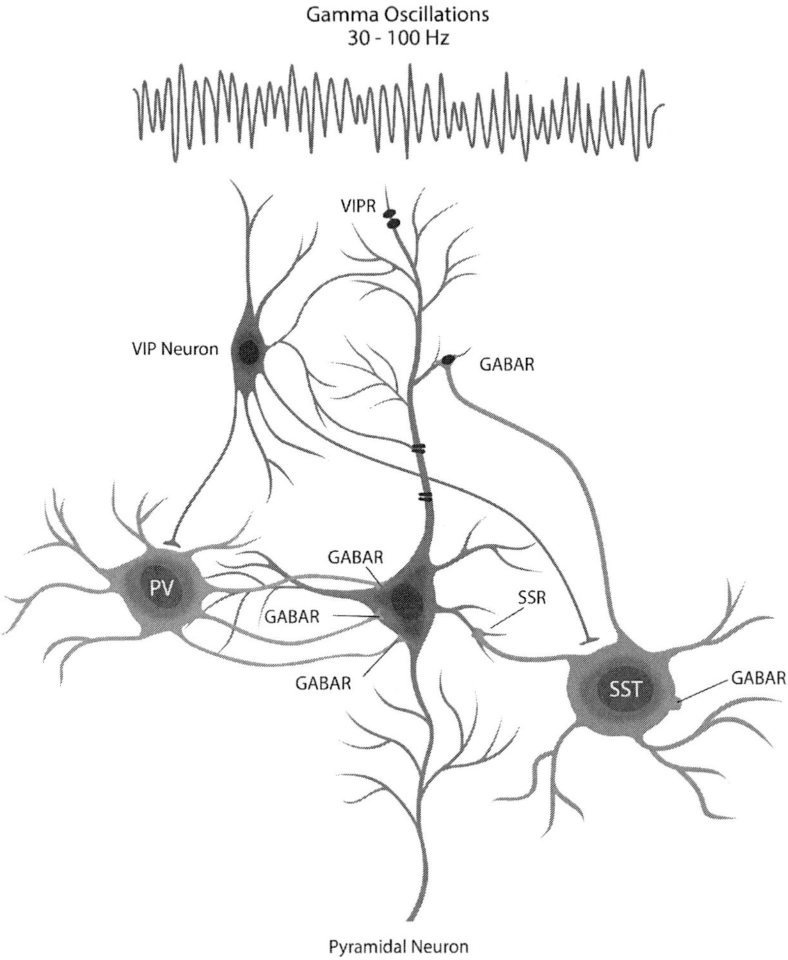


**Figure 3: Gamma oscillations comprise a rapid rhythm believed to be generated by the synaptic "chatter" of inhibitory GABAergic interneurons, such as PV-expressing and somatostatin (SST)-expressing cells which interact with GABA receptors. When inhibitory neurons fail to suppress the pyramidal cells, the first psychotic episode may become manifest. In the figure, a VIP neuron inhibits PV and SST cells, disinhibiting the pyramidal neuron.**

the senescent phenotype to the neighboring healthy cells, promoting inflammation. Upregulated npGH may be the cause of senescent cells' resistance to apoptosis as well as the neuronal reattempts at mitosis.

Augmenting gamma oscillatory band may improve insight in patients with SCZ, likely by promoting neurite growth, opening novel treatment opportunities [93,94]. For example, several studies have found that 40 Hz intranasal photobiomodulation or transcranial magnetic stimulation (TMS) at 40 Hz were beneficial for negative symptoms and cognition in SCZ [95-99]. Aside from gamma oscillations, anosognosia correlates directly with the loss of both gray matter and SST [100-102]. Can gray matter loss be restored? Studies are contradictory in this area and much more research is needed.

## The Good Vibes and The Bad Vibes

Oscillations or vibrations are fundamental properties of all matter, including the living organisms [103,104]. For example, auditory cortex not only responds to the exogenous oscillatory input but also generates its own spontaneous oscillations, likely utilizing these waves as a signaling platform [105]. In addition, pancreatic β-cells utilize electrical and metabolic oscillations to signal with other cells, suggesting that this communication tool is used routinely for intercellular crosstalk [106]. In the CNS, astrocytes communicate via calcium (Ca2+) waves evoked by the GH-activated NMDA channels, implicating this hormone in glial homeostasis [107,108]. This is significant as SCZ, marked by impoverished gamma spectrum, has also been associated with abnormal Ca2+ signaling, further implicating SST in this pathology [109]. Simple organisms, including yeast, were shown to communicate with their counterparts via partially synchronized glycolytic oscillations, indicating that this mechanism is highly conserved in nature [110, 111]. Moreover, microbial community in the GI tract was demonstrated to oscillate in synchrony with the metabolism, suggesting that the enteric nervous system (ENS) may sense these signals and relays them to the CNS [104].

Oscillation synchronization via "traveling waves", can transfer information to distant brain regions, likely driving human awareness. In contrast, desynchronization, observed during general anesthesia, induces unconsciousness, emphasizing the role of this signaling platform for the higher order of brain functions [112,113]. Indeed, it is believed that gamma waves, drive both the interoceptive awareness and cognition, contributing to a highly specialized form of information processing [114,115]. Interoceptive awareness refers the individual's ability to direct attention to the endogenous sensory information, discerning visceral cues on well-being, pain, discomfort, or ownership of limbs and body parts. In SCZ, anosognosia was associated with more frequent decompensations, worse psychotic or negative symptoms, and aggressive behavior, emphasizing the importance of insight for the outcome of this illness neuropsychiatric disorders, including SCZ, are often associated with anosognosia, neglect, or unawareness of the illness presence. For example, strokes of the right hemisphere can cause left-sided neglect with denial of left extremities [118]. Another example of anosognosia is failure to acknowledge one's own memory impairment, a phenomenon observed in cognitive disorders as well as in viral infections, including HIV and COVID-19 [119,120]. These findings have rekindled the interest of researchers and clinicians in the mental illness-associated anosognosia. Several neuroimaging studies have linked interoceptive awareness to insight as well as the abundance of GABAergic interneurons in the insular cortex (IC), a brain area associated with insight.

GABAergic interneurons are comprised of PV—expressing neurons, SST-expressing cells and 5-hydroxytryptamine (5HTRs) cells which include VIP-generating neurons (Figure 4). Interestingly, SST interneurons and some VIP neurons express muscarinic receptors, which are currently targeted in SCZ [121]. For example, xanomeline, a muscarinic M1/M4 agonist, exerts antipsychotic properties despite very low affinity for DA receptors, suggesting that non-dopaminergic transmission may be implicated in SCZ [122]. Therefore, enhancing GABAergic signaling to ameliorate anosognosia could likely be accomplished by inhibiting VIP-expressing GABAergic interneurons (Figure 4) [123]. Ameliorating anosognosia may significantly improve the long-term prognosis of SCZ, therefore, searching for therapeutics in this area is of paramount importance [124]. Along this line, a recent preclinical study has identified SST interneurons in anterior insula, suggesting that depletion of this hormone may impair insight by driving neuronal senescence [125].

Taken together, SCZ characteristics, including decreased gray matter volume, anosognosia, and impaired gamma oscillations may mirror the loss of inhibitory SST interneurons. Absent SST, npGH is upregulated, leading to cellular senescence and likely, the negative symptoms of SCZ [126,127].

## HERVs, Ancient Viruses Causing Contemporary Illness

DNA damage-associated cellular senescence was shown to activate HERV-W, an ancient retroviral element, associated with SCZ [128-133). HERV-W is encoded in the regulatory region of GABA receptor B1 (GABBR1), linking these pathogens to the inhibitory interneurons. HERV-W encodes for syncytin-1, a placental protein known for fusing individual trophoblasts into the syncytiotrophoblast, enabling placentation. Excessive syncytin-1 may trigger pathology by fusing healthy neurons, a phenomenon observed in neurodegenerative disorders as well as in normal aging [134-136]. Most HERVs are incomplete genes, which are never transcribed, however, some of these elements were "domesticated" in time and had assumed physiological functions. Several studies have shown that HERVs can lay dormant in host DNA until activated by infections, cellular senescence, or placental hormones [137,138]. Upregulated by the damaged DNA, npGH induces cellular senescence and disseminates this phenotype via SASP. Damaged DNA upregulates p53, which in turn, induces further npGH transcription [6]. Recent studies have revealed that p53 can activate HERVs, utilizing them as tools against various cancers, suggesting that these dormant pathogens may destabilize the genome [139-141]. Elevated HERV-W levels were previously documented in SCZ, linking these viral relics to the genetics of SCZ [142].

In our previous work, we have discussed SARS-CoV-2 inhibition of p53 and HERV-W activation, pathological cell-cell fusion and virus-induced neurocognitive deficits [143] (Figure 5). For this reason, we will not discuss HERVs in more detail here. Taken together, contemporary viruses can activate HERVs to enhance their own infection. Neurocognitive deficits, autoimmune disorders and SCZ were associated with reactivated HERVs.

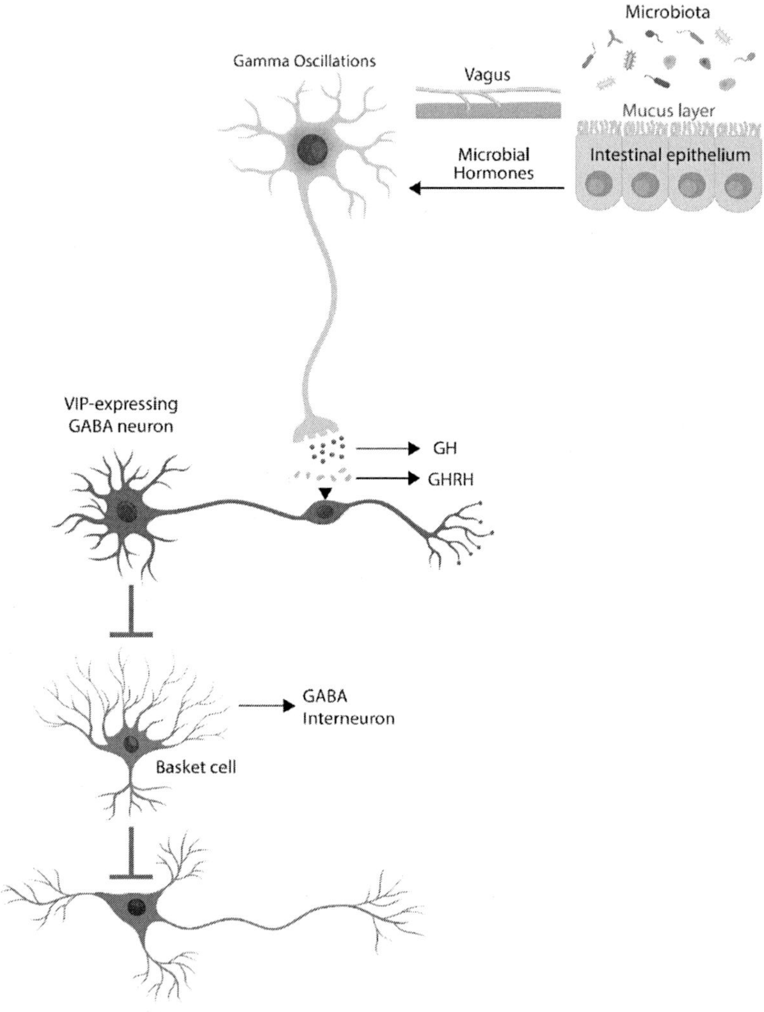


**Figure 4: The ENS gastrin neurons sense microbial input from the gut lumen and relay these signals to the CNS via vagal, humoral, and oscillatory pathway. Gastrin neurons secrete GH to activate the VIP-expressing GABA cells. These cells inhibit (the inhibitory) GABA and SST neurons, releasing the pyramidal cells' inhibitory brakes.**

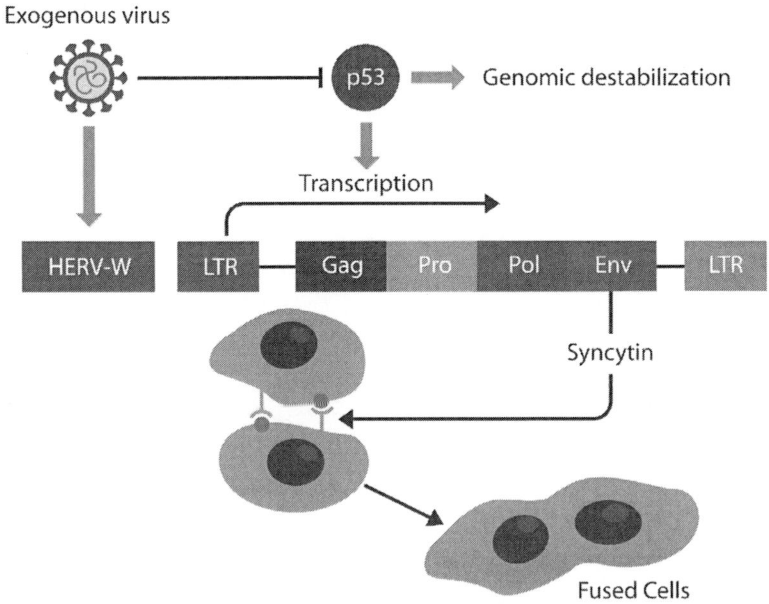


**Figure 5: Contemporary viruses, including COVID-19, activate HERV-W gene, while inhibiting p53. Both actions allow for the transcription of HERV envelope (ENV) gene, producing excessive syncyctin-1. This protein drives pathological cell-cell fusion in various organs, including the brain. Fusion of postmitotic neurons may predispose to the development of cognitive or negative symptoms of SCZ.**

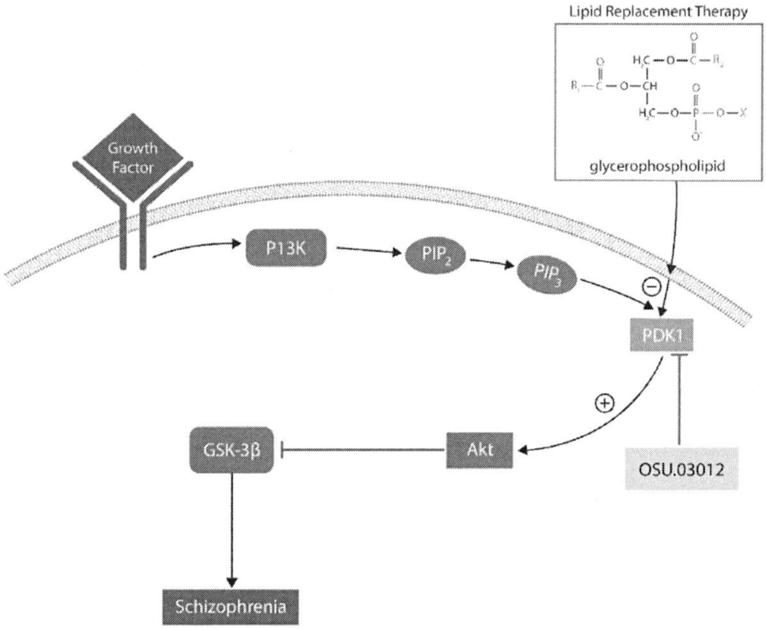


**Figure 6: LRT exerts neuroprotective action in SCZ via PDK1/AKT/ GSK3β axis. PS (part of glycerophospholipids) binds PDK1, recruiting this kinase to the cell membrane. Natural or synthetic PDK1 inhibitors, enhance AKT-blockade of GSK3β, ameliorating the negative symptoms of SCZ.**

# Novel, Natural Antipsychotic Strategies for Schizophrenia

Membrane and serum lipids are altered in SCZ, suggesting that a better understanding of neurolipidomics, could lead to the development of novel therapies for negative and cognitive symptoms [144]. These include natural lipids with plant-derived PDK1 inhibitors, aiming at replacing the oxidized membrane lipidome with natural phospholipids.

## Lipid replacement Therapy (LRT) adapted for schizophrenia (LRT+K)

LRT refers to the oral intake of natural glycerophospholipids to which we added kaempferol (3,4′,5,7-tetrahydroxyflavone), a natural flavonoid. The aim of LRT+K is to gradually replace damaged lipids in neuronal cell membranes with natural glycerides, containing phosphatidylserine (PS) and plant-derived kaempferol.

LRT interacts with a pathway previously implicated in SCZ: PDK1/ AKT/GSK3β (3-phosphoinositide-dependent kinase 1/ protein kinase B/ glycogen synthase kinase 3). PDK1, found upstream of AKT and GSK3β, contains a pleckstrin homology (PH) domain, which binds PS in the cytoplasmic leaflet of cell membranes. PS/PDK1 attachment has two beneficial effects: 1) recruitment of PDK1 at the cell membrane, and 2) maintaining PDK1 in inactive conformation (Figure 6) [145,146]. This modulates the downstream phosphorylome, inhibiting, GSK3β. Uninhibited GSK3β promotes psychosis and several antipsychotic drugs and lithium are inhibitors of this enzyme [147].

AKT also contains a PH domain which binds PS in the lipid rafts. However, unlike PDK1, upon attachment to PS, AKT becomes active (probably via autophosphorylation). Activated AKT suppresses the downstream GSK3β, lowering the risk of psychosis (Figure 6) [145,146]. In contrast, kaempferol inhibits PDK1 (by a non-PH mechanism), probably via regulating the phosphorylation of AKT and GSK3β. Therefore, unlike antipsychotics and lithium, kaempferol, blocks PDK1 in a totally natural manner [148]. In addition, OSU-03012, a synthetic PDK1 inhibitor, is currently being evaluated for anticancer efficacy. OSU-03012 may help LRT by inactivating PDK1 by a mechanism different than PS (Figure 6). Taken together, PS, a component of LRT, inactivates PDK1 by recruiting it to the cell membrane. Conversely, PS attachment, activates AKT effectively suppressing GSK3β and psychosis.

## Lipid Rafts: Hubs of Cellular Senescence

Lipids play a key role in the pathogenesis of negative and cognitive symptoms of SCZ not only because of lipid oxidation but also because of decreased membrane cholesterol [149]. For example, a study found that external radiofrequencies-induced cell membrane oscillations depend on the lipid composition (the more cholesterol, the more fluid the membrane) [150]. Cholesterol modulates the bilayer structure of cell membrane by altering not only the fluidity, but also the thickness, compressibility, exocytosis of secretory vesicles, and oscillatory activity. Suggesting that in the absence of this lipid, cell membrane vibrations are attenuated [151]. In this regard, ceramide has a more rigid molecular structure and restrains the oscillatory activity [152].

In senescent neurons, lipid rafts contain a disproportionate amount of ceramide compared to cholesterol, suggesting that old membranes are much less flexible and resistant to synchronization [153,154]. Indeed, earlier studies have implicated ceramide and sphingosine-1-phosphate in SCZ, further linking neuronal senescence to the biophysical properties of cell membranes [155-158]. Interestingly, several antipsychotic drugs intercalate themselves in the lipid bilayer, altering the biophysical properties of cell membranes. This suggests that antipsychotics may exert their actions by dopaminergic and non-dopaminergic mechanisms, the latter, including biophysical [159]. For example, cell membrane sterols were found altered in individuals at ultra-high risk of psychosis (UHR), suggesting that the membrane lipidome may be crucial for the pathogenesis of SCZ [160]. Likewise, in older individuals, the lipid composition of neuronal plasma membrane is altered in favor of ceramide, as cholesterol is replaced with this lipid in older individuals [161-163]. Indeed, loss of cholesterol may reduce gamma frequencies, predisposing to cognitive deficit [164]. Moreover, npGH was demonstrated to upregulate cell membrane ceramides, suggesting that aside from the genome, this hormone may also damage the cell membranes [165]. Taken together, as LRT provides healthy natural lipids to neuronal lipid rafts, this intervention may rehabilitate not only the lipidome but also the gray matter and the oscillatory gamma activity.

## Natural and synthetic PDK1 inhibitors

Protein kinases are enzymes that transfer phosphate groups from adenine triphosphate (ATP) to specific proteins. PDK1 inhibitors exert their beneficial effects by inhibiting GSK3β. Natural PDK1 inhibitors are ubiquitous, being present in numerous fruits and vegetables and for this reason, have no known adverse effects (Table 1).

| PDK1 inhibitor | Plant | References |
|---|---|---|
| Kaempferol | fruits, vegetables, and herbs | 166 |
| Quercetin | Onions, kale, broccoli | 167 |
| Myricetin | Oranges, berries, tomatoes, nuts, tea | 168 |
| Epigallcatechin-3 gallate | Green tea | 169 |
| Lupiwighteone isoflavone | Glycyrrhiza glabra; Lotus pedunculatus | 170 |
| Delphinidin | Citrus fruits | 171 |
| Honokiol | Cherries, berries, grapes | 172 |
| Delphinidin | Cranberries, Concord grapes, Pomegranates | 173 |

## Synthetic PDK1 inhibitors

Several synthetic PDK1 inhibitors have been developed, but few can cross the BBB. The exception is OSU-03012, a celecoxib derivative without cyclooxygenase-2 inhibitory activity, which exerts antiviral properties and is currently being evaluated for glioblastoma (Figure 6) [174,175]. OSU-03012 may be a suitable candidate for SCZ with negative and cognitive symptoms. At present, several other PDK1 inhibitors are in clinical trials for in AD.

## Conclusions

For the past 70 years, psychiatry has been obsessed with the postsynaptic dopaminergic blockade and paid much less attention to the gray matter loss, enlargement of lateral ventricles, and the paucity of gamma oscillations. Novel SCZ studies have started to emphasize the importance of local hormones, GABAergic interneurons, as well as the lipid composition of neuronal membranes. The therapeutic strategies derived from these models may, for the first time, improve SCZ outcomes. Limiting gray matter loss, restoring the homeostasis of SST interneurons, and npGH inhibition, may address the root cause of SCZ. Biophysical approaches, including TMS or photobiomodulation at 40 Hz, may promote healthy oscillatory activities, restoring the integrity of the connectome and the synchronization of brain areas. Acknowledging brain oscillations as a unique communication platform has the advantage of influencing the connectome in a noninvasive manner. Together, these approaches may address the etiopathogenesis, rather than SCZ symptoms, bringing for the first time, remission instead of symptom reduction.

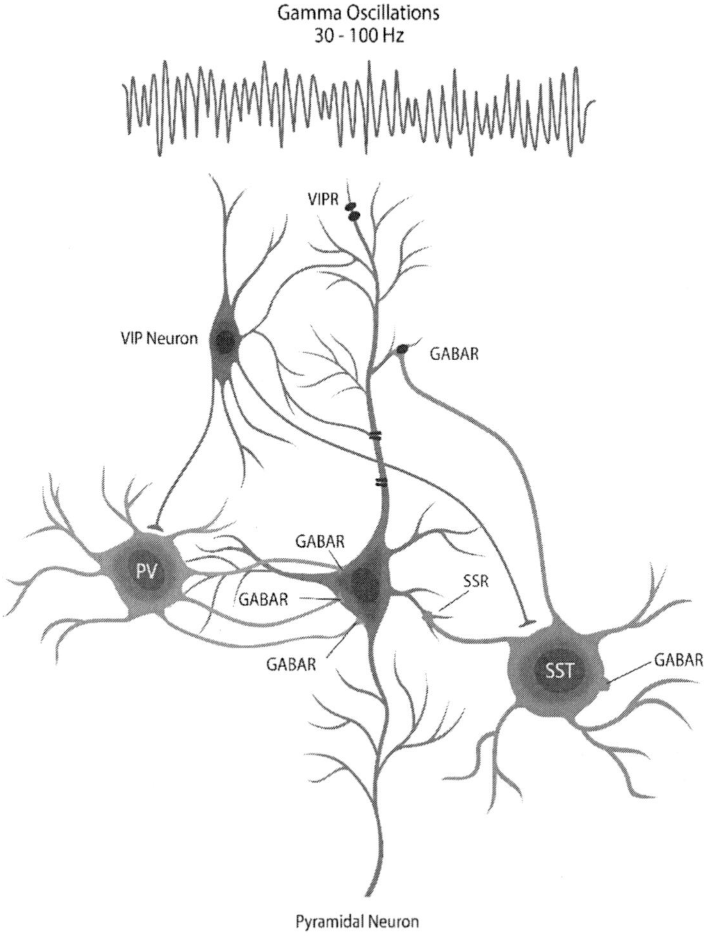


**The mechanism of gamma oscillations: Gamma oscillations comprise a rapid brain rhythm believed to be generated by the synaptic "chatter" of inhibitory GABAergic interneurons, such as PV-expressing and somatostatin (SST)-expressing cells which signal with the GABA receptors. Loss of inhibitory neurons disinhibits pyramidal cells, leading to psychosis. VIP neurons counteract inhibition by inhibiting the inhibitory neurons, which leads to the disinhibition of pyramidal neurons.**

## References


1. Rose MF, Ahmad KA, Thaller C, Zoghbi HY. Excitatory neurons of the proprioceptive, interoceptive, and arousal hindbrain networks share a developmental requirement for Math1. Proc Natl Acad Sci U S A. 2009 Dec 29;106(52):22462-7. doi: 10.1073/pnas.0911579106.
2. Fujimoto H, Matsuoka T, Kato Y, Shibata K, Nakamura K, Yamada K, Narumoto J. Brain regions associated with anosognosia for memory disturbance in Alzheimer's disease: a magnetic resonance imaging study. Neuropsychiatr Dis Treat. 2017 Jul 5;13:1753-1759. Doi: 10.2147/NDT.S139177.
3. Einstein, Albert (1905). "Über die von der molekularkinetischen Theorie der Wärme geforderte Bewegung von in ruhenden Flüssigkeiten suspendierten Teilchen" [On the Movement of Small Particles Suspended in Stationary Liquids Required by the Molecular-Kinetic Theory of Heat] (PDF). Annalen der Physik (in German). 322 (8): 549-560. Bibcode:1905AnP...322..549E. doi:10.1002/andp.19053220806. We have archived (PDF) from the original on 9 October 2022.
4. Bazargani N, Attwell D. Astrocyte calcium signaling: the third wave. Nat Neurosci. 2016 Feb;19(2):182-9. doi: 10.1038/nn.4201. PMID: 26814587.
5. Rulands S, Lee HJ, Clark SJ, Angermueller C, Smallwood SA, Krueger F, Mohammed H, Dean W, Nichols J, Rugg-Gunn P, Kelsey G, Stegle O, Simons BD, Reik W. Genome-Scale Oscillations in DNA Methylation during Exit from Pluripotency. Cell Syst. 2018 Jul 25;7(1):63-76.e12. doi: 10.1016/j.cels.2018.06.012.
6. Heltberg MS, Lucchetti A, Hsieh FS, Minh Nguyen DP, Chen SH, Jensen MH. Enhanced DNA repair through droplet formation and p53 oscillations. Cell. 2022 Nov 10;185(23):4394-4408.e10. Doi: 10.1016/j.cell.2022.10.004
7. Stiefel, K. M., and Ermentrout, G. B. (2016). Neurons as oscillators. J. Neurophysiol. 116, 2950–2960. doi: 10.1152/Jn.00525.2015
8. Lin, H. R., Wang, C. H., Deng, Q. L., Xu, C., Deng, Z. K., and Zhou, C. (2021). Review on chaotic dynamics of memristive neuron and

neural network. Nonlinear Dyn. 106, 959–973. doi: 10.1007/s11071-021-06853-x

9. Grossberg, S. (2013). Adaptive Resonance Theory: how a brain learns to attend, learn, and recognize a changing world consciously. Neural. Netw. 37, 1–47. doi: 10.1016/j.neunet.2012.09.017
10. Pérez-Cervera, A., Seara, T. M., and Huguet, G. (2020). Phase-locked states in oscillating neural networks and their role in neural communication. Commun. Nonlinear. Sci. Numer. Simul. 80, 104992. doi: 10.1016/j.cnsns.2019.104992
11. Cao L, Thut G, Gross J. The role of brain oscillations in predicting self-generated sounds. Neuroimage. 2017 Feb 15;147:895-903. doi: 10.1016/j.neuroimage.2016.11.001. Epub 2016 Nov 3. PMID: 27818209; PMCID: PMC5315057.
12. Hussain T, Murtaza G, Kalhoro DH, Kalhoro MS, Metwally E, Chughtai MI, Mazhar MU, Khan SA. Relationship between gut microbiota and host-metabolism: Emphasis on hormones related to reproductive function. Anim Nutr. 2021 Mar;7(1):1-10. doi: 10.1016/j.aninu.2020.11.005.
13. Martinez-Corral R, Liu J, Prindle A, Süel GM, Garcia-Ojalvo J. Metabolic basis of brain-like electrical signaling in bacterial communities. Philos Trans R Soc Lond B Biol Sci. 2019 Jun 10;374(1774):20180382. doi: 10.1098/rstb.2018.0382.
14. Martinez-Corral R, Liu J, Süel GM, Garcia-Ojalvo J. Bistable emergence of oscillations in growing Bacillus subtilis biofilms. Proc Natl Acad Sci USA. 2018 Sep 4;115(36): E8333-E8340. doi: 10.1073/pnas.1805004115.
15. Prindle A, Liu J, Asally M, Ly S, Garcia-Ojalvo J, Süel GM. Ion channels enable electrical communication in bacterial communities. Nature. 2015 Nov 5;527(7576):59-63. Doi: 10.1038/nature15709.
16. Liu J, Prindle A, Humphries J, Gabalda-Sagarra M, Asally M, Lee DY, Ly S, Garcia-Ojalvo J, Süel GM. Metabolic co-dependence gives rise to collective oscillations within biofilms. Nature. 2015 Jul 30;523(7562):550-4. doi: 10.1038/nature14660.
17. Lenz P, Søgaard-Andersen L. Temporal and spatial oscillations in bacteria. Nat Rev Microbiol. 2011 Aug 15;9(8):565-77. doi: 10.1038/nrmicro2612.

18. Erkin Şeker, Bacterial Vibrations.Sci. Transl. Med.5,196ec126-196ec126(2013).DOI:10.1126/scitranslmed.3007046
19. Raskin DM, de Boer PA. Rapid pole-to-pole oscillation of a protein required for directing division to the middle of Escherichia coli. Proc Natl Acad Sci U S A. 1999 Apr 27;96(9):4971-6. doi: 10.1073/pnas.96.9.4971.
20. Mojica-Benavides M, van Niekerk DD, Mijalkov M, Snoep JL, Mehlig B, Volpe G, Goksör M, Adiels CB. Intercellular communication induces glycolytic synchronization waves between individually oscillating cells. Proc Natl Acad Sci USA. 2021 Feb 9;118(6): e2010075118. doi: 10.1073/pnas.2010075118.
21. Weber A, Prokazov Y, Zuschratter W, Hauser MJ. Desynchronization of glycolytic oscillations in yeast cell populations. PLoS One. 2012;7(9):e43276. doi: 10.1371/journal.pone.0043276
22. Aggarwal A, Brennan C, Shortal B, Contreras D, Kelz MB, Proekt A. Coherence of Visual-Evoked Gamma Oscillations Is Disrupted by Propofol but Preserved Under Equipotent Doses of Isoflurane. Front Syst Neurosci. 2019 May 8;13:19. doi: 10.3389/fnsys.2019.00019.
23. Dipoppa, M., Ranson, A., Krumin, M., Pachitariu, M., Carandini, M., and Harris, K. D. (2018). Vision and Locomotion Shape the Interactions between Neuron Types in Mouse Visual Cortex. Neuron 98, 602–615.e8. doi: 10.1016/j.neuron.2018.03.037
24. Amir, A., Headley, D. B., Lee, S.-C., Haufler, D., and Paré, D. (2018). Vigilance-associated gamma Oscillations Coordinate the Ensemble Activity of Basolateral Amygdala Neurons. Neuron 97, 656–669.e7. doi: 10.1016/j.neuron.2017.12.035
25. Besserve M, Lowe SC, Logothetis NK, Schölkopf B, Panzeri S. Shifts of Gamma Phase across Primary Visual Cortical Sites Reflect Dynamic Stimulus-Modulated Information Transfer. PLOS Biology. 2015;13:e1002257. doi: 10.1371/journal.pbio.1002257.
26. Davis ZW, Muller L, Martinez-Trujillo J, Sejnowski T, Reynolds JH. Spontaneous traveling cortical waves gate perception in behaving primates. Nature. 2020;587:432–436. doi: 10.1038/s41586-020-2802-y.

27. Gallotto S, Sack AT, Schuhmann T, de Graaf TA. Oscillatory Correlates of Visual Consciousness. Front Psychol. 2017 Jul 7;8:1147. Doi: 10.3389/fpsyg.2017.01147.
28. Başar E. A review of gamma oscillations in healthy subjects and cognitive impairment. Int J Psychophysiol. 2013 Nov;90(2):99-117. doi: 10.1016/j.ijpsycho.2013.07.005
29. Pelkey, K. A., Chittajallu, R., Craig, M. T., Tricoire, L., Wester, J. C., and McBain, C. J. (2017). Hippocampal GABAergic Inhibitory Interneurons. Physiol. Rev. 97, 1619–1747. doi: 10.1152/physrev.00007.2017
30. Murueta-Goyena, A., Ortuzar, N., Lafuente, J.V. et al. Enriched Environment Reverts Somatostatin Interneuron Loss in MK-801 Model of Schizophrenia. Mol Neurobiol 57, 125–134 (2020). https://doi.org/10.1007/s12035-019-01762-y
31. Petrie KA, Schmidt D, Bubser M, Fadel J, Carraway RE, Deutch AY. Neurotensin activates GABAergic interneurons in the prefrontal cortex. J Neurosci. 2005 Feb 16;25(7):1629-36.
32. doi: 10.1523/JNEUROSCI.3579-04.2005.
33. Chen CM, Stanford AD, Mao X, Abi-Dargham A, Shungu DC, Lisanby SH, Schroeder CE, Kegeles LS. GABA level, gamma oscillation, and working memory performance in schizophrenia. Neuroimage Clin. 2014 Mar 20;4:531-9. doi: 10.1016/j.nicl.2014.03.007
34. Antonoudiou P, Tan YL, Kontou G, Upton AL, Mann EO. Parvalbumin and Somatostatin Interneurons Contribute to the Generation of Hippocampal Gamma Oscillations. J Neurosci. 2020 Sep 30;40(40):7668-7687. doi: 10.1523/JNEUROSCI.0261-20.2020.
35. Vendemia JMC, Caine KE, Evans JR. Quantitative EEG Findings in Convicted Murderers (2005), Vol 9 No 3. doi: https://doi.org/10.1300/J184v09n03_02
36. James R. Evans Ph.D. & Nan-Sook Park M.A. (1997) Quantitative EEG Findings Among Men Convicted of Murder, Journal of Neurotherapy: Investigations in Neuromodulation, Neurofeedback and Applied Neuroscience, 2:2, 31-39, doi: 10.1300/J184v02n02_05

37. Raine A, Meloy JR, Bihrle S, Stoddard J, LaCasse L, Buchsbaum MS. Reduced prefrontal and increased subcortical brain functioning assessed using positron emission tomography in predatory and affective murderers. Behav Sci Law. 1998 Summer;16(3):319-32. doi: 10.1002/(sici)1099-0798(199822)16:3<319::aid-bsl311>3.0.co;2-g.

38. Schug RA, Yang Y, Raine A, Han C, Liu J, Li L. Resting EEG deficits in accused murderers with schizophrenia. Psychiatry Res. 2011 Oct 31;194(1):85-94. doi: 10.1016/j.pscychresns.2010.12.017.

39. J. R. Evans, Quantitative EEG findings in a group of death row inmates, Archives of Clinical Neuropsychology, Volume 12, Issue 4, 1997, Pages 315–316, https://doi.org/10.1093/arclin/12.4.315a

40. Zomorrodi, R., Loheswaran, G., Pushparaj, A., et al. Pulsed Near Infrared Transcranial and Intranasal Photobiomodulation Significantly Modulates Neural Oscillations: A Pilot Exploratory Study. Sci Rep 9, 6309 (2019). https://doi.org/10.1038/s41598-019-42693-x

41. Dompe C, Moncrieff L, Matys J, Grzech-Leśniak K, Kocherova I, Bryja A, Bruska M, Dominiak M, Mozdziak P, Skiba THI, Shibli JA, Angelova Volponi A, Kempisty B, Dyszkiewicz-Konwińska M. Photobiomodulation-Underlying Mechanism and Clinical Applications. J Clin Med. 2020 Jun 3;9(6):1724. doi: 10.3390/jcm9061724. PMID: 32503238; PMCID: PMC7356229.

42. Liu J, Prindle A, Humphries J, Gabalda-Sagarra M, Asally M, Lee DY, Ly S, Garcia-Ojalvo J, Süel GM. Metabolic co-dependence gives rise to collective oscillations within biofilms. Nature. 2015 Jul 30;523(7562):550-4. doi: 10.1038/nature14660.

43. Pathak H, Sreeraj VS, Venkatasubramanian G. Transcranial Alternating Current Stimulation (tACS) and Its Role in Schizophrenia: A Scoping Review. Clin Psychopharmacol Neurosci. 2023 Nov 30;21(4):634-649. Doi: 10.9758/cpn.22.1042.

44. Koshiyama, D. et al. Auditory gamma oscillations predict global symptomatic outcome in the early stages of psychosis: a longitudinal investigation. Clin. Neurophysiol. 129, 2268–2275 (2018).

45. Griskova-Bulanova I, Dapsys K, Melynyte S, Voicikas A, Maciulis V, Andruskevicius S, Korostenskaja M. 40Hz auditory steady-state response in schizophrenia: Sensitivity to stimulation type (clicks

versus flutter amplitude-modulated tones). Neurosci Lett. 2018 Jan 1;662:152-157. doi: 10.1016/j.neulet.2017.10.025.

46. Zhang Y, Zhang Z, Luo L, Tong H, Chen F, Hou ST. 40 Hz Light Flicker Alters Human Brain Electroencephalography Microstates and Complexity Implicated in Brain Diseases. Front Neurosci. 2021 Dec 13;15:777183. doi: 10.3389/fnins.2021.777183.

47. Chan D, Suk HJ, Jackson BL, Milman NP, Stark D, Klerman EB, Kitchener E, Fernandez Avalos VS, de Weck G, Banerjee A, Beach SD, et al. Gamma frequency sensory stimulation in mild probable Alzheimer's dementia patients: Results of feasibility and pilot studies. PLoS One. 2022 Dec 1;17(12):e0278412. doi: 10.1371/journal.pone.0278412.

48. Jang HJ, Chung H, Rowland JM, Richards BA, Kohl MM, Kwag J. Distinct roles of parvalbumin and somatostatin interneurons in gating the synchronization of spike times in the neocortex. Sci Adv. 2020 Apr 22;6(17):eaay5333. Doi: 10.1126/sciadv.aay5333.

49. Liguz-Lecznar M, Urban-Ciecko J, Kossuth M. Somatostatin and Somatostatin-Containing Neurons in Shaping Neuronal Activity and Plasticity. Front Neural Circuits. 2016 Jun 30;10:48. doi: 10.3389/fncir.2016.00048.

50. Murty DVPS, Manikandan K, Kumar WS, Ramesh RG, Purokayastha S, Javali M, Rao NP, Ray S. Gamma oscillations weaken with age in healthy elderly in human EEG. Neuroimage. 2020 Jul 15;215:116826. doi: 10.1016/j.neuroimage.2020.116826.

51. Karrasch M, Laine M, Rapinoja P, Krause CM. Effects of normal aging on event-related desynchronization/synchronization during a human memory task. Neurosci Lett. 2004 Aug 5;366(1):18-23. doi: 10.1016/j.neulet.2004.05.010.

52. Chesnokova V, Zonis S, Apostolou A, Estrada HQ, Knott S, Wawrowsky K, Michelsen K, Ben-Shlomo A, Barrett R, Gorbunova V, Karalis K, Melmed S. Local non-pituitary growth hormone is induced with aging and facilitates epithelial damage. Cell Rep. 2021 Dec 14;37(11):110068. doi: 10.1016/j.celrep.2021.110068. PMID: 34910915

53. Nelson Espinosa, Alejandra Alonso, Cristian Morales, Pedro Espinosa, Andrés E Chávez, Pablo Fuentealba, Basal Forebrain

Gating by Somatostatin Neurons Drives Prefrontal Cortical Activity, Cerebral Cortex, Volume 29, Issue 1, January 2019, Pages 42–53, https://doi.org/10.1093/cercor/bhx302

# CHAPTER 7

# SLEEPLESS IN CAPTIVITY: INSOMNIA KILLS THE VON ECONOMO NEURONS

## Highlights

- The salience network is likely the common pathway of insomnia, severe mental illness, and neurodegenerative disorders.
- Selective loss of Von Economo Neurons in frontotemporal dementia behavioral variant manifests clinically as an acquired psychopathy.
- Insomnia-driven lipid peroxidation, ferroptosis, and mitochondrial loss selectively eliminate the Von Economo Neurons.
- Damaged mitochondria and oxidized lipids activate aryl hydrocarbon receptors, worsening insomnia.
- Novel phenazine and phenothiazine derivatives, as well as mitochondrial transplantation, can reverse this pathology.

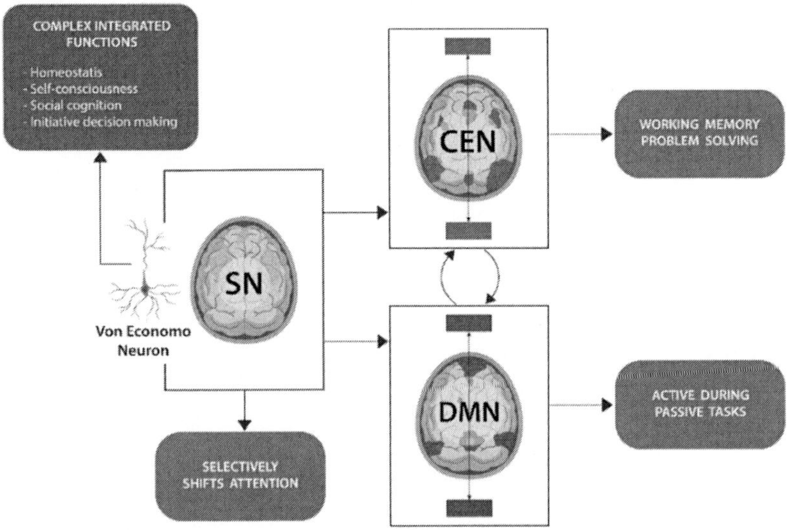


## Visual Abstract

**The salience network (SN), comprised of the insular cortex (IC), anterior cingulate cortex (ACC), and several subcortical nodes, has recently been implicated in the etiopathogenesis of insomnia, chronic psychosis, and neurodegenerative disorders. SN is a dynamic switch between interoception and exteroception, driven by the Von Economo neurons (VENS). VENs are crucial in empathy, social awareness, alertness, and morality. Selective loss of VENS occurs in frontotemporal dementia behavioral variant (bvFTD), engendering an acquired psychopathy.**

Forensic hospitals throughout the country house individuals with severe mental illness and a history of criminal violations. Insomnia affects 67.4% of hospitalized patients with chronic neuropsychiatric disorders, indicating that these conditions may hijack human somnogenic pathways. Conversely, somnolence is a common adverse effect of many antipsychotic drugs, further highlighting a common etiopathogenesis.

The role of dysfunctional mitochondria in psychopathology is well-established. However, the association of these organelles with sleep physiology is novel. Indeed, reducing neuronal oxidative stress by importing mitochondria from astrocytes may be the purpose of human slumber. This model may explain mitochondrial dysfunction during anesthesia as well as in the rare genetic disease, fatal familial insomnia (FFI).

One of the most common sleep disorders in the United States, primary insomnia, is usually defined as long sleep latency, difficulty staying asleep, prolonged nighttime wakefulness, and early morning awakening (1). In incarcerated individuals, over 60% of inmates experience insomnia, a prevalence 6-10 times higher than in the general population (2). Moreover, insomnia is present in 67.4% of hospitalized patients with severe mental illness, suggesting that pathways of sleep and neuropathology are highly intertwined (3). Insomnia is common in forensic psychiatric detainees, and failure to address this condition may increase healthcare expenditure due to medical complications, including metabolic, cardiovascular, and neurodegenerative disorders.

The salience network (SN), comprised of the insular cortex (IC), anterior cingulate cortex (ACC), and several subcortical nodes, has recently been implicated in the etiopathogenesis of insomnia, SCZ, and neurodegenerative disorders (4)(5)(6)(7)(8)(9). VENS, a particular class of large, spindle-shaped cells found only in humans and superior mammals, are found primarily in IC and ACC and have been involved in empathy and fairness, connecting sleep with higher brain functions (10)(11). In addition, VENS play a crucial role in shifting the attentional focus from interoception to exteroception as required by each situation.

At the molecular level, incarceration, insomnia, and severe mental illness have been associated with premature cellular senescence, a phenotype marked by increased intracellular iron and mitochondrial depletion (11)(12)(13)(14)(15)(16)(17)(18). Premature cellular senescence is likely triggered by the activation of AhR, the master regulator of cellular aging (19)(20)(21). Senescent cells upregulated intracellular iron, increasing the risk of lipid peroxidation and neuronal demise by ferroptosis (22)(23)(24). Ferroptosis is a programmed cell death induced by iron in the context of antioxidant failure marked by depletion of glutathione peroxidase-4 (GPX-4)(25)(26). GPX-4 is a mitochondrial enzyme that repairs oxidized phospholipids and cholesterol in neuronal and mitochondrial membranes (27).

Antipsychotic drugs are known for causing drowsiness, indicating interference with the human sleep pathways. For example, phenothiazines induce sleep by antagonizing histamine H1 and alpha1 adrenergic receptors (28). Clozapine, an AhR-activating ligand, may cause drowsiness by altering the expression of circadian clock genes, some of which are controlled by the AhR (29)(30).

The phenothiazine class of antipsychotic drugs is a potent inhibitor of cholesterol metabolism as they lower 7-dehydrocholesterol reductase (7DHC), upregulating 7-dehydrocholesterol (7DHC), a plasma membrane lipid that strengthens the lipid bilayer (31). For example, trifluoperazine upregulates 7DH, protecting the mitochondrion by preventing pore formation and organelle demise (32). Moreover, phenothiazines enter the lipid bilayer of plasma and mitochondrial membranes, inhibiting peroxidation and thus protecting the neurons from ferroptosis (33)(34)(35). Interestingly, chlorpromazine was found effective against prion diseases, emphasizing a likely beneficial role in fatal familial insomnia (FFI), a genetic mutation of the prion protein (PRNP) gene (36).

Dysfunctional mitochondria and impaired oxidative phosphorylation (OXPHOS) increase glycolysis and lactic acid levels, a metabolic pattern characteristic of SCZ or SLDs (37). Indeed, increased lactate, considered a marker of sleep deprivation, likely activates mitochondrial AhR (mitoAhR), disrupting the organelle (38)(39)(40). This is significant as lactate and neuro-metabolism likely comprise another sleep pathway hijacked by mental illness.

To compensate for dysfunctional mitochondria, neurons import these organelles from glial cells, especially the astrocyte (41)(42). In large cells, such as VENS, mitochondria are more vulnerable to damage and autophagic elimination as they undergo more wear and tear during their journey through the long axons of these neurons (43). Due to their small number (around 193,000) and large size, VENS are more susceptible to plasma membrane oxidation, which may explain their selective loss in bvFTD.

Since mitochondria are crucial for neuronal function, preserving the integrity of these organelles via membrane lipid replacement (MLR) is of utmost importance. Microbial phenazines and the novel antioxidant phenothiazine derivatives offer new opportunities to combat insomnia, psychosis, and neurodegeneration at the level of cell and mitochondrial membranes.

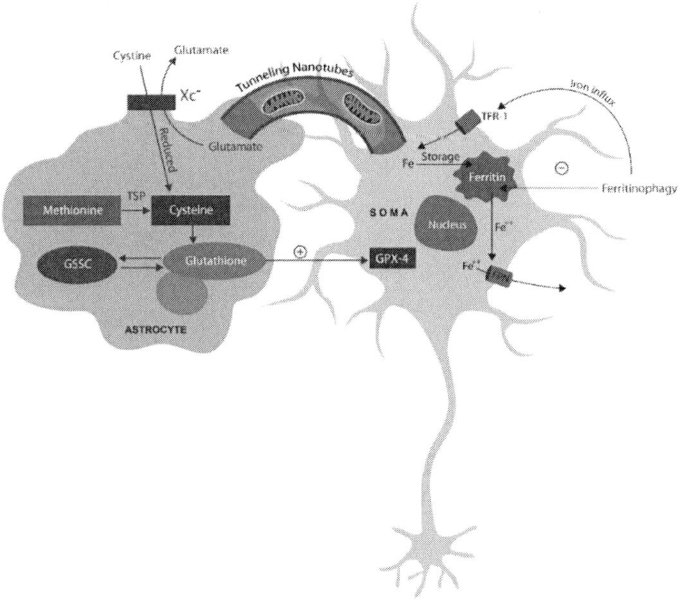


**Astrocytes support the postmitotic, long-lived neurons by helping them avert death by ferroptosis and loss of mitochondria. The former is accomplished by exporting GPX-4 to neurons (to repair oxidized lipids), while the latter is by exporting healthy mitochondria to neuronal cells (via tunneling nanotubules. Interestingly, selective serotonin reuptake inhibitors (SSRIs) promote mitochondrial transfer from astrocytes to neurons, suggesting a non-synaptic mechanism of action.**

## Four cases of bvFTD from our hospital and community

### *Case #1 The teacher who shot her neighbor*

Ms. KS (initials changed), a Caucasian female, age 68, divorced, retired elementary school teacher, lived alone before admission to Patton State Hospital. Ms. KS did not have a psychiatric history until the age of 56, when she purchased a gun and shot her neighbor in the shoulder. She stated that she attacked the man because he was spying on her and intruded into her house during the night. She was convicted of attempted murder and sent to prison, where her condition deteriorated, prompting her transfer to our forensic institution. KS was diagnosed with SCZ and admitted as a forensic detainee.

During her hospital stay, KS was treated with various antipsychotic drugs with minimal symptomatic relief. She was unaware that she did anything wrong, and her poor insight and impulsivity were documented during her six years of hospital stay. Because of poor insight, KS never met the criteria for the conditional release program (CONREP).

In 2014, KS became more forgetful, required assistance with most activities of daily living (ADLs), and changed her dietary preferences. For example, she asked for ice cream daily, although earlier in her life, she detested ice cream. In time, KS became more apathetic and often refused to get out of bed. The internal medicine consultant performed a dementia workup, but the laboratory studies came back normal, except for mild anemia and a vitamin D level of 29.3 nmol/L. KS scored 25/30 on the Mini-Mental Status Exam (MMSE), and when a Montreal Cognitive Assessment (MoCA) was administered, the score was 23/30, consistent with executive dysfunction. A neuropsychology consult was called, and after a battery of tests, bvFTD was diagnosed.

With this information, the treatment team petitioned the Court, arguing that KS did not benefit from hospitalization in a forensic institution as she was not expected to recover. The judge agreed with the treating clinicians and ordered placement in a facility specialized in dementia.

Due to the numerous clinical and legal ramifications (discussed below), this case was featured in the mass media at the time:
https://www.reuters.com/article/us-crime-dementia-idUSKBN0KE1Q020150105/
https://www.foxnews.com/health/breaking-the-law-may-be-a-sign-of-dementia

https://clbb.mgh.harvard.edu/when-frontotemporal-dementia-leads-to-crime-prosecution-or-protection/

### *Case #2 The attorney with a sweet tooth*

An outpatient we treated in 2013 was a 72-year-old retired attorney arrested because he stole chocolate from a grocery store while casually conversing with the owner. When confronted, he replied: "What's the problem? I have a sweet tooth". According to the family, the patient came across as careless and indifferent to his children and the spouse, being either apathetic or angry and irritable. For example, when he learned that his son-in-law died unexpectedly, he responded by saying, "Let's go out to eat." According to his wife, his eating habits had changed dramatically, mainly consuming sweets he had previously avoided. When told to eat more nutritious food, he often became angry.

### *Case #3 The psychiatrist turned a drug dealer*

Dr. Joel Stanley Dreyer was a well-respected psychiatrist who practiced in Riverside, California. In the 1990s, Dr. Dreyer was diagnosed with bvFTD but continued to practice psychiatry, and in 2010 was convicted for prescribing, selling, and distributing large amounts of addictive painkillers. As a result of careless prescribing, one person died of an overdose, and Dr. Dreyer was convicted and served ten years in prison despite having been diagnosed with bvFTD before his crime. This case emphasizes that some jurisdictions do not recognize bvFTD as an attenuating circumstance. The court ruling was based on the testimony of the prison psychiatrist, who did not challenge the diagnosis of bvFTD but stated that since not all individuals with this disorder engage in criminal behavior, "direct causality" between Dr. Dreyer's crime and bvFTD could not be established. A detailed history of this case can be found at the link below:
https://story.californiasunday.com/joel-dreyer-criminal-psychiatrist/.

### *Case #4 The Buick murderer*

On July 16, 2003, Mr. GRW, an 83-year-old man, crashed his Buick LeSabre in an open-air market in Santa Monica, California, killing ten and injuring 63 individuals. Despite the catastrophic event he caused, GRW did not express remorse and showed indifference, callousness, and lack of empathy. In the court, he appeared numb, angry, and unapologetic, stating that he was sorry the dead and injured could not "enjoy the value of their purchases." No psychiatric evaluation was ordered because there was no previous history. However, criminal behavior may often represent the first symptom of bvFTD. Despite never being diagnosed with a neurodegenerative disorder, people who knew GRW noticed a drastic personality change in the years before this event, indicative of bvFTD. His neighbors, friends, and pastor described GRW as caring, pleasant, and friendly. He had been married for over 60 years, was compassionate, involved in people's lives, and, after retirement, volunteered with various civic organizations. Although GRW was never officially diagnosed with bvFTD, this case illustrates the difficulty clinicians encounter because this neurodegenerative disorder affects executive function, leaving memory intact for many years. Indeed, shortly before his crime, GRW was able to pass his DMV license renewal test, suggesting that his memory was unaffected. Since in California, drivers who are 70 or older must renew their driver's license in person, GRW did not raise a dementia red flag with the DMV worker.

## Discussion

Since bvFTD comprises 2.7% of all dementias and is in its early stages, patients retain their cognitive abilities; this condition is often misdiagnosed as SCZ, depression, or bipolar disorder and frequently admitted to psychiatric institutions. Patients with bvFTD respond poorly to antipsychotic drugs, are usually labeled "treatment resistant," and are prescribed additional psychotropics (157). Moreover, as criminal behavior is frequently the initial manifestation of bvFTD, clinicians rarely suspect this condition when examining an incarcerated individual. However, several characteristics of this disorder should prompt the clinician to think of a neurodegenerative condition. These include absence of psychiatric history at a younger age, first legal violation after the age of 55, poor insight despite a previously successful life, sudden change in eating habits, altered sleep pattern, lack of empathy, and engaging in criminal acts despite the presence of witnesses.

## Conclusions

Forensic institutions throughout the country house individuals with severe mental illness and often comorbid insomnia, suggesting overlapping pathogeneses. Loss of neurons due to impaired sleep, along with SCZ or SLDs-related gray matter depletion, may trigger the premature development of dementias and other medical complications. These comorbidities increase healthcare expenditures and shorten patients' lifespans; therefore, identifying and treating these conditions early is essential.

YOD, a category of neurodegenerative disorders that include bvFTD, has been on the rise over the past few decades, as evidenced by the increased number of first offenders younger than 65. Selective loss of VENS in bvFTD is likely due to the large size of these cells, predisposing to peroxidation of plasma membrane lipids and mitochondrial loss by autophagy.

At the molecular level, AhR is the equivalent of cerebral VENS, as this protein responds to both endogenous and exogenous ligands, including lipid peroxides and other insomnia and psychosis-related molecules.

Novel AhR ligands, phenazine and phenothiazine derivatives, as well as mitochondrial transfer or transplantation, are potential new strategies for treating psychosis, insomnia, and neurodegeneration without additional loss of brain volume.

**Mitochondria-protective treatments and novel phenazines are discussed in the article below.**

# ARTICLE FOR CHAPTER 7: INSOMNIA IN FORENSIC DETAINEES: IS SALIENCE NETWORK THE COMMON PATHWAY FOR SLEEP, NEUROPSYCHIATRIC, AND NEURODEGENERATIVE DISORDERS?

## ADONIS SFERA[1,2], KYLE A. THOMAS[1], ISAAC A. OGUNJALE[1], NYLA JAFRI[1] AND PETER G. BOTA[2]

*1. Department of Psychiatry, Patton State Hospital, University of California, Riverside, CA 92521, USA*
*2. School of Medicine, California University of Science and Medicine, Colton, CA 92324, USA*

## Highlights

**What are the main findings?**

- SN dysfunction is the common denominator of insomnia, schizophrenia (SCZ), and frontotemporal dementia behavioral variant (bvFTD).

**What is the implication of the main finding?**

- The diagnosis of bvFTD is often missed or misdiagnosed in forensic institutions.
- To ensure adequate placement and treatment planning, courts and clinicians require education to differentiate bvFTD from SCZ.

## Abstract

Forensic hospitals throughout the country house individuals with severe mental illness and history of criminal violations. Insomnia affects 67.4% of hospitalized patients with chronic neuropsychiatric disorders, indicating that these conditions may hijack human somnogenic pathways. Conversely, somnolence is a common adverse effect of many antipsychotic drugs, further highlighting a common etiopathogenesis. Since the brain salience network is likely the common denominator for insomnia, neuropsychiatric and neurodegenerative disorders, here, we focus on the pathology of this neuronal assembly and its likely driver, the dysfunctional neuronal and mitochondrial membrane. We also discuss potential treatment strategies ranging from membrane lipid replacement to mitochondrial transplantation. The aims of this review are threefold: 1. Examining the causes of insomnia in forensic detainees with severe mental illness, as well as its role in predisposing them to neurodegenerative disorders. 2. Educating State hospital and prison clinicians on frontotemporal dementia behavioral variant, a condition increasingly diagnosed in older first offenders which is often missed due to the absence of memory impairment. 3. Introducing clinicians to natural compounds that are potentially beneficial for insomnia and severe mental illness.

**Keywords:** Von Economo neuron; interoceptive awareness; frontotemporal dementia behavioral variant; phenazines.

## 1. Introduction

One of the most common sleep disorders in the United States, primary insomnia, is usually defined as long sleep latency, difficulty staying asleep, prolonged nighttime wakefulness, and/or early morning awakening [1]. In prison, approximately 60% of inmates experience insomnia, a prevalence 6–10 times higher than in the population at large [2]. Moreover, insomnia is present in 67.4% of hospitalized patients with severe mental illness, suggesting that the pathways of sleep and neuropathology are highly intertwined [3].

Forensic psychiatric hospitals admit patients with schizophrenia (SCZ) or schizophrenia-like disorders (SLDs) and criminal violations. Insomnia is common in this population and failure to address this condition may increase healthcare expenditure due to medical complications, including metabolic, cardiovascular, and neurodegenerative disorders.

The salience network (SN), comprised of the anterior insular cortex (AIC), anterior cingulate cortex (ACC) and several subcortical nodes, has recently been implicated in the etiopathogenesis of insomnia, SCZ, and neurodegenerative disorders [4–9]. SN is comprised of Von Economo neurons (VENs), a special class of large, spindle-shaped cells found only in humans and superior mammals that are believed to drive empathy, social awareness, and emotional intelligence [10].

At the molecular level, incarceration, insomnia, and severe mental illness have been associated with premature cellular senescence, a phenotype marked by increased intracellular iron and mitochondrial damage [11–18]. Premature cellular senescence is driven by the aryl hydrocarbon receptor (AhR), expressed in neuronal cytosol and mitochondria [19–21]. Senescent cells upregulate intracellular iron which, in the proximity of cytosolic fats, increases the risk of lipid peroxidation and neuronal demise by ferroptosis [22–24]. Ferroptosis is a programmed cell death induced by iron in the context of antioxidant failure marked by the depletion of glutathione peroxidase-4 (GPX-4) [25,26]. GPX-4 is a mitochondrial enzyme which averts ferroptosis by repairing the oxidized phospholipids and cholesterol in mitochondrial and neuronal membranes [27]. Ferroptosis causes mitochondrial swelling, loss of cristae, dissipation of the membrane potential, as well as an increase in membrane permeability, changes that ultimately lead to mitochondrial loss [28]. Mitochondrial dysfunction and loss drive cellular senescence, a phenotype found in insomnia, severe mental illness and frontotemporal lobar degeneration (FTLD) [29–32]. In addition, insomnia, SCZ, and frontotemporal dementia (FTD) have been connected to impaired phagocytosis of senescent cells by natural killer cells (NKCs) [33–35]. Accumulation of senescent cells due to accelerated aging and impaired removal leads to inflammation, a pathology encountered in sleep deprivation, severe mental illness and FTD [36–38]. Since mitochondria is a key driver of inflammation, dysfunction or loss of these organelles likely account for these pathologies [39,40].

To compensate for dysfunctional mitochondria, neurons import these organelles from glial cells, especially the astrocyte [41,42]. In large cells, such as VENs, mitochondria are more vulnerable to damage and autophagic elimination as they undergo more wear and tear during their journey through the long axons of these neurons [42]. Due to their small number (around 193,000) and their large sizes, VENs are more susceptible to plasma membrane oxidative stress, which may trigger significant pathology even after a limited neuronal loss, a pathology encountered in frontotemporal dementia behavioral variant (bvFTD) [43].

Since mitochondria are crucial for neuronal function, preserving the integrity of these organelles via membrane lipid replacement (MLR) and other natural strategies is of utmost importance. Microbial phenazines and the novel antioxidant phenothiazine derivatives offer new opportunities to combat insomnia, psychosis, and neurodegeneration at the level of cell and mitochondrial membranes.

### *1.1. Salienve Network in Sleep and Neuropathology*

The SN is comprised of ACC and AIC which, along with subcortical nodes in the hypothalamus, thalamus, striatum, and midbrain, process salient stimuli [44,45]. SN functions as a switch between exteroception and interoception or central executive network (CEN) and default mode network (DMN), depending on stimulus relevance [46]. Switching from CEN to DMN and vice versa is impaired in severe mental illness, insomnia, and neurodegenerative disorders [47]. Several antipsychotic drugs are known to lower the salience assignment to objects and events, likely restoring SN function, which, in turn, may ameliorate insomnia and psychosis [48].

The SN harbors VENs, which are large, corkscrew neurons located in layer V of the AIC and ACC. These non-telencephalic cells are believed to drive prosocial cognition, empathy, and emotional intelligence. As parts of the SN, VENs respond to endogenous or exogenous stimuli in the order of priority. VENs are selectively eliminated in bvFTD, a disorder marked by criminal violations, lack of empathy, poor insight, and sleep impairment [49–53]. In forensic institutions, bvFTD is increasingly diagnosed in older first offenders with no previous criminal history and often coexists with insomnia and altered eating habits.

Under physiological circumstances, sleep is driven by the ventrolateral preoptic nucleus (VLPO) of the anterior hypothalamus which releases inhibitory neurotransmitters, including γ-aminobutyric acid (GABA), and galanin [54]. The opposing system, orexin (hypocretin) neurons in the lateral hypothalamus, inhibits VLPO [55–57]. In addition, orexin/hypocretin neurons induce wakefulness by blocking melanin concentrating hormone (MCH), a somnogen released by the hypothalamus and zona incerta [58,59]. Orexin and DA, the key players of saliency, have been implicated in the neuropsychiatric disorders associated with sleep disturbances, including narcolepsy, attention-deficit/hyperactivity disorder (ADHD), and Parkinson's disease (PD) [60]. Histamine is another wakefulnesspromoting neurotransmitter implicated in SCZ and a novel target for treating negative and cognitive symptoms [61].

To better comprehend the pathogenesis of insomnia, it is necessary to study the pathways of wakefulness, a brain state driving self-awareness and probably consciousness [62]. Early studies on this subject have focused on the locus coeruleus, midbrain tegmentum, pons, and parabrachial nucleus, as neurons in these regions are active during wakefulness [63,64]. In the early 1900s, while studying encephalitis lethargica, Constantin von Economo found that lesions in the posterior hypothalamus were associated with sleep, hypothesizing that this area contained the "center of wakefulness" [65–67].

Fatal familial insomnia (FFI), a rare autosomal dominant disease, is marked by hypometabolism and neuronal loss in the thalamus and ACC, linking this condition to the SN [68–72]. The role of SN in sleep physiology and pathology is further highlighted by the anesthetics, especially propofol, which lower salience processing, inducing sleep [68–78]. Moreover, recent studies on sleep-deprived human volunteers and patients with primary insomnia demonstrated altered connectivity in AIC, further linking SN to sleep and wakefulness [79,80]. Furthermore, several preclinical studies are in line with the findings in humans, implicating the SN in slumber homeostasis [74,81].

Aside from insomnia and neuropsychiatric pathology, the SN connectivity is disrupted in neurodegenerative disorders, including Alzheimer's disease (AD), Parkinson's disease (PD), and bvFTD, suggesting that insomnia and neuropathology are highly intertwined [82–86]. Indeed, dysfunctional AIC and ACC connectivity may account for the criminal violations in patients with bvFTD, in which breaking the law may often be the initial dementia symptom [87,88].

### *1.2. Salience Network in Frontotemporal Dementia Behavioral Variant*

The second most common neurodegenerative disorder after AD, bvFTD, is marked by inappropriate emotional responses and disinhibited behaviors, often leading to criminal violations, as this pathology targets VENs selectively [52,89]. In forensic institutions, individuals with first incarceration after the age of 55 may suffer from bvFTD, an entity difficult to diagnose as the memory may remain intact for longer periods of time. As a result, bvFTD is often missed or misdiagnosed as antisocial personality disorder (APD), SCZ, or even major depressive disorder [90].

Over the past two decades, the number of senior first offenders has grown in parallel with the prevalence of young-onset dementia (YOD, emergence of symptoms before age 65), a subgroup of neurodegenerative disorders, which may include bvFTD [91,92]. Indeed, recent studies have revealed that the prevalence of bvFTD has increased from 15/100,000 in 2013 to 119 per 100,000 in 2021, mirroring the growing number of forensic detainees with this diagnosis [92,93].

Compared to AD, in which 12% of patients exhibit criminal behavior, bvFTD is associated with a crime rate of 54%, suggesting an acquired psychopathy [94]. Frontotemporal lobar degeneration (FTLD), the pathology driving bvFTD, is associated with impulsivity and criminal violations due to the paucity of "honesty cells", VENs [95]. The latter is likely due to the autophagy of damaged organelles traveling through the long VENs axons. Indeed, lysosomal aggregates, hallmarks of hyperactive autophagy, were demonstrated in the VENs derived from patients with bvFTD and SCZ, suggesting excessive mitophagy [95–97]. Depletion of VENs has been associated with a lack of empathy, aggressive behavior, and criminal violations documented in bvFTD and severe mental illness [51,52]. For example, homicide or attempted homicide have been documented in bvFTD, indicating that criminal behavior and murder can sometimes be the earliest manifestation of this disorder [98,99]. Since VENs are only present in large mammals, including humans, great apes, macaques, cetaceans, and elephants, but not in rodents, these cells are difficult to study in vivo [10]. VENs are larger than pyramidal neurons and drive interoceptive awareness, which is the ability to detect and process internal cues such as heartbeat, respiration and the overall visceral state [100,101]. VENs are components of the SN, an attention-shifting large neuronal assembly that can activate or silence CEN to DMN [102,103].

Recent transcriptomic studies found that VENs express monoaminergic proteins, including vesicular monoamine transporter 2 (VMAT2) and adrenergic receptor α-1A (ADRA1A), suggesting involvement in autonomic functions, including the circadian rhythm [104–106]. Indeed, impaired monoaminergic signaling has been documented in insomnia, bvFTD, SCZ, and SLDs, implicating VENs in these pathologies [107–111].

### *1.3. Sleep and Glial Cells*

Astrocytes, the most numerous brain cells, communicate with each other via calcium waves, attaining synchronization with neurons and supporting slow-wave sleep [112,113]. Moreover, astrocytes release molecules, including adenosine, lactate, glutamate, GABA, and interleukin-1 (IL-1), which may indirectly influence the status of neuronal cells, inducing sleep [114].

Astrocytes are central to the neurovascular unit (NVU) and bridge the gap between the neuron and brain microvessels, regulating the flow of interstitial fluid through the aquaporin 4 (AQP-4) receptors [115] (Figure 1). The volume of the brain interstitial fluid (ISF) fluctuates in a circadian manner as it flows through the glymphatic system, a mechanism for clearing misfolded proteins during sleep [116]. The glymphatic system can also carry extracellular vesicles containing mitochondria from astrocytes to neurons [117]. Astrocytes support the neurons by generating GPX-4 to avert neuronal death by ferroptosis. GPX-4 functions to repair oxidized lipids and oxysterols, including 7-ketocholesterol (7KCl), toxins that disrupt plasma and mitochondrial membranes, triggering neuronal death [118]. Ferroptosis has been associated with sleep deprivation, indicating that neurons likely import GPX-4 during sleep [119]. As mitochondria play a key role in sleep homeostasis, insomnia may be the result of plasma or mitochondrial membrane oxidation. Indeed, it has been suggested that sleep is necessary for abrogating neuronal oxidative stress [120].

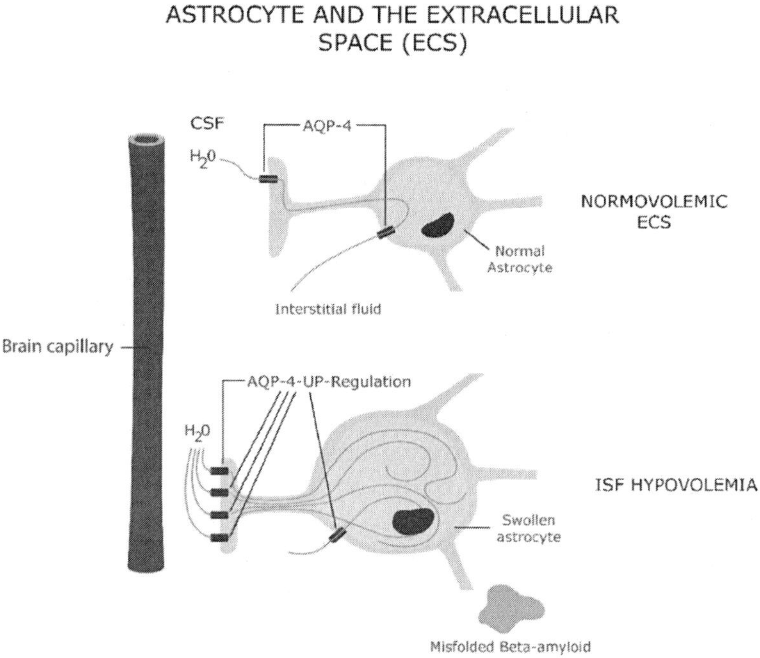


**Figure 1. Astrocytes contact cerebral microvessels with their end-feet processes, delineating a pathway for the flow of extracellular fluid, known as the glymphatic system. The volume of interstitial fluid (ISF) in the brain parenchyma varies with the brain work. During high intensity work, AQP-4 water receptors are upregulated in the end-feet, pumping the ISF into astrocytes. This results in low ISF (hypovolemia). During sleep (low-intensity brain work), less ISF enters the astrocyte. The circulation of ISF clears the molecular debris (including beta amyloid) from the extracellular space.**

Intracellular iron is stored in ferritin and released for intracellular needs via ferritinophagy (ferritin autophagy) in lysosomes. Several antipsychotic drugs, including haloperidol, accumulate in lysosomes disrupting ferritinophagy, which, in turn, lowers intracellular iron, averting ferroptosis [121,122] (Figure 2). This may highlight a DAindependent, antipsychotic

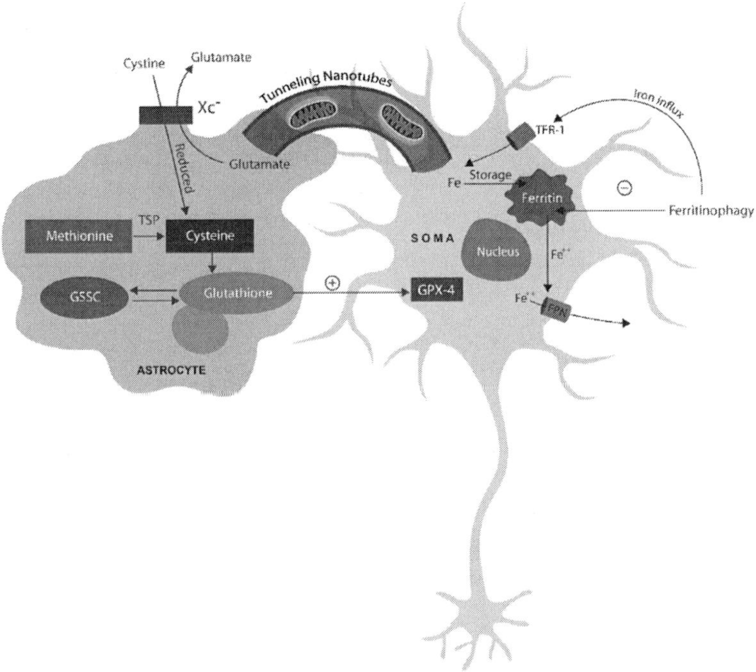


**Figure 2. Astrocytes support the postmitotic, long-lived neurons by helping them avert death by ferroptosis and loss of mitochondria. The former is accomplished by exporting GPX-4 to neurons (to repair oxidized lipids), while the latter by exporting healthy mitochondria to neuronal cells (via tunneling nanotubules, extracellular vesicles, or cell–cell fusion). Astrocytes import cystine via cystine/glutamate antiporter (Xc-). Cystine is reduced to cysteine and generates glutathione and GPX-4 (which is transferred to neurons). Cysteine can also be derived from methionine, while glutathione can be generated from cysteine and glutathione disulfide (GSSC). In neurons, iron is stored in ferritin and, when needed, ferritin undergoes ferritinophagy (autophagy) in lysosomes, releasing free iron. Iron ingresses the neuron via transferrin receptor 1 (TRF-1), while the excess intracellular iron is eliminated via ferroportin.**

action of haloperidol, suggesting that dopaminergic blockade is not the only psychosis-deterring mechanism of this drug. Indeed, ferroptosis of hippocampal neurons, documented in AD and severe mental illness, is the likely cause of cognitive impairment and negative symptoms in these conditions [123,124]. Prolonged insomnia has been demonstrated to damage the astrocyte which, in turn, may trigger neuronal demise [125].

Moreover, chronic sleep loss was demonstrated to activate both astrocytes and microglia, turning these cells into neurotoxic phenotypes capable of eliminating healthy neurons and synapses [126–128].

## 2. Mitochondria and Aryl Hydrocarbon Receptor

Recent studies have implicated mitochondria in the pathophysiology of sleep and neurodegenerative disorders, while the role of these organelles in severe mental illness, including SCZ and SLDs, has been previously established [129,130]. AhR is the master regulator of cellular senescence, a phenotype conducive to aging and neurodegeneration and is expressed by the mitochondrion [19–21]. Oxidized lipids in the mitochondrial membrane are AhR ligands, which in conjunction with senescence-upregulated intracellular iron, can trigger ferroptosis and organelle demise [131–134]. Indeed, lipid peroxides and oxysterols, such as 7KCl, are mitoAhR ligands, contributing to mitochondrial dysfunction and autophagic elimination [135].

AhR is a xenobiotic sensor which regulates cytochrome p450 and binds the environmental toxin, dioxin (2,3,7,8-tetrachlorodibenzo-p-dioxin). Other AhR ligands include somnogens, such as phenazines, melatonin, and tryptophan derivatives, which participate in the physiology of sleep, wakefulness, and the circadian rhythm [136–138]. In addition, reactive oxygen species (ROS), known to induce sleep via a redox-sensitive potassium channel, are AhR ligands, bringing this transcription factor in the arena of slumber, mental illness, and neurodegeneration [131,139]. Indeed, microbial phenazines, including pyocyanin and 1-hydroxyphenazine, activate AhR, influencing the transcription of many genes, including those involved in sleep regulation [140,141].

The importance of mitochondria in sleep physiology is further substantiated by the organelle involvement in FFI, as well as in general anesthesia [142,143]. Indeed, general anesthetics are known to inhibit N-methyl-d-aspartate (NMDA) and α-amino-3-hydroxy-5methyl-4-isoxazolepropionic acid (AMPA) glutamate receptors while stimulating GABA. NMDA and AMPA upregulate intracellular and mitochondrial calcium, inducing cell and organelle demise [144]. Interestingly, elevated mitochondrial calcium, a characteristic of prion diseases, may link these organelles to FFI [145,146]. Indeed, the prion peptide causes calcium inflow via L-type calcium channels, triggering neuronal damage and apoptosis [147]. In contrast, the typical antipsychotic, chlorpromazine, not only induces sleep, but also exerts anti-prion properties, probably by promoting autophagy of the misfolded protein [148–150].

Mitochondrial trafficking from astrocytes to neurons supports neuronal bioenergetic needs, especially in large pyramidal cells or VENs. Mitochondria can be imported via cell– cell fusion, tunneling nanotubes (cytoskeletal protrusions reaching to other cells), as well as transported by extracellular vesicles [151,152] (Figure 2). Moreover, astrocytes generate GPX-4 from cysteine obtained via the cystine/glutamate antiporter system (Xc) or by transmethylation of methionine. Glutathione is generated from cysteine and glutathione disulfide (GSSC) [153] (Figure 2).

Mitochondrial trafficking as well as autophagy (mitophagy) occur during sleep, probably explaining the reason most living beings require rest [154]. Interestingly, serotonin (5-HT) promotes mitochondrial transport in hippocampal neurons, suggesting that antidepressant drugs, serotonin reuptake inhibitors (SSRIs), may "exert their action by supplying healthy mitochondria to stressed neurons [155]. This may imply that ROS accumulation during wakefulness may induce slumber to repair oxidized lipids and import mitochondria from glial cells [120,131,139]. In addition, the accumulation of intracellular microtubuleassociated protein tau (MAPT) in VENs likely impairs mitochondrial transport, contributing to bvFTD pathogenesis [156].

### *2.1. Mitochondria-Protective Treatments*

The key role of mitochondria in sleep disorders, SCZ, SLDs, and neurodegeneration, highlights the importance of mitoprotective approaches to resuscitate, replace, or increase the import of mitochondria from glial cells [157]. For example, treatment with SSRIs during the early stages of dementia may delay the onset of cognitive decline. Along this line, a recent study found that treatment with SSRIs slowed the conversion of mild cognitive impairment to frank dementia, suggesting that prophylactic treatment with these agents may be beneficial [158]. In addition, natural anti-ferroptosis drugs and iron chelators, such as halogenated phenazines, may improve the course of neurodegenerative disorders, suggesting novel therapeutic strategies [159,160].

### 2.2. Membrane Lipid Replacement (MLR)

MLR refers to the oral supplementation with natural cell membrane glycerophospholipids and kaempferol (3,4′,5,7-tetrahydroxyflavone), a natural flavonoid found in tea, broccoli, cabbage, kale, beans, endive, leek, tomato, strawberries, and grapes [161]. Kaempferol is a glycogen synthase kinase-3β (GSK-3β) inhibitor which prevents sleep deprivation-induced cognitive decline [162,163]. Like lithium and several antipsychotic drugs, kaempferol blocks GSK-3β, an enzyme previously implicated in SCZ and circadian rhythm disorders, suggesting that this natural compound may exert antipsychotic properties without the adverse effects of conventional therapeutics [164–167].

The aim of MLR + kaempferol is the gradual replacement of damaged phospholipids and oxysterols from neuronal and/or mitochondrial membranes with natural glycerophospholipids and a polyphenol. Indeed, oxidized membrane lipids have been implicated in SCZ, SLDs, insomnia, and neurodegeneration, while MLR and kaempferol offer a dual mechanism of action: (1) elimination of lipid peroxides and (2) GSK-3β inhibition [168]. Replacing oxidized plasma and/or mitochondrial membrane fats with healthy natural lipids averts deformation of the neuronal membrane and misalignment of neuroreceptors. Conversely, oxidized membrane lipids and ferroptosis alter the biophysical properties of membranes, disrupting neuronal functions [169].

### 2.3. Phenazines and Phenothiazine Derivatives

Several natural phenazines and phenothiazines are neuroprotective, improve sleep, and delay neurodegenerative processes. For example, geranyl-phenazine is a naural acetylcholinesterase inhibitor which exerts antipsychotic effects via muscarinic receptors. Indeed, a new class of antipsychotic drugs is currently being developed for SCZ and a patent exists for treating sleep disorders by upregulating acetylcholine [170–172] (WO2005016327A2). Other natural phenazines with neuroprotective functions include baraphenazines A–G fused compounds derived from Streptomyces sp. PU-10A which likely possess antipsychotic properties [173]. Moreover, several natural phenazines, including baraphenazines, leucanicidin and endophenasides, exert antimicrobial, anticancer activity, and very likely possess antipsychotic properties [173–175].

Natural antipsychotic and phytotherapeutic compounds are not only devoid of extrapyramidal adverse effects but more accepted by many patients who often dread or distrust pharmaceuticals.

**Synthetic phenazine derivatives** consist of over 6000 compounds, exerting antimicrobial, antiparasitic, neuroprotective, anti-inflammatory, and anticancer activities [176–178]. To the best of our knowledge, natural or synthetic phenazines have not been tested for SCZ, insomnia, or neurodegeneration. Pontemazines A and B are neuroprotective phenazine derivatives that, in animal studies, have rescued hippocampal neurons from glutamate cytotoxicity, highlighting their pro-cognitive properties which could benefit patients with negative symptoms of SCZ or neurodegenerative disorders [176].

Synthetic phenazines exert antioxidant and radical-scavenging properties, and inhibit lipid peroxidation, suggesting beneficial effects in severe insomnia, mental illness and neurodegeneration [179,180] (Figure 3). Moreover, halogenated phenazines act as iron chelators, likely preventing neuronal ferroptosis [181]. We believe that pontemazines and halogenated phenazines should be assessed for antipsychotic/anti-neurodegenerative properties.

From the biochemical standpoint, phenazines are almost identical to phenothiazine antipsychotics and likely possess similar properties (Figure 4). Phenothiazines are typical antipsychotic drugs utilized primarily for SCZ and SLDs, which block dopaminergic transmission at the level of postsynaptic neuron. Several phenothiazines influence other receptors, including adrenergic, histaminergic, and cholinergic, exerting various clinical effects as well as adverse reactions. Aside from psychotic disorders, phenothiazines are also used for the treatment of migraine headaches, hiccups, nausea, vomiting, and cancer [182]. Like phenazines, phenothiazines intercalate themselves into the lipid bilayer of plasma and mitochondrial membranes, disrupting the curvature and receptor alignment on neuronal/mitochondrial surfaces [183] (Figure 3). In contrast, oxidized lipids, including 7-ketocholesterol (7KCl), form looped structures, generating membrane curvatures and pores that may trigger cell death [184].

**Antioxidant phenothiazine and their derivatives** have recently been developed for cancer, cardiovascular disease (CVD), Mycobacterium leprae and other antibiotic-resistant microbes [185,186].

Phenothiazine derivatives exert anti-peroxidation properties and protect against lipid pathology and ferroptosis, suggesting efficacy as antipsychotic drugs [187]. In addition, antioxidant phenothiazines are likely beneficial for insomnia and neurodegenerative disorders, suggesting that these compounds should be tested for neuropsychiatric pathology [186].

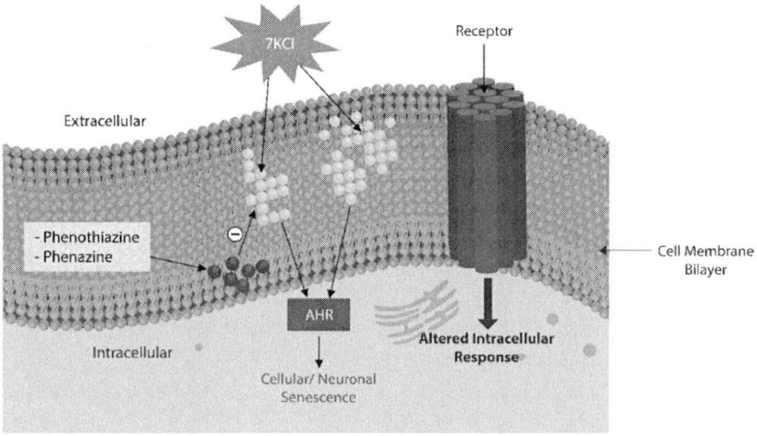


**Figure 3. The lipid bilayer of neuronal membrane is easily oxidated when intracellular iron is upregulated. Oxysterols, including 7-Ketocholesterol (a toxic oxide), and oxidated phospholipids alter the biophysical properties of cell membranes, disrupting neurotransmission. In addition, oxidized lipids activate AhR, triggering premature neuronal senescence. Phenazines, phenothiazines, and their derivatives, intercalate themselves into the lipid bilayer, repairing the lipids in cellular and/or mitochondrial membranes.**

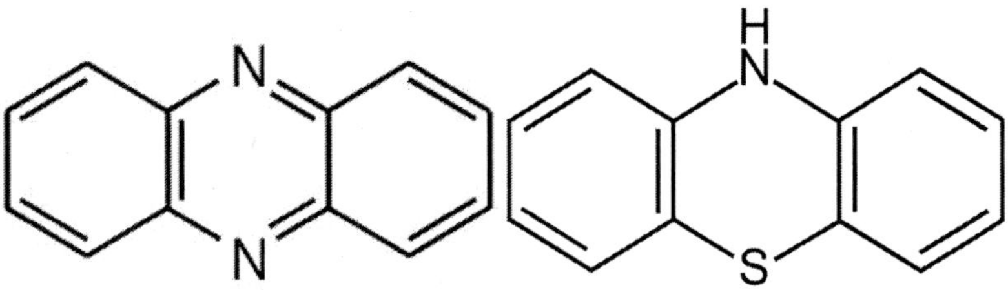


**Figure 4. Phenazine vs. phenothiazine: similarities and differences**

Propenylphenothiazine is a potent antioxidant with electron-donor capability that could prevent gray matter loss, a hallmark of SCZ and SLDs [188,189]. Electron-donating psychotropic drugs have been known to preserve the brain volume, suggesting that propenylphenothiazine may treat psychosis without reducing the gray matter volume. The majority of conventional antipsychotic drugs are electron-acceptors which often lower the brain volume as documented by many neuroimaging studies [190]. An even newer category of tetracyclic and pentacyclic phenothiazines with antioxidant properties has recently been developed, suggesting likely efficacy for cognitive impairment and negative SCZ symptoms. Moreover, the N10-carbonyl-substituted phenothiazines were demonstrated to inhibit lipid peroxidation, suggesting superior antipsychotic efficacy [191].

Natural and some synthetic phenazines and novel antioxidant phenothiazines have not been tested for SCZ, insomnia or neurodegenerative disorders but are likely efficient somnogens and antipsychotics. For example, synthetic phenazines, known as pontemazines A and B, rescued hippocampal neurons from glutamate cytotoxicity in rodents, highlighting their pro-cognitive properties which could benefit patients with negative symptoms of SCZ [192].

## *2.4. Natural Antioxidants*

SCZ and SLDs have been associated with premature cellular senescence, a phenotype marked by shortened telomeres, accumulation of macromolecular aggregates, increased level of senescence-associated β-galactosidase (SA-β-gal) and a detrimental secretome known as senescence-associated secretory phenotype (SASP).

**Natural Antioxidant Foods**

Antioxidants are major players in repairing damages to macromolecules, opposing pathological events associated with cellular senescence (Table 1). Since AhR is the master regulator of cellular senescence and responds to external pollutants (such as polycyclic aromatic hydrocarbons (PAHs) as well as internal toxins, including oxidized lipids, antioxidants likely have the opposite effect.

**Table 1. SCZ-relevant antioxidants and sources.**

| Antioxidants | Source | References |
|---|---|---|
| Lycopene | Grape skin, guava, grapefruit, blueberries, tomatoes | [193] |
| Apigenin | Cabbage, blueberries, acai berries | [194] |
| Phenolic acid | Oilseeds, cereals, grains | [195] |
| Curcumin | chicken, beef, tofu, vegetables | [196] |
| Epigallocatechin gallate | Apples, blackberries, broad beans, cherries, black grapes, pears, raspberries, and chocolate | [197] |
| Berberine | Oregon grape, phellodendron, and tree turmeric. | [198] |
| Quercetin | Fruits, apples, onions, parsley, sage, tea, and red wine | [199] |
| Kempferol | Fruits and vegetables. | [200] |
| Tocopherols | Oilseed, cereals, eggs, deary products | [201] |

## *2.5. Mitochondrial Transfer and Transplantation*

Early studies on mitochondrial transplantation from the 1980s utilized co-incubation of various cell types with naked mitochondria, hoping that cells would internalize the organelles from the extracellular environment [202–204]. Later, HeLa cells and mesenchymal stem cells were used as mitochondrial sources and found that successful organelle uptake occurred in a short time interval of 1–2 h [205–207]. At present, mitochondrial transplantation into cardiomyocytes has been accomplished successfully and confirmed by mitochondrial DNA (mtDNA) detected in host cells [208,209].

Mitochondrial transplantation and neuronal rescue from ferroptosis have been performed successfully in both animals and humans, suggesting a novel strategy for neurometabolic disorders [210]. To our knowledge, mitochondrial transplantation has not been attempted in sleep disorders, while in mental illness, it has been tried in animal models only [132]. Trafficking mitochondria from astrocytes and microglia to neurons can take place spontaneously after brain injuries, reflecting a likely compensatory mechanism to preserve neuronal viability [211]. In addition, it has been established that SSRIs, GJA1-20K, and CD38 signaling can facilitate mitochondrial transfer, emphasizing potential strategies for insomnia, severe mental illness, and neurodegeneration [210,211].

## 3. Conclusions

Forensic detainees with severe mental illness and comorbid insomnia age at an accelerated pace, suggesting that premature cellular senescence, a characteristic of SCZ, may comprise the common pathway where sleep and mental illness intersect. Loss of neurons due to impaired sleep may trigger the premature development of dementia and other age-related conditions, known to occur earlier in life compared to the general population. These comorbidities increase healthcare expenditures and shorten patients' lifespan; thus, identifying and treating these conditions early is crucial. YOD, a category of neurodegenerative disorders which include bvFTD, has been on the rise over the past few decades, as evidenced by the increased number of first offenders before the age of 65. Selective loss of VENs in bvFTD is likely due to the large size of these cells, predisposed to peroxidation of plasma membrane lipids and mitochondrial loss by dysfunctional autophagy.

At the molecular level, AhR is the equivalent of VENs, as this protein responds to both endogenous and exogenous ligands, including lipid peroxides and other insomnia and psychosis-related molecules.

Antioxidants and phenazine and phenothiazine derivatives are AhR ligands, highlighting potential natural treatment strategies against psychosis, insomnia, and neurodegeneration.

**Author Contributions**: Conceptualization, A.S. and P.G.B.; methodology, N.J.; validation, K.A.T. and I.A.O.; writing—review and editing, P.G.B. All authors have read and agreed to the published version of the manuscript.

**Funding:** This research received no external funding.

**Institutional Review Board Statement:** Not applicable.

**Informed Consent Statement:** Not applicable.

**Data Availability Statement:** Not applicable.

**Conflicts of Interest:** The authors declare no conflicts of interest.

## References

1. Sateia MJ, Doghramji K, Hauri PJ, Morin CM. Evaluation of chronic insomnia. An American Academy of Sleep Medicine review. Sleep. 2000;23:243–308.
2. Lindsay H Dewa, Bethan Thibaut, Natalie Pattison, Sean James Campbell, Thomas Woodcock, Paul Aylin, Stephanie Archer, Treating insomnia in people who are incarcerated: a feasibility study of a multi-component treatment pathway, SLEEP Advances, 2024; zpae003, https://doi.org/10.1093/sleepadvances/zpae003
3. Talih F, Ajaltouni J, Ghandour H, Abu-Mohammad AS, Kobeissy F. Insomnia in hospitalized psychiatric patients: prevalence and associated factors. Neuropsychiatr Dis Treat. 2018 Apr 10;14:969-975. Doi: 10.2147/NDT.S160742.
4. Wang Y, Li M, Li W, Xiao L, Huo X, Ding J, Sun T. Is the insula linked to sleep? A systematic review and narrative synthesis. Heliyon. 2022 Nov 5;8(11):e11406.
doi: 10.1016/j.heliyon.2022.e11406. PMID: 36387567; PMCID: PMC9647461

5. Li C, Dong M, Yin Y, Hua K, Fu S, Jiang G. Aberrant Effective Connectivity of the Right Anterior Insula in Primary Insomnia. Front Neurol. 2018 May 8;9:317. doi: 10.3389/fneur.2018.00317. PMID: 29867727; PMCID: PMC5951943.
6. Wylie KP, Tregellas JR. The role of the insula in schizophrenia. Schizophr Res. 2010 Nov;123(2-3):93-104. doi: 10.1016/j.schres.2010.08.027.
7. Fathy, Y.Y., Hoogers, S.E., Berendse, H.W. et al. Differential insular cortex sub-regional atrophy in neurodegenerative diseases: a systematic review and meta-analysis. Brain Imaging and Behavior 14, 2799–2816 (2020). https://doi.org/10.1007/s11682-019-00099-3
8. Koutsouleris N, Pantelis C, Velakoulis D, McGuire P, Dwyer DB, Urquijo-Castro MF, Paul R, Dong S, Popovic D, Oeztuerk O, Kambeitz J, et al. Exploring Links Between Psychosis and Frontotemporal Dementia Using Multimodal Machine Learning: Dementia Praecox Revisited. JAMA Psychiatry. 2022 Sep 1;79(9): 907-919. doi: 10.1001/jamapsychiatry.2022.2075.
9. Triarhou LC. The percipient observations of Constantin von Economo on encephalitis lethargica and sleep disruption and their lasting impact on contemporary sleep research. Brain Res Bull. 2006 Apr 14;69(3):244-58. doi: 10.1016/j.brainresbull.2006.02.002. Epub 2006 Mar 3. PMID: 16564419.
10. Allman JM, Tetreault NA, Hakeem AY, Manaye KF, Semendeferi K, Erwin JM, Park S, Goubert V, Hof PR. The von Economo neurons are in the frontoinsular and anterior cingulate cortex in great apes and humans. Brain Struct Funct. 2010 Jun;214(5-6):495-517. doi: 10.1007/s00429-010-0254-0.
11. Berg MT, Rogers EM, Lei MK, Simons RL. Losing Years Doing Time: Incarceration Exposure and Accelerated Biological Aging among African American Adults. J Health Soc Behav. 2021 Dec;62(4):460-476. doi: 10.1177/00221465211052568.
12. Kaiksow FA, Brown L, Merss KB. Caring for the Rapidly Aging Incarcerated Population: The Role of Policy. J Gerontol Nurs. 2023 Mar;49(3):7-11. doi: 10.3928/00989134-20230209-02.
13. Papanastasiou E, Gaughran F, Smith S. Schizophrenia as segmental progeria. J R Soc Med. 2011 Nov;104(11):475-84.

doi: 10.1258/jrsm.2011.110051.

14. Killilea DW, Wong SL, Cahaya HS, Atamna H, Ames BN. Iron accumulation during cellular senescence. Ann N Y Acad Sci. 2004 Jun;1019:365-7. Doi: 10.1196/annals.1297.063.
15. Urrutia PJ, Mena NP, Núñez MT. The interplay between iron accumulation, mitochondrial dysfunction, and inflammation during the execution step of neurodegenerative disorders. Front Pharmacol. 2014 Mar 10;5:38. Doi: 10.3389/fphar.2014.00038. PMID: 24653 700; PMCID: PMC3948003.
16. Carvalhas-Almeida C, Cavadas C, Álvaro AR. The impact of insomnia on frailty and the hallmarks of aging. Aging Clin Exp Res. 2023 Feb;35(2):253-269. doi: 10.1007/s40520-022-02310-w.
17. Carroll JE, Prather AA. Sleep and Biological Aging: A Short Review. Curr Opin Endocr Metab Res. 2021 Jun;18:159-164. doi: 10.1016/j.coemr.2021.03.021
18. Skonieczna-Żydecka K, Jamioł-Milc D, Borecki K, Stachowska E, Zabielska P, Kamińska M, Karakiewicz B. The Prevalence of Insomnia and the Link between Iron Metabolism Genes Polymorphisms, TF rs1049296 C>T, TF rs3811647 G>A, TFR rs7385804 A>C, HAMP rs10421768 A>G and Sleep Disorders in Polish Individuals with ASD. Int J Environ Res Public Health. 2020 Jan 8;17(2):400. doi: 10.3390/ijerph17020400.
19. Nacarino-Palma A, Rico-Leo EM, Campisi J, Ramanathan A, González-Rico FJ, Rejano-Gordillo CM, Ordiales-Talavero A, Merino JM, Fernández-Salguero PM. Aryl hydrocarbon receptor blocks aging-induced senescence in the liver and fibroblast cells. Aging (Albany, NY). 2022 May 26;14(10):4281-4304. doi: 10.18632/aging.204103.
20. Panda SK, Peng V, Sudan R, Ulezko Antonova A, Di Luccia B, Ohara TE, Fachi JL, Grajales-Reyes GE, Jaeger N, Trsan T, Gilfillan S, Cella M, Colonna M. Repression of the aryl-hydrocarbon receptor prevents oxidative stress and ferroptosis of intestinal intraepithelial lymphocytes. Immunity. 2023 Apr 11;56(4):797-812.e4. doi: 10.1016/j.immuni.2023.01.023.
21. Hwang HJ, Dornbos P, Steidemann M, Dunivin TK, Rizzo M, LaPres JJ. Mitochondrial-targeted aryl hydrocarbon receptor and the

impact of 2,3,7,8-tetrachlorodibenzo-p-dioxin on cellular respiration and the mitochondrial proteome. Toxicol Appl Pharmacol. 2016 Aug 1;304:121-32. doi: 10.1016/j.taap.2016.04.005.

22. Dietrich-Muszalska A, Kontek B. Lipid peroxidation in patients with schizophrenia. Psychiatry Clin Neurosci. 2010 Oct;64(5):469-75. doi: 10.1111/j.1440-1819.2010.02132.x. PMID: 20923426.
23. Feng S, Chen J, Qu C, Yang L, Wu X, Wang S, Yang T, Liu H, Fang Y, Sun P. Identification of Ferroptosis-Related Genes in Schizophrenia Based on Bioinformatic Analysis. Genes (Basel). 2022 Nov 20;13(11):2168. Doi: 10.3390/genes13112168.
24. Gulec M, Ozkol H, Selvi Y, Tuluce Y, Aydin A, Besiroglu L, Ozdemir PG. Oxidative stress in patients with primary insomnia. Prog Neuropsychopharmacol Biol Psychiatry. 2012 Jun 1;37(2):247-51. doi: 10.1016/j.pnpbp.2012.02.011.
25. Liang H, Van Remmen H, Frohlich V, Lechleiter J, Richardson A, Ran Q. Gpx4 protects mitochondrial ATP generation against oxidative damage. Biochem Biophys Res Commun. 2007 May 18;356(4):893-8. doi: 10.1016/j.bbrc.2007.03.045.
26. Seibt TM, Proneth B, Conrad M. Role of GPX4 in ferroptosis and its pharmacological implication. Free Radic Biol Med. 2019 Mar;133:144-152. Doi: 10.1016/j.freeradbiomed.2018.09.014. Epub 2018 Sep 13. PMID: 30219704.
27. Cole-Ezea P, Swan D, Shanley D, Hesketh J. Glutathione peroxidase 4 is major in protecting mitochondria from oxidative damage and maintaining oxidative phosphorylation complexes in gut epithelial cells. Free Radic Biol Med. 2012 Aug 1;53(3):488-97. doi: 10.1016/j.freeradbiomed.2012.05.029
28. Fujii R, Hasuo H, Sakuma H, Okada M, Uchitani K. The efficacy and safety of intravenous chlorpromazine treatment for sleep disturbance in patients with incurable cancer, with oral administration difficulty: a 1-week, prospective observational study. Ann Palliat Med. 2021 Aug;10(8):8547-8556. doi: 10.21037/apm-21-948.
29. Tischkau SA. Mechanisms of circadian clock interactions with aryl hydrocarbon receptor signaling. Eur J Neurosci. 2020 Jan;51(1):379-395. doi: 10.1111/ejn.14361. Epub 2019 Feb 25.

30. Fehsel K, Schwanke K, Kappel BA, Fahimi E, Meisenzahl-Lechner E, Esser C, Hemmrich K, Haarmann-Stemmann T, Kojda G, Lange-Asschenfeldt C. Activation of the aryl hydrocarbon receptor by clozapine induces preadipocyte differentiation and contributes to endothelial dysfunction. J Psychopharmacol. 2022 Feb;36(2):191-201. doi: 10.1177/02698811211055811.
31. Korade Ž, Liu W, Warren EB, Armstrong K, Porter NA, Konradi C. Effect of psychotropic drug treatment on sterol metabolism. Schizophr Res. 2017 Sep;187:74-81. doi: 10.1016/j.schres.2017.02.001.
32. Kiani A, Nik SH, Khodadoost A, Salimi A, Pourahmad J. Trifluoperazine an Antipsychotic Drug and Inhibitor of Mitochondrial Permeability Transition Protects Cytarabine and Ifosfamide-Induced Neurotoxicity. Drug Res (Stuttg). 2020 Jun;70(6):265-272. doi: 10.1055/a-1154-8672
33. Roy D, Pathak DN, Singh R. Effects of chlorpromazine on the activities of antioxidant enzymes and lipid peroxidation in the various regions of aging rat brain. J Neurochem. 1984 Mar;42(3): 628-33. Doi: 10.1111/j.1471-4159.1984.tb02728.x.
34. Ficarra S, Russo A, Barreca D, Giunta E, Galtieri A, Tellone E. Short-Term Effects of Chlorpromazine on Oxidative Stress in Erythrocyte Functionality: Activation of Metabolism and Membrane Perturbation. Oxid Med Cell Longev. 2016;2016:2394130. doi: 10.1155/2016/2394130.
35. Chen JY, Brunauer LS, Chu FC, Helsel CM, Gedde MM, Huestis WH. Selective amphipathic nature of chlorpromazine binding to plasma membrane bilayers. Biochim Biophys Acta. 2003 Sep 22;1616(1):95-105. doi: 10.1016/s0005-2736(03)00229-3
36. Korth C, May BC, Cohen FE, Prusiner SB. Acridine and phenothiazine derivatives as pharmacotherapeutics for prion disease. Proc Natl Acad Sci U S A. 2001 Aug 14;98(17):9836-41. doi: 10.1073/pnas.161274798.
37. Henkel, N.D., Wu, X., O'Donovan, S.M. et al. Schizophrenia: a disorder of broken brain bioenergetics. Mol Psychiatry 27, 2393–2404 (2022). https://doi.org/10.1038/s41380-022-01494-x

38. Hartmann C, Kempf A. Mitochondrial control of sleep. Curr Opin Neurobiol. 2023 Aug;81:102733. doi: 10.1016/j.conb.2023.102733.
39. Richardson RB, Mailloux RJ. Mitochondria Need Their Sleep: Redox, Bioenergetics, and Temperature Regulation of Circadian Rhythms and the Role of Cysteine-Mediated Redox Signaling, Uncoupling Proteins, and Substrate Cycles. Antioxidants (Basel). 2023 Mar 9;12(3):674. doi: 10.3390/antiox12030674.
40. A. A. Denis, D. Toledo, Q. A. Hakim, A. A. Quintana, C. R. Escobar, S. A. Oluwole, A. Costa, E. G. Garcia, A. R. Hill, C. Agatemor, Ligand-Independent Activation of Aryl Hydrocarbon Receptor and Attenuation of Glutamine Levels by Natural Deep Eutectic Solvent. ChemBioChem 2023, 24, e202300540.
41. Hayakawa, K., Esposito, E., Wang, X. et al. Transfer of mitochondria from astrocytes to neurons after stroke. Nature 535, 551–555 (2016). https://doi.org/10.1038/nature18928

# CHAPTER 8

# THE NEUROBIOLOGY OF HOMICIDE: GRAY MATTER VOLUME LOSS

Gray matter loss is a marker of chronic mental illness as well as dementia and was documented by multiple neuroimaging studies. GMV loss was associated with poor insight and homicidal behavior (1)(2)(3). At the cellular level, this phenomenon reflects premature brain aging.

In the past, patients with chronic SCZ or SLDs lived, on average, 15-20 years shorter than the general population and, for this reason, rarely exhibited dementia. Currently, due to improved medical care, hygiene, and nutrition, this group lives long enough to develop age-related diseases, including neurocognitive disorders.

## Central pathology: premature cellular senescence and gray matter volume loss

SCZ and SLDs, as well as dementia, are marked by premature cellular senescence, gray matter loss, and shorter telomeres (4)(5). The stable phase of SCZ, marked by cognitive and negative symptoms, is likely a prodromal dementia (6).

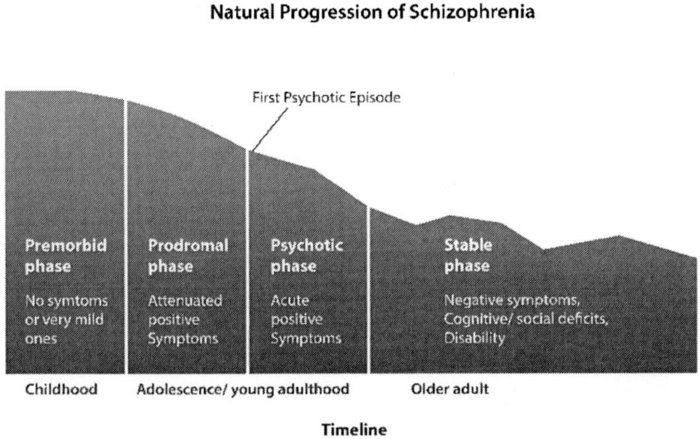


**The natural course of SCZ: the disorder starts in childhood with a premorbid phase with no or very mild symptoms. Attenuated symptoms, such as social isolation, anxiety, and insomnia, mark the prodromal phase. This blends gradually into the psychotic phase, during which patients are usually hospitalized numerous times for exhibiting positive symptoms. Around midlife, the positive symptoms gradually subside and are replaced by the negative and cognitive symptoms.**

Taking into consideration premature cellular senescence and gray matter loss brings forth the following treatment dilemmas:

## Treatment Dilemma #1

People living with SCZ (PLWS) require maintenance antipsychotic treatment to prevent recurrences, which may precipitate violent behavior, including homicide. On the other hand, antipsychotic drugs may cause cardiovascular and cerebrovascular events, phenomena poorly defined a generation ago (7).

Questions: should psychotropic drugs be decreased in elderly with lifelong SCZ and newly acquired dementia? Could the addition of a D1R agonist lower both the risk of these adverse reactions and aggressive behavior?

## Treatment Dilemma #2

Since DA plays a crucial role in learning and memory, do DAblocking agents precipitate dementia? (8). In this regard, several neuroimaging studies have revealed accelerated GMV reduction in SCZ patients treated with antipsychotic drugs (9)(10). In younger adults with SCZ, hippocampal, insular, and temporal lobe gray matter depletion was associated with an increased risk for homicide (3). In this regard, a recent study has suggested that the reduction of antipsychotic medication in chronic SCZ patients may be feasible, mainly when a selective DA 1R agonist is prescribed (11).

Question: can antipsychotic drugs precipitate aggressive behaviors?

## Treatment Dilemma #3

To delay premature brain aging, would older people living with SCZ (PLWS) benefit from senotherapeutic drugs? Senotherapeutics are divided into senolytics (selectively eliminate senescent cells) and senomorphics (delete senescence markers in old cells).

Question: Should senotherapeutic drugs be administered in conjunction with antipsychotics in PLWS?

## Antipsychotics and sustained recovery

Antipsychotic drugs are very effective for the treatment of acute psychosis and are likely to remain the golden standard of care for the foreseeable future. However, in chronic psychosis, these agents are less helpful and only marginally improve the overall outcome, suggesting that other options may need to be explored to prevent gray matter atrophy (12). For example, 13.5% of SCZ patients meet recovery criteria at any point in time during an initial psychotic episode (13). These outcome studies align with a large meta-analysis by Warner, R., who looked at the entire 20th century and found that today's prognosis is not different from that of the first decades of the past century (12)(14).

| Interval | Sustained Recovery | Employed |
|---|---|---|
| 1901-1920 | 20% | 4.7% |
| 1921-1940 | 12% | 11.9% |
| 1941-1955 | 23% | 4.1% |
| 1956-1975 | 20% | 5.1% |
| 1976-1995 | 20% | 6.9% |

**Sustained recovery in SCZ patients during the 20th century, including employment (Table adapted from Warner R data)**

## Take home message

As antipsychotic drugs do not address the core pathology of SCZ, SLDs, or dementia, novel strategies are urgently needed to address premature cellular senescence and the subsequent gray matter loss.

At the level of the gut barrier and BBB, premature cellular senescence alters the permeability, allowing gut microbes to translocate into host tissues and organs, including the brain, triggering neuropathology.

**The following articles discuss noncanonical approaches to SCZ, dementia, and aggressive behavior.**

# Article for Chapter 8: Novel Insights into Psychosis and Antipsychotic Interventions: From Managing Symptoms to Improving Outcomes

Adonis Sfera[1,2,3], Hassan Imran[1,2,3], Dan O. Sfera[1,2,3], Jacob J. Anton[4], Zisis Kozlakidis[5] and Sabine Hazan[6]

*1. Patton State Hospital, 3102 Highland Ave., Patton, CA 92369, USA; hassan.inran@dsh.ca.gov (H.I.)*
*2. University of California Riverside, Riverside 900 University Ave., Riverside, CA 92521, USA*
*3. Loma Linda University, 11139 Anderson St., Loma Linda, CA 92350, USA*
*4. California Baptist University, Riverside, CA 92521, USA*
*5. International Agency for Research on Cancer, 69372 Lyon, France*
*6. ProgenaBiome, Ventura, CA 93003, USA*

## Abstract

For the past 70 years, the dopamine hypothesis has been the key working model in schizophrenia. This has contributed to the development of numerous inhibitors of dopaminergic signaling and antipsychotic drugs, which led to rapid symptom resolution but only marginal outcome improvement. Over the past decades, there has been limited research on the quantifiable pathological changes in schizophrenia, including premature cellular/neuronal senescence, brain volume loss, the attenuation of gamma oscillations in electroencephalograms, and the oxidation of lipids in the plasma and mitochondrial membranes. We surmise that the aberrant activation of the aryl hydrocarbon receptor by toxins derived from gut microbes or the environment drives premature cellular and neuronal senescence, a hallmark of schizophrenia. Early brain aging promotes secondary changes, including the impairment and loss of mitochondria, gray matter depletion, decreased gamma oscillations, and a compensatory metabolic shift to lactate and lactylation. The aim of this narrative review is twofold: (1) to summarize what is known about premature cellular/neuronal senescence in schizophrenia or schizophrenia-like disorders, and (2) to discuss novel strategies for improving longterm outcomes in severe mental illness with natural senotherapeutics, membrane lipid replacement, mitochondrial transplantation, microbial phenazines, novel antioxidant phenothiazines, inhibitors of glycogen synthase kinase-3 beta, and aryl hydrocarbon receptor antagonists.

**Keywords:** aryl hydrocarbon receptor; dopamine; antipsychotic drugs; naturally occurring antipsychotics; senotherapeutics.

## 1. Introduction

The discovery of chlorpromazine in the 1950s revolutionized psychiatry and contributed to the deinstitutionalization of people with severe mental illness. Subsequently, the homelessness and incarceration of individuals with schizophrenia (SCZ) and schizophrenialike disorders (SLDs) dramatically increased, suggesting that symptomatic relief in these conditions rarely translates into sustained recovery [1,2].

Although most patients treated with antipsychotic drugs attain partial remission or amelioration of symptoms, few return to premorbid levels of functioning, measured by stable employment, attending school, raising a family, and being independent in all activities of daily living (ADLs) [3]. For this reason, large public institutions for the treatment of mental illness, such as state hospitals, are still in existence, while sanatoria for tuberculosis or leprosy were closed almost a century ago.

The early antipsychotic drugs were derived from methylene blue (MB), a phenothiazine synthesized in 1876 in Germany. The interest in this agent dramatically surged after the realization that it exerts antidepressant actions by inhibiting monoamine oxidase A (MAO-A), a surreptitious discovery that commenced the era of modern psychopharmacology [4]. Upon chlorpromazine's approval in the US, over 40 dopamine-blocking antipsychotic drugs were developed, aiming at restoring premorbid functioning by targeting major symptoms.

Although antipsychotic drugs are extremely efficacious for acute psychosis as the symptoms are often cleared within hours or days, sustained recovery is achieved by only 13.5% of patients after an initial psychotic episode [5]. Moreover, looking at the entire 20th century, in the early decades, long-term recovery was at 20%, not differing from the end of the century when antipsychotic drugs were being widely utilized [6]. At present, 33% of patients with SCZ relapse within 12 months after an initial psychotic episode, 26% remain homeless at the 2-year follow-up, and 5 years after the first psychotic outbreak, only 10% are employed [7–9]. Together, these data indicate that the blockade of dopamine (DA) receptors seldom improves the outcomes of SCZ or SLDs. Moreover, some antipsychotic drugs, including clozapine and aripiprazole, upregulate DA, suggesting that this neurotransmitter may play an indirect role in the etiopathogenesis of severe mental illness [10,11].

The aims of this narrative review are as follows:

1. To summarize what is known about the role of premature cellular/neuronal senescence in the pathogenesis of SCZ and SLDs.
2. To discuss potential strategies for improving sustained recovery in SCZ and SLDs via natural senotherapeutics, microbial phenazines, aryl hydrocarbon receptor (AhR) antagonists, membrane lipid replacement (MLR), and mitochondrial transplantation.

## 2. Premature Cellular Senescence in Schizophrenia

Patients with SCZ and SLDs live, on average, 15–20 years less than the general population, exhibit shortened telomeres, and develop age-related diseases earlier in life, suggesting that premature cellular senescence plays an important role in this pathology [12–15]. Indeed, many researchers and clinicians refer to SCZ as a "segmental progeria" to highlight the accelerated aging of tissues and organs, including the brain, in this disorder [12].

Cellular senescence is a program of permanent cell cycle arrest with an active metabolism, shortened telomeres, accumulation of macromolecular aggregates, increased levels of senescence-associated β-galactosidase (SA-β-gal), and a toxic secretome, known as the senescence-associated secretory phenotype (SASP), which can spread senescence to neighboring healthy cells [16]. It is believed that cellular senescence defends against tumorigenesis by preventing oncogene-driven malignant transformation. However, the accumulation of aged cells and the subsequent inflammation may paradoxically promote cancer and disrupt biological barriers, facilitating the dissemination of metastases [16,17]. Inflammation and senescent cells increase the permeability of the gut barrier, facilitating the translocation of the gastrointestinal (GI) tract bacteria (or their molecules) into the systemic circulation, a phenomenon encountered in neuropsychiatric and neurodegenerative disorders [18]. In another example, microbiota-derived gallic acid converts p53, the key anticancer protein, into an oncogene that drives tumorigenesis [19–21]. As p53, an SCZ risk gene, also promotes cellular senescence, it likely connects microbial translocation to severe mental illness [22,23]. Indeed, bacterial molecules were demonstrated to induce cellular senescence in neurons and microglia, as documented in SCZ [24–27]. For example, Escherichia coli (E. coli)-induced psychosis was reported in epidemics as well as in urinary tract infections (UTI), connecting bacteria to SCZ and SLDs [28].

Recent studies have found that downregulated DA receptors and transporters induce premature neuronal senescence, suggesting that dopaminergic signaling is required to avert early brain aging [29]. These findings were further substantiated by virus-induced senescence (VIS), a phenotype documented during the COVID-19 pandemic, marked by brain aging due to the infection of DA neurons [29,30]. Clostridium sp. are gut microbes also known for interfering with dopaminergic signaling, further linking cellular senescence to insufficient DA [31,32]. This is significant since both treated and untreated SCZ patients were found to exhibit body-wide premature cellular/neuronal aging, linking this condition to abnormal intestinal permeability [33,34]. Indeed, SCZ has been associated with increased microbial migration into the host's systemic circulation [35–37]. Furthermore, premature cellular senescence may contribute to the other

SCZ markers, including gray matter loss, decreased mitochondrial abundance, the attenuation of gamma (γ)-oscillations in EEGs, and the peroxidation of cell membrane lipids.

## *2.1. Ferrosenescence vs. Ferroptosis*

Fe2+ is an essential nutrient for both hosts and pathogens. It is also a cofactor in the biosynthesis of tyrosine hydroxylase and tryptophan hydroxylase, enzymes involved in the synthesis of DA and serotonin (5-HT), respectively. In the gut, DA acts as a microbial siderophore, which clears Fe2+ from the microenvironment, lowering the risk of ferroptosis [38,39].

Senescent cells, including neurons, upregulate intracellular Fe2+, which in the vicinity

of cytosolic lipids, may increase the risk of peroxidation and neuronal death by ferroptosis. In addition, senescence-upregulated lactate may also increase intracellular Fe2+ levels further, predisposing to neuronal demise [40]. Moreover, Fe2+ and lactate are known to enhance the biosynthesis of ceramide, a cell membrane lipid, which, in excess, can cause neurotoxicity [41,42]. Ferroptosis has been documented in SCZ; however, senescent cells are often resistant to programmed cell death, suggesting that impaired autophagy may drive iron-mediated brain aging [43–45]. Conversely, inducing ferroptosis in senescent cells precipitates their clearance by the immune system, indicating that this mechanism may be compensatory [46].

In our previous work, we introduced the concept of ferrosenescence, senescent cells, including neurons, with damaged DNA and dysfunctional p53-mediated genomic repair, as well as defective NKCs that are incapable of clearing senescent cells [47–49]. Ferrosenescent cells are resistant to ferroptosis due to impaired ferritin autophagy as well as the upregulation of ferroptosis inhibitors [glutathione peroxidase 4 (GPX-4) and apolipoprotein E (APOE)] [50–53]. For example, in SCZ, upregulated APOE, low ferritin levels, and increased intracellular Fe2+ levels likely reflect ferrosenescence [43,54]. Consequently, we believe that ferrosenescence may be more prevalent in SCZ than ferroptosis. Moreover, ferrosenescence may account for the other SCZ markers, including a decreased brain volume, γ-oscillations in EEGs, and mitochondrial dysfunction [55–58].

### 2.2. Senescent Gut Barrier

The relationship between the gut microbiome and senescent intestinal epithelial cells (IECs) is an emerging field that likely plays a major role in SCZ and SLDs [59,60]. For example, antibodies against translocated microbes, such as Hafnei alvei, Pseudomonas aeruginosa, Pseudomonas putida, and Klebsiella pneumoniae, were demonstrated in SCZ with negative symptoms, connecting microbial translocation to this pathology [61]. Moreover, translocated gut microbes may trigger nutritional immunity and iron sequestration in macrophages to withhold it from microbes, decreasing total circulatory Fe2+ levels [62]. In conditions of low circulatory Fe2+ levels, translocated bacteria may adopt a dormant state in human tissues, including the brain, awaiting increased Fe2+ availability to be reactivated [63,64].

The gut microbiota is immunologically tolerated in the gut lumen; however, upon translocation into the systemic circulation, the immune system is activated, triggering inflammation and, often, antibodies against microbial molecules. Since the microorganisms populating the GI tract express receptors identical or structurally related to human proteins, antibodies against these molecules may be construed as autoantibodies. Moreover, translocated microbes elicit inflammation, promoting cellular senescence, engendering a vicious circle in which senescent IECs facilitate the translocation of bacteria across the lamina propria, while inflammation triggered by these pathogens promotes further senescence [65–67].

Senescent cells were recently found to play a major role in the pathogenesis of inflammatory bowel disease (IBD), a condition marked by the translocation of microbes from the GI tract into the host tissues, including the brain [68]. This is further enhanced by the increased prevalence of SCZ in patients with IBD, emphasizing the role of the GI tract in severe mental illness [68,69]. Microbial translocation has been extensively studied in human immunodeficiency virus (HIV) infection, a condition marked by the massive exit of microbes from the GI tract due to interleukin-22 (IL-22) deficiency [70,71]. For this reason, we believe that recombinant IL-22 may comprise a new SCZ treatment [72].

## 3. Aryl Hydrocarbon, the Master Regulator of Cellular Senescence

The AhR is a ligand-activated transcription factor originally characterized as the receptor for dioxin (2,3,7,8-tetrachlorodibenzo-p-dioxin). Later, it was revealed that the AhR is also activated by various endogenous and exogenous ligands, driving multiple physiological processes and pathologies, likely including SCZ [73,74]. Aside from being the master regulator of cellular senescence, the AhR negatively regulates lactate and, by extension, the posttranslational modification, lactylation. As such, a dysfunctional AhR may drive both premature neuronal and glial aging as well as the excessive lactylation documented in SCZ and SLDs [75,76].

Several AhR ligands are molecules of interest in neuropsychiatry, including DA, phenazines, phenothiazines, serotonin, melatonin, and clozapine, suggesting that this transcription factor may play a significant role in the etiopathogenesis of SCZ (Figure 1) [77–79]. In prokaryotes, DA exerts iron-chelating properties; therefore, depletion in this neurotransmitter may upregulate intracellular Fe2+, leading to ferroptosis or ferrosenescence [39,43]. In addition, DA enhances the phagocytic properties of NKCs, facilitating the elimination of senescent and damaged cells [80]. Moreover, DA, via the DA 1 receptor (D1R), enhances the generation of acetylcholine (ACh), a neurotransmitter required for maintaining both the gray matter volume and rapid brain oscillations [81]. Conversely, lowering DA levels may promote inflammation by the accumulation of aged cells.

Compared with young neurons, senescent neuronal cells downregulate most surface receptors, including the dopaminergic and cholinergic ones, contain fewer mitochondria, and undergo metabolic and epigenetic reprogramming via lactate and lactylation, respectively [82]. Indeed, the lactylation of histone 3 (H3) lysine opposes neuronal senescence and restores the pre-senescent cellular status, suggesting that harnessing lactylation may comprise a potential neuropsychiatric therapy [83]. However, dysfunctional lactylation was shown to induce cell cycle reentry in senescent neurons, as

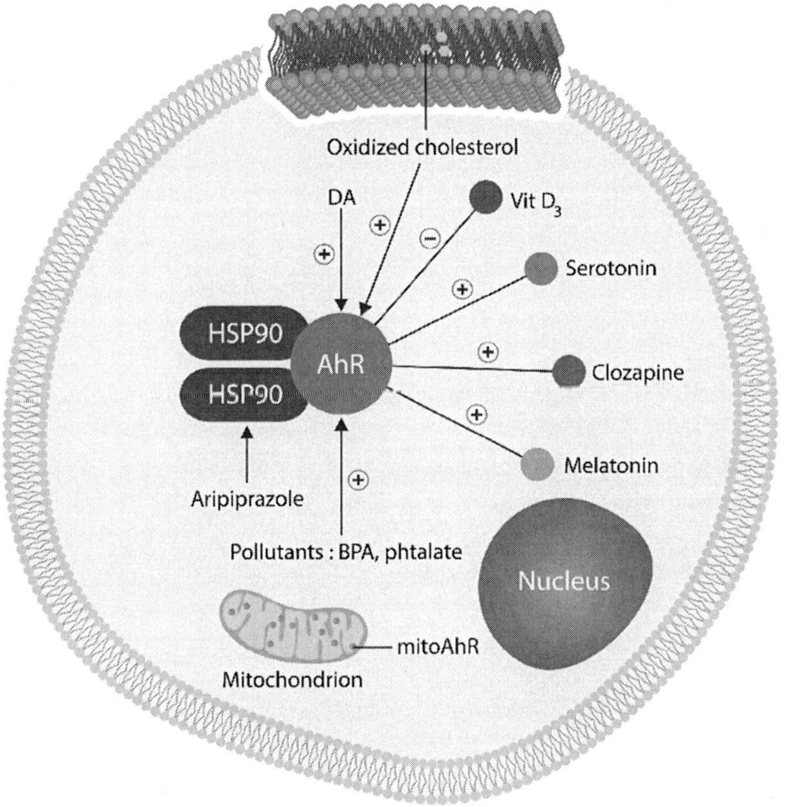


**Figure 1. In the cytosol, the AhR is stabilized by two HSP90 molecules. DA, oxidized lipids (and toxic ceramide), clozapine, serotonin, melatonin, and vitamin D3 are AhR ligands [95,96]. Pollutants, such as phthalate and bisphenol A (BPA), are also AhR ligands. In contrast, aripiprazole binds to the AhR chaperone, HSP90. HSP90 prevents AhR's entry into the nucleus where it drives the transcription of genes, including those for cellular senescence.**

demonstrated in Alzheimer's disease (AD) and other neurodegenerative disorders [84]. Moreover, senescent microglia with histone 3 (H3K18) lactylation were demonstrated to adopt a neurotoxic phenotype, engaging in the elimination of healthy synapses and neurons, a phenomenon documented in SCZ and neurodegeneration [85–89]. Following this line of research, preclinical studies have revealed that neuronal excitation and social stress enhance the lactylation of histones, further linking this posttranslational modification to the pathogenesis of SCZ and SLDs [90]. Furthermore, previous studies have associated SCZ with increased brain lactate levels and the alteration of histone proteins, suggesting that lactylated neurotoxic microglia may be more detrimental to severe mental illness than previously thought [91–94].

### *3.1. Gray and White Matter Loss*

The data on sustained remission in SCZ match with neuroimaging studies, showing life-long gray matter loss in both medicated and unmedicated patients. This is significant, as preventing or restoring brain volume homeostasis likely improves outcomes in severe mental illness [97–101]. Indeed, preclinical studies have shown that AhR homeostasis is directly correlated with brain volume, suggesting that DA/AhR binding is critical for averting parenchymal loss [95]. The AhR also preserves the gray matter volume by regulating the availability of ACh, which, like DA, acts as a brain volume guardian [102]. Low brain DA levels also induce white matter loss, but to a lesser extent in SCZ compared with demyelinating disorders [103, 104]. This is significant, as microbial toxins, including lipopolysaccharide (LPS), as well as environmental pollutants, such as plasticizers, are AhR ligands associated with SCZ. For example, the high comorbidity between SCZ and IBD may be the result of bacterial molecules "escaping" through the hyperpermeable intestinal barrier, a hallmark of IBD [105–107]. In addition, the higher prevalence of SCZ in northern regions of the world compared with the equatorial countries may be explained by AhR binding to vitamin D3 [96].

Taken together, DA is an indispensable neurotransmitter that prevents gray matter depletion by acting as an AhR ligand. Conversely, DA-blocking antipsychotic drugs may induce iatrogenic gray matter loss. This is further substantiated by the fact that clozapine, the most effective antipsychotic drug, is an AhR ligand that also upregulates DA levels [77,78,108].

### *3.2. Dopamine-Sparing Antipsychotics*

Like SCZ itself, treatment with firstand second-generation antipsychotic drugs is associated with gray matter loss, suggesting that brain DA levels are strictly regulated so that minimal fluctuations in this neurotransmitter may cause brain volume depletion [99,100,109–114].

Novel studies have found that antipsychotic drugs transfer positive or negative electrical charges to their substrates, donating or accepting electrons. For example, DA, lithium, clozapine, novel phenothiazines, and aripiprazole give away electrons, preserving the gray matter volume, while most other antipsychotics are electron acceptors and associated with brain volume loss [115–117]. More studies are needed to identify and develop DA-sparing, electron-donor antipsychotics.

## 4. Mitochondrial Dysfunction and Loss of Gamma-Band Oscillations

According to the endosymbiotic hypothesis, mitochondria are derived from ancestral bacteria and can communicate with the gut microbes via chemical messengers, such as ROS and sphingolipids [118–120]. Ceramide, one of the sphingolipids, is secreted by the microbiome and, in excess, can be toxic to mitochondria [121]. Senescent cells, including neurons, upregulate ceramide, probably accounting for the paucity of mitochondria in the aging brain [122–124]. Moreover, senescence-upregulated intracellular Fe2+ disrupts ceramide metabolism, further contributing to mitochondrial loss [125]. Indeed, ceramideinduced mitochondrial damage has been associated with atherosclerosis and SCZ, disorders associated with premature cellular senescence [126,127].

Acid sphingomyelinase (ASM), the enzyme catalyzing the conversion of sphingomyelin into ceramide, has been identified as an SCZ target, and ASM inhibitors, such as fluvoxamine and rosuvastatin, appear to ameliorate clinical outcomes in this disorder [128]. In addition, a natural alkaloid, berberine, decreases ceramide levels as well as inflammation, indicating a potentially beneficial effect on SCZ and SLDs [129,130].

Neurons have the capability of replacing defective mitochondria by importing them from microglia and astrocytes via tunneling nanotubules or extracellular vesicles (EVs) (Figure 2) [131,132]. Indeed, preventing neuronal loss by supplying mitochondria to neurons is one of the main functions of astrocytes.

Interestingly, antidepressant drugs in the class of serotonin reuptake inhibitors (SSRIs), including fluvoxamine, facilitate mitochondrial export to neuronal cells, emphasizing the neuroprotective role of these agents (Figure 3) [133]. Indeed, SSRIs were demonstrated to delay the conversion of mild cognitive impairment (MCI) into dementia, indicating that mitochondrial import contributes to neuronal rescue [134]. In addition, ferroptosisblocking drugs and iron chelators, including halogenated phenazines, may delay or prevent neurodegenerative disorders, suggesting a novel therapeutic approach (see the section on phenazines and phenothiazines) [135,136].

Aside from supplying healthy mitochondria to neurons, astrocytes also export antioxidants, including GPX-4, an enzyme involved in rescuing neuronal cells from ferroptosis. Additionally, ASM inhibitors, such as fluvoxamine, facilitate GPX-4 biosynthesis, averting ferroptosis. Indeed, fluvoxamine and other SSRIs preserve neuronal cells by both inhibiting ferroptosis and facilitating mitochondrial transfer [137,138]. GPX-4 is derived from cysteine, which enters astrocytes via the cystine/glutamate antiporter (Xc−) and enables the biosynthesis of glutathione and GPX-4 (Figure 2).

Given that γ-band frequencies are energy-consuming, mitochondria are essential for the generation of these rapid brain oscillations [139]. In this regard, preclinical studies have shown that lost γ-oscillations can be restored by inhibiting GSK-3β, an enzyme previously implicated in SCZ and SLDs [140,141]. Several antipsychotic drugs, including lithium, and natural compounds, kaempferol, are GSK-3β inhibitors and, therefore, capable of restoring the γ-rhythm (Figure 3).

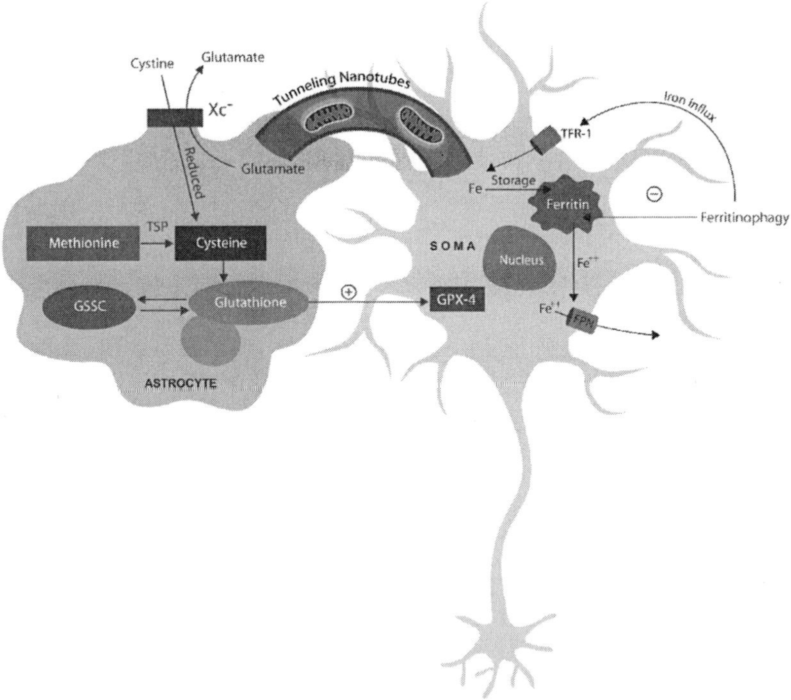


**Figure 2. Glial cells, including astrocytes, supply neurons with healthy mitochondria via tunneling nanotubules, preventing apoptosis [137,138]. In addition, astrocytes prevent neuronal ferroptosis by transferring antioxidants, including GPX-4. Astrocytes uptake cystine via the cystine/glutamate antiporter (Xc−). Cysteine can also be obtained from methionine via glutathione. Fe2+ enters neurons through the transferrin receptor-1 (TRF-1), which is stored in ferritin and requires ferritinophagy to be released. Excess Fe2+ exits the neurons via ferroportin (FPT) channels.**

## *Entrainment of Gamma-Band Oscillations in Schizophrenia*

Oscillations in the γ-range are rhythmic patterns of high-frequency (25 Hz to 100 Hz) EEG waves, playing a key role in cognition, attention, perception, and movement [142]. Under normal circumstances, this neuronal activity is synchronized across numerous brain regions, while in SCZ, there are γ-rhythm abnormalities, especially those elicited by auditory stimuli [143,144].

Interneurons, including parvalbumin (PV), vasoactive intestinal polypeptide (VIP), and somatostatin (SST), are the main drivers of γ-rhythms, indicating that the defective inhibition of pyramidal cells may trigger the loss of rapid rhythms [145,146]. Regarding neurotransmitters, γ-oscillations are dependent on ACh, an AhR-regulated biomolecule controlled by acetylcholinesterase (AChE), a direct AhR ligand [147].

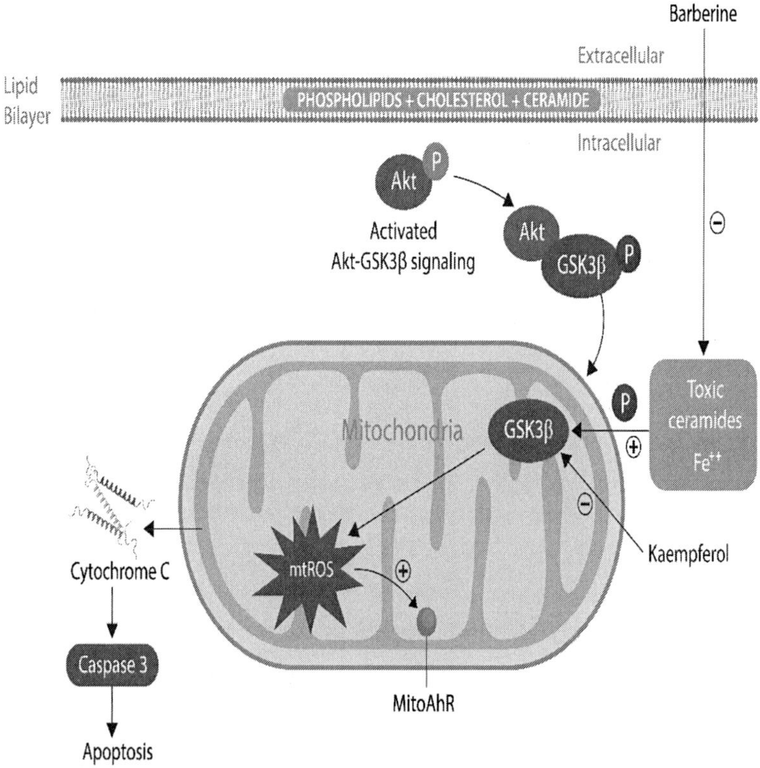


**Figure 3. The AhR is represented in the cytosol and mitochondria (mitoAhR). Akt negatively phosphorylates GSK-3β, inhibiting its function. Toxic ceramides and iron activate GSK-3β, resulting in excessive mitochondrial ROS (mtROS) levels, which activate the mitoAhR, triggering organelle death. mtROS can also cause mitochondrial demise by activating cytochrome-C and caspase-3. The natural compounds berberine and kaempferol inhibit GSK-3β, averting organelle death.**

Several studies have connected γ-oscillations to the microbiome-derived ACh, linking rapid EEG rhythms to intestinal microbes [148,149]. This is significant, as decreased brain ACh levels in SCZ have been associated with gray matter loss, emphasizing the key role of the AhR and AChE in maintaining both brain volume and rapid oscillations [150,151]. Given the important role of the cholinergic system in SCZ, it is not surprising that novel ACh-based antipsychotics have been developed [130,152].

Aside from ACh and mitochondrial import, lost γ-oscillations may be restored by entrainment with sensory stimuli, such as ultrasound or transcutaneous vagal nerve stimulation (tVNS) at 40 Hz, emphasizing a potential strategy for SCZ and SLDs [149,153]. Interestingly, tVNS improves not only neuronal function but also optimizes gut permeability, decreasing microbial translocation [149,154].

## 5. Senotherapeutics

It is currently established that severe mental illness is associated with cellular/neuronal senescence, indicating that endogenous or exogenous toxins may play a key role in this pathology [155–157]. For example, viral or bacterial infections induce premature aging in brain cells by eliciting immune responses, likely triggering psychosis [158,159]. Indeed, new-onset psychosis was documented in infections with senescence-inducing viruses including HIV and SARS-CoV-2 [160,161].

Senotherapeutics are natural or synthetic compounds that can delay, prevent, or reverse cellular/neuronal senescence. Senotherapeutics comprise senolytic agents that facilitate the elimination of senescent cells, and senomorphic compounds capable of deleting senescence markers, including SASP and SA-β-gal [162]. While, in the past, it was thought that cellular senescence could not be reversed, newer studies have found that inhibiting 3-phosphoinositide-dependent protein kinase-1 (PDK1) can revert cellular senescence in humans [163]. Interestingly, PDK1 is an upstream modulator of SCZ-linked GSK-3β.

Senolytic antibiotics belong to a distinct class of agents that include azithromycin, minocycline, and roxithromycin and possess neuroprotective, anti-inflammatory, and senolytic properties [164]. For example, it has been known for some time that minocycline may be beneficial for SCZ, suggesting that senolytics have a place in the treatment of SCZ and SLDs, probably by clearing neurotoxic glial cells [165].

Other senolytic agents relevant to SCZ and SLDs are summarized in Table 1.

**Table 1. Natural senolytics and their sources.**

| Senolytics | Sources | Reference |
|---|---|---|
| Lycopene | Grape skin, guava, grapefruit, blueberries, and tomatoes | [166] |
| Apigenin | Cabbage, blueberries, and acai berries | [167] |
| Fisetin | Strawberries, onions, apples, mangoes, persimmons, and kiwis | [168] |
| Curcumin and EF24 analog | Chicken, beef, tofu, and vegetables | [169] |
| Epigallocatechin gallate | Apples, blackberries, broad beans, cherries, black grapes, pears, raspberries, and chocolate | [170] |
| Berberine | Oregon grape, phellodendron, and tree turmeric | [171] |
| Quercetin | Fruits, apples, onions, parsley, sage, tea, and red wine | [172] |
| Kaempferol | Fruits and vegetables | [173] |

A senolytic vaccine recently tested in progeroid mice may usher in a new era of neuropsychiatry, raising the possibility of vaccination or serum treatment for SCZ and SLDs [174]. Another immunological intervention, an antibody–drug conjugate against a membrane senescence marker, was demonstrated to clear senescent, damaged, or infected cells, emphasizing a new therapeutic strategy [175].

## 6. Membrane Lipid Replacement (MLR)

MLR refers to the oral administration of natural cell membrane glycerophospholipids, along with kaempferol (3,4′,5,7-tetrahydroxyflavone), a flavonoid found in tea, broccoli, cabbage, kale, beans, endive, leek, tomato, strawberries, and grapes [176]. Like lithium and some antipsychotics, kaempferol is an inhibitor of GSK-3β, suggesting that it may exert antipsychotic properties without the typical adverse effects of psychotropic drugs [177,178]. The administration of MLR + kaempferol gradually replaces damaged phospholipids, ceramides, and oxysterols from neuronal and/or mitochondrial membranes with natural glycerophospholipids and a polyphenol.

Oxidized membrane lipids are AhR ligands that have previously been implicated in the pathogenesis of SCZ (Figure 1). MLR and kaempferol exert a dual mechanism of action: the elimination of lipid peroxides and GSK-3β inhibition [179]. Replacing oxidized plasma and/or mitochondrial membrane fats with healthy natural lipids averts ferroptosis and optimizes neurotransmission by correcting membrane distortion. Conversely, oxidized membrane lipids can trigger neuronal demise by ferroptosis [180]. Indeed, MLR reverses biophysical changes in the plasma and mitochondrial membrane induced by oxidized lipids. This action is not different from that of phenothiazines, which insert themselves into the lipid bilayer, lowering the curvature of cell membranes (Figure 4). In contrast, oxidized lipids form looped structures and generate membrane curvatures and pores, which leads to cell death [181].

## 7. Phenazines and Antioxidant Phenothiazines

Phenazines are microbial metabolites produced by various soil and water microorganisms that exert antibacterial, anticancer, antimalarial, and antipsychotic properties [184].

### *7.1. Natural Phenazines*

Natural phenazines are synthesized by bacteria, including Streptococcus species and Pseudomonas aeruginosa, the latter known for generating pyocyanin(5-N-methyl-1-hydroxyphenazine), a compound with electron-shuttling properties [185,186].

Neuroprotective natural phenazines such as geranyl-phenazine, an AChE inhibitor, upregulate ACh, exerting antipsychotic effects via muscarinic receptors [187,188]. Another natural phenazine with neuroprotective functions, bara-phenazines A–G, are fused molecules with antipsychotic properties derived from Streptomyces sp. PU-10A [189].

### *7.2. Synthetic Phenazine Derivatives*

Synthetic phenazine derivatives consist of over 6000 compounds, exerting antimicrobial, antiparasitic, neuroprotective, anti-inflammatory, and anticancer activities. Pontemazines A and B are neuroprotective phenazines derived from Streptomyces sp. UT1123, which, in animal studies, rescued hippocampal neurons from glutamate cytotoxicity, highlighting their pro-cognitive properties that could benefit patients with negative SCZ symptoms [190]. Pontemazines exert antioxidant, radical-scavenging properties and inhibit lipid peroxidation, suggesting beneficial effects on SCZ [191]. Halogenated phenazines act as iron chelators and are probably helpful against ferroptosis [192,193]. We believe that pontemazines and halogenated phenazines should be assessed for their antipsychotic and anti-neurodegenerative properties (Figure 4).

From a biochemical standpoint, phenazines are almost identical to phenothiazine antipsychotics and likely possess similar properties (Figure 5). Phenothiazines are typical antipsychotic drugs utilized primarily for SCZ and SLDs that block dopaminergic transmission at the level of postsynaptic neurons. They also correct the curvature and receptor alignment on neuronal/mitochondrial surfaces, restoring signaling homeostasis (Figure 4) [182]. In contrast, oxidized lipids, toxic ceramides, and 7-ketocholesterol (7KCl) form looped structures, generating membrane curvatures and pores that may lead to neuronal death [183].

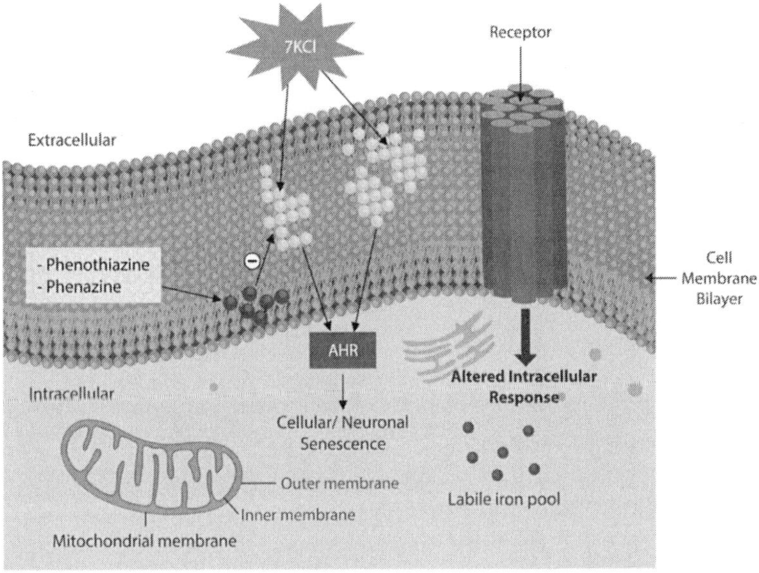


**Figure 4. The lipid bilayer of neuronal membranes is easily oxidated when intracellular iron is upregulated [182]. Oxysterols, including 7-ketocholesterol (a toxic oxide), and oxidated phospholipids alter the biophysical properties of cell membranes, disrupting neurotransmission [183]. In addition, oxidized lipids activate the AhR, triggering premature neuronal senescence. Phenazines, phenothiazines, and their derivatives intercalate themselves into the lipid bilayer, repairing the lipids in cellular and/or mitochondrial membranes.**

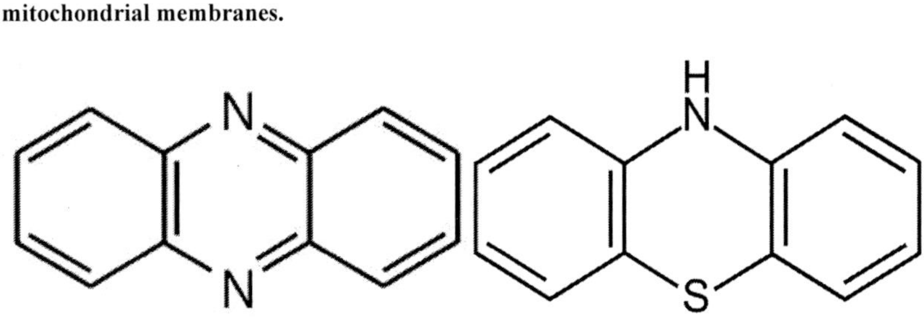


**PHENAZINE** **PHENOTHIAZINE**

**Figure 5. Phenazine vs. phenothiazine: similarities and differences.**

### *7.3. Antioxidant Phenothiazines and Their Derivatives*

Antioxidant phenothiazines and their derivatives have recently been developed for cancer, cardiovascular disease (CVD), Mycobacterium leprae, and other antibiotic-resistant microbes [194].

Phenothiazine derivatives exert anti-peroxidation properties and protect against lipid pathology and ferroptosis, suggesting their efficacy as antipsychotic drugs [195]. Phenothiazine nuclei possess hydrophobic properties that facilitate their insertion into the plasma or mitochondrial membranes [196].

Propenyl-phenothiazine is a potent antioxidant with electron-donor capabilities that likely prevents gray matter loss in patients with SCZ or SLDs. Moreover, a new category of tetracyclic and pentacyclic phenothiazines with antioxidant properties have recently been developed, suggesting their likely efficacy for cognitive impairment and negative SCZ symptoms [197,198]. Furthermore, N10-carbonyl-substituted phenothiazines were demonstrated to inhibit lipid peroxidation, suggesting their enhanced antipsychotic efficacy [100].

## 8. Mitochondrial Transfer and Transplantation

Mitochondrial transplantation experiments started in the 1980s, wherein naked organelles were co-incubated with various cell types, attempting to facilitate internalization [199]. Using HeLa cells and mesenchymal stem cells as mitochondrial sources, this transplantation technique takes only 1–2 h to supply organelles to mitochondria-depleted cells [200–202]. At present, mitochondrial transplantation in cardiomyocytes is possible and can be confirmed by the presence of mitochondrial DNA (mtDNA) in the heart [203,204].

Mitochondrial transplantation to rescue neurons from ferroptosis is currently possible and has been successfully performed in both animals and humans; however, to the best of our knowledge, it has not been attempted as a treatment for mental illness [205].

Rescuing the mitochondria with MLR, kaempferol, and berberine (Figure 6) is a strategy for averting GSK-3β overactivation by toxic ceramides, oxysterols, or oxidized phospholipids [130,206]. In addition, SSRIs, GJA1-20K, and CD38 signaling were demonstrated to facilitate mitochondrial transfer, emphasizing potential strategies for restoring neurometabolic homeostasis in severe mental illness and neurodegeneration [207,208].

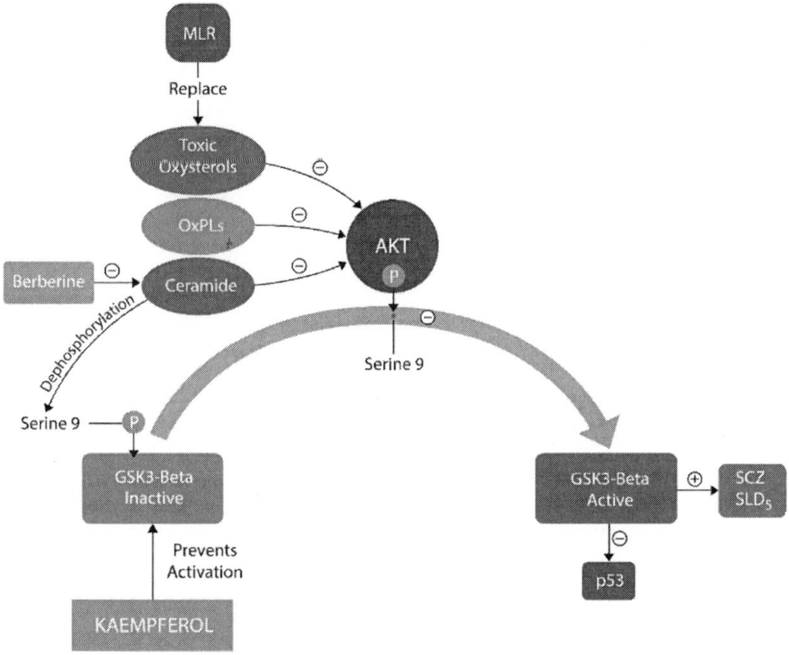


**Figure 6. Membrane lipid replacement (MLR) replenishes oxidized lipids from the plasma and mitochondrial membrane, such as oxysterols, ceramide, and oxidized phospholipids (OxPLs) with natural glycerophospholipids. Oxidized lipids inhibit AKT (by serine-9 phosphorylation), activating GSK-3β, an enzyme associated with SCZ, SLDs, and cancer (by p53 inhibition). Berberine and kaempferol inhibit GSK-3β activation by different mechanisms, generating beneficial effects. Ceramide activates GSK-3β by the dephosphorylation of serine-9.**

## 9. Using AhR Antagonists as Antipsychotics

Aberrant AhR overactivation has been associated with psychosis, while several antagonists of this receptor exert antipsychotic properties. The following natural and synthetic AhR inhibitors were found to be therapeutic for SCZ:

1. Quercetin is a natural flavonoid and plant pigment that exerts antioxidant and anticancer properties. In the CNS, quercetin is a negative allosteric modulator of GABARs as well as an enhancer of glutamatergic neurotransmission, a signaling pathway deficient in SCZ [209]. In addition, quercetin inhibits the apoptosis of cortical neurons, likely preventing gray matter loss.
2. Apigenin is a plant-based remedy extract from Elsholtzia rugulosa used by traditional practitioners from Africa for treating mental illness. Aside from antagonizing the AhR, apigenin exhibits vasorelaxant, antioxidant, and antipsychotic properties [209].
3. Alstonine is an indole alkaloid with antipsychotic effects that increases serotonergic, but not dopaminergic, signaling, possibly facilitating mitochondrial transfer [209,210].
4. Luteolin is a natural antipsychotic that exerts its beneficial actions by reducing microglial inflammation [202]. Luteolin is currently under clinical trials for SCZ treatment (NCT05204407).

## 10. Synthetic AhR Antagonists

Synthetic AhR antagonists are anti-inflammatory and anticancer compounds that likely exert antipsychotic properties.

IK-175 (structure undisclosed) was shown to block ligand-mediated AhR activation in preclinical studies. IK-175 was recently approved for cancer treatment, and it may possess antipsychotic properties [211].

HBU651 is a novel synthetic AhR antagonist developed primarily for cancer treatment that appears to be a suitable candidate for SCZ treatment [212]. Figure 7 summarizes AhR agonists/antagonists relevant for neuropsychiatry.

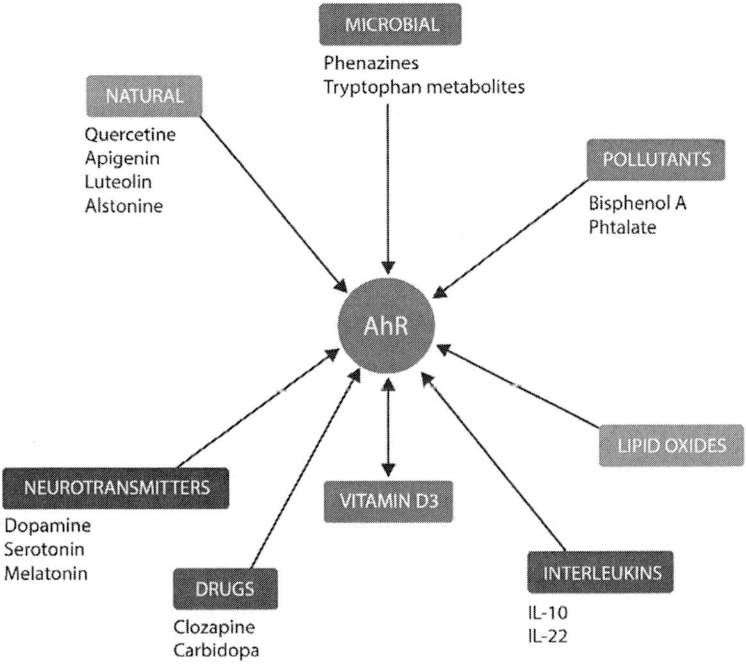


**Figure 7. AhR agonists and antagonists relevant for neuropsychiatry [74,213–222].**

## 11. Recombinant Interleukin-22

Recombinant interleukin-22 (IL-22) is a pleiotropic cytokine known for facilitating tissue regeneration and protecting the GI tract barrier. Recombinant IL-22, comprising two molecules connected by a fusion protein, exerts better efficacy with reduced systemic side effects [223].

In our previous work, we hypothesized that SCZ and SLDs may be initiated by aberrant AhR hyperactivation by endogenous or exogenous ligands, including intestinal or environmental toxins, such as LPS or plasticizers, respectively [224].

This hypothesis is supported by the following findings:

1. SCZ is often comorbid with IBD, conditions associated with increased gut barrier permeability and microbial translocation from the GI tract into host tissues, including the brain.
2. Translocation markers, including soluble CD14 (sCD14) and lipopolysaccharidebinding protein (LBP), are elevated in SCZ, suggesting bacterial translocation.
3. Increased BBB permeability in SCZ enables translocated gut microbes to reach the brain. The following are examples of pathogens triggering psychosis:
   i. The Escherichia coli (E. coli) outbreak in 2011 in Germany has been associated with cases of new-onset psychosis.
   ii. New-onset psychosis, or its exacerbation, has been identified in E. coli-associated UTIs.

IL-22 has been successfully used to restore the integrity of the gut barrier in various conditions, including IBD, HIV, and nonalcoholic fatty liver disease [225,226]. We construe that recombinant IL-22 would be effective for SCZ by limiting the translocation of bacteria and/or their molecules.

Table 2 summarizes the major representatives from the categories discussed above with potential therapeutic properties for SCZ and SLDs.

**Table 2. Naturally occurring and synthetic compounds with potential benefits for SCZ and SLDs.**

| Compound | Naturally Occurring | Synthetic |
|---|---|---|
| Phenazines | Geranyl-phenazine and bara-phenazines A | Pontemazines A and B and halogenated phenazines |
| Phenothiazines | | Propenyl-phenothiazine and N10-carbonyl-substituted phenothiazines |
| GSK-3β inhibitors | Kaempferol and curcumin | Lithium, valproic acid, clozapine, and olanzapine. |

| | | |
|---|---|---|
| AhR inhibitors | Quercetin, apigenin, alstonine and luteolin | IK-175 and HBU651 |
| Acid sphingomyelinase (ASM) inhibitors | | Fluvoxamine, rosuvastatin, and tricyclic antidepressants. |
| Dopamine D1R agonists | | Fluvoxamine, rosuvastatin, and dihydrexidine |
| Mitochondrial export | | SSRIs |
| ACh agonists | Catharanthus roseus and Salvia spp. (Lamiaceae) | Cholinesterase inhibitors: donepezil, galantamine, and rivastigmine |
| Senotherapeutics | Quercetin, apigenin, alstonine and luteolin | Senotherapeutic antibiotics |
| Ferroptosis inhibitors | Natural flavonoids and berberine | Fluvoxamine, SSRIs, and N acetyl cysteine (NAC) |
| | Recombinant IL-22 | |
| | Membrane lipid replacement | |
| | Mitochondrial transplantation | |
| | 40 HZ entrainment with sensory stimuli | |

## 12. Vehicles: Lipid Nanoparticles

The COVID-19 pandemic has accelerated the development of lipid nanoparticles (LNPs), vehicles for drug delivery. As LNPs are liposoluble, they can access specific body niches, including the brain [227].

The COVID-19 messenger RNA (mRNA) vaccines, Pfizer-BioNTech and Moderna, are incorporated in LNPs comprising four lipids: 1,2-distearoyl-sn-glycero-3-phosphocholine (DSPC), PEG, an alternative cholesterol, and ionizable lipids such as SM-102 or ALC0315 [228]. SM-102, ALC-0315, and the alternative cholesterol are proprietary molecules and have not been revealed. However, looking at the previous LNP research, the ionizable lipids likely resemble DLin-MC3-DMA, which was approved by the Food and Drug Administration (FDA) for transthyretin-mediated amyloidosis [229–231]. Like phenothiazines, LNPs enter cells, including neurons, through the endocytic pathway (EP). Subsequently, LNPs travel from the early to late endosomes, but not to lysosomes because the organelle pH of 4.5–5.0 could degrade the nanoparticles. Therefore, "lysosomal escape" into the cytosol must occur from the late endosomes without interfering with autophagy, as most antipsychotic drugs do.

Utilizing LNPs not for vaccination, but as a vehicle for transporting psychotropic drugs directly to the neuronal networks could revolutionize psychopharmacology. As nano-doses of antipsychotics or mood stabilizers would be utilized for the treatment of psychotic symptoms or affective disorders, systemic adverse effects would be avoided. We surmise that LNPs would be extremely efficacious as vehicles for psychotropic drugs.

## 13. Conclusions

Antipsychotic drugs are extremely helpful for the acute symptoms of SCZ or SLDs; however, sustained recovery (measured by the ability to hold a job, go to school, raise a family, or be independent in ADLs) is rarely achieved. For this reason, the next chapter in neuropsychopharmacology will have to improve functionality rather than symptom resolution. Over the past 70 years, it has become obvious that lowering dopaminergic transmission does not restore premorbid functions in patients with SCZ and SLDs. DA is an indispensable neurotransmitter that maintains the integrity of the brain parenchyma, a physiological function disrupted by both SCZ and its treatment.

The study of neuronal senescence-induced neuropsychiatric disorders is in its infancy but is rapidly developing, especially after the advent of age-accelerating viruses, such as HIV and COVID-19. Aberrantly activated AhR, the master regulator of cellular senescence, explains not only how gut microbes and/or their molecules trigger psychosis but also how environmental pollutants precipitate SCZ or SLDs. AhR hyperactivation likely accounts for gray matter reduction, the loss of rapid brain oscillations, and oxidized lipids in the plasma and mitochondrial membranes. The recent discovery that DA, serotonin, vitamin D3, clozapine, and melatonin are AhR ligands has opened new horizons in the management of chronic psychosis. Novel strategies, such as natural senotherapeutics, MLR, GSK-3β, ceramide inhibitors, recombinant IL-22, mitochondrial transplantation or transfer, and AhR antagonists, could improve long-term recovery in SCZ or SLDs. Senescence-associated downregulation of ACh and DA likely reduces brain volume and rapid oscillations, contributing to deficit symptoms.

The utilization of natural compounds, such as kaempferol or berberine, alone or in conjunction with LNP-delivered DA-sparing antipsychotic drugs, may improve sustained recovery in patients with severe mental illness.

**Author Contributions:** A.S. conceptualization, S.H. writing—review and editing, D.O.S. data curation, H.I. methodology and software, J.J.A. draft preparation, Z.K. supervision. All authors have read and agreed to the published version of the manuscript.

**Funding:** This research received no external funding.

**Institutional Review Board Statement:** Not applicable.

**Informed Consent Statement:** Not applicable.

**Data Availability Statement:** Not applicable.

**Conflicts of Interest:** The authors declare no conflicts of interest. Where authors are identified as personnel of the International Agency for Research on Cancer/WHO, the authors alone are responsible for the views expressed in this article and they do not necessarily represent the decisions, policy or views of the International Agency for Research on Cancer/WHO.

## References

1. Lincoln TM, Hodgins S. Is lack of insight associated with physically aggressive behavior among people with schizophrenia living in the community? J Nerv Ment Dis. 2008 Jan;196(1):62-6. doi: 10.1097/NMD.0b013e31815faa4d.
2. Cooke MA, Fannon D, Kuipers E, Peters E, Williams SC, Kumari V. Neurological basis of poor insight in psychosis: a voxel-based MRI study. Schizophr Res. 2008 Aug;103(1-3):40-51. doi: 10.1016/j.schres.2008.04.022.
3. Cope LM, Ermer E, Gaudet LM, Steele VR, Eckhardt AL, Arbabshirani MR, Caldwell MF, Calhoun VD, Kiehl KA. Abnormal brain structure in youth who commit homicide. Neuroimage Clin. 2014 May 10;4:800-7. Doi: 10.1016/j.nicl.2014.05.002.
4. Constantinides, C., Han, L.K.M., Alloza, C. et al. Brain aging in schizophrenia: evidence from 26 international cohorts via the ENIGMA Schizophrenia consortium. Mol Psychiatry 28, 1201–1209 (2023). https://doi.org/10.1038/s41380-022-01897-w
5. Yu WY, Chang HW, Lin CH, Cho CL. Short telomeres in patients with chronic schizophrenia who show a poor response to treatment. J Psychiatry Neurosci. 2008 May;33(3):244-7. Erratum in: J Psychiatry Neurosci. 2008 Jul;33(4):343.
6. Lieberman JA. Neurobiology and the natural history of schizophrenia. J Clin Psychiatry. 2006 Oct;67(10):e14. PMID: 17107237.
7. Zivkovic S, Koh CH, Kaza N, Jackson CA. Antipsychotic drug use and risk of stroke and myocardial infarction: a systematic review and meta-analysis. BMC Psychiatry. 2019 Jun 20;19(1):189. doi: 10.1186/s12888-019-2177-5.
8. Tsetsenis T, Broussard JI, Dani JA. Dopaminergic regulation of hippocampal plasticity, learning, and memory. Front Behav Neurosci. 2023 Jan 27;16:1092420. doi: 10.3389/fnbeh.2022.1092420
9. Fusar-Poli P, Smieskova R, Kempton MJ, et al.: Progressive brain changes in schizophrenia related to antipsychotic treatment? A meta-analysis of longitudinal MRI studies. Neurosci Biobehav Rev 2013; 37:1680–1691

10. Ho B-C, Andreasen NC, Ziebell S, et al.: Long-term antipsychotic treatment and brain volumes: a longitudinal study of first-episode schizophrenia. Arch Gen Psychiatry 2011; 68:128–137
11. Huhn M, Leucht C, Rothe P, Dold M, Heres S, Bornschein S, Schneider-Axmann T, Hasan A, Leucht S. Reducing antipsychotic drugs in stable patients with chronic schizophrenia or schizoaffective disorder: a randomized controlled pilot trial. Eur Arch Psychiatry Clin Neurosci. 2021 Mar;271(2):293-302. doi: 10.1007/s00406-020-01109-y.
12. Warner, R. (2009). Recovery from schizophrenia and the recovery model. Current Opinion in Psychiatry, 22(4), 374–380. https://doi.org/10.1097/YCO.0b013e32832c920b
13. Jääskeläinen, E.; Juola, P.; Hirvonen, N.; McGrath, J.J.; Saha, S.; Isohanni, M.; Veijola, J.; Miettunen, J. A Systematic Review and Meta-Analysis of Recovery in Schizophrenia. Schizophr. Bull. 2012, 39, 1296–1306.
14. Kotov, R.; Fochtmann, L.; Li, K.; Tanenberg-Karant, M.; Constantino, E.A.; Rubinstein, J.; Perlman, G.; Velthorst, E.; Fett, A.-K.J.;

# CHAPTER 9

# OF FAT AND WRATH: HYPOCHOLESTEROLEMIA AND AGGRESSION

Most patients with SCZ do not exhibit violent behaviors and are more likely to be victims rather than perpetrators of aggressive acts. However, a subgroup of forensic detainees with untreated mental illness exhibits tendencies to engage in criminal violations. For example, it has been reported that 10% of all homicides and approximately 50% of mass shootings are committed by individuals with untreated SCZ or SCZ-like disorders (1)(2).

Vitamin D deficiency was demonstrated in over 95% of forensic patients with SCZ, emphasizing the critical role of this nutrient in neuropathology (3). Low levels of cholesterol, a vitamin D precursor, were associated with both violent crime and suicide, implicating the dysfunctional lipidome in this pathology (4)(5)(6)(7).

We hypothesize that low cholesterol and hypovitaminosis D contribute to gray matter volume (GMV) reduction, a hallmark of SCZ, aggression, and neurocognitive disorders. We hypothesize further that a subgroup of patients with SCZ is more vulnerable to cholesterol-lowering drugs, including statins, due to upregulated ATP-Binding Cassette Transporter A1 (ABCA1), a cholesterol efflux pump.

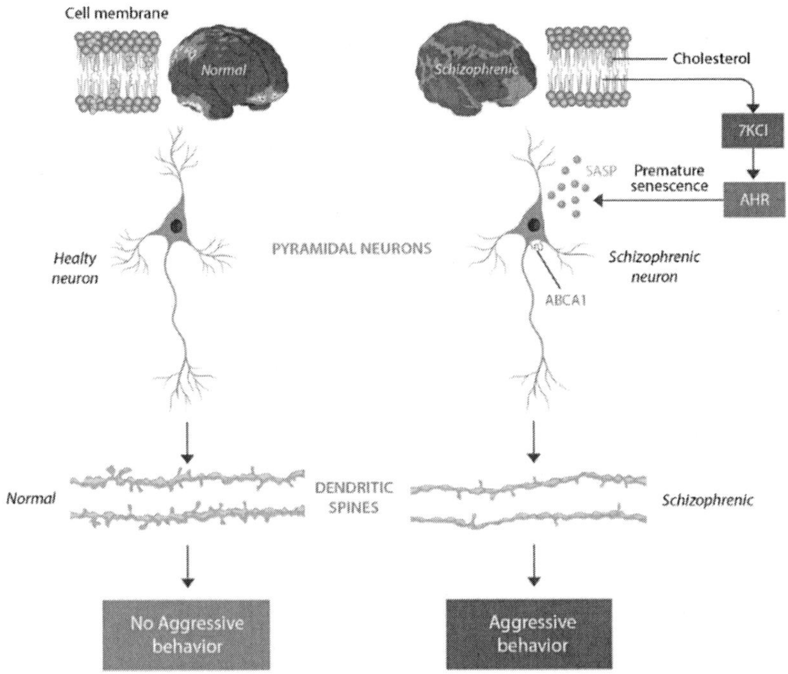


**Left: normal brain with adequate cholesterol in cell membranes (yellow). Right: schizophrenic brain with upregulated ABCA1 and low cholesterol in neuronal membranes. Upregulated ABCA1 lowers cholesterol content in cellular and mitochondrial membranes, contributing to GMV loss and subsequent aggressive behaviors. This may lead to decreased dendritic arborizations and lower dendritic spine density (also linked to aggressive behavior). Cholesterol oxide, 7KCl, induces premature cellular senescence via AhR. Senescent neurons release a toxic secretome, the senescence-associated secretory phenotype (SASP), which enhances the oxidation of membrane phospholipids and cholesterol, contributing further to GMV loss.**

# A quick reminder of cholesterol and vitamin D physiology and pathology

The brain, the cholesterol-richest organ in the human body, stores this lipid in two pools: the lipid bilayer of cell membranes and the axonal myelin sheath (8)(9). Cholesterol, the primary vitamin D precursor, is decreased in a subgroup of SCZ patients with uncontrolled aggression, probably accounting for the increased prevalence of hypovitaminosis D in this population (10)(11)(12).

Aggressive and violent behaviors in forensic patients with SCZ are directly correlated with the GMV reduction in four regions of the brain: the right superior frontal cortex, left inferior parietal (LIP) region, insular cortex (IC), and ventromedial prefrontal (VMPF) cortex (10)(13)(14)(15). For example, suicidal behavior (self-aggression) was associated with faulty remyelination, while aggression directed at others was linked to the dysfunctional lipidome in cell and mitochondrial membranes (16).

Cholesterol depletion was previously demonstrated to disrupt glutamatergic α-amino-3-hydroxy-5-methyl-4-isoxazole propionic acid (AMPA) receptors, leading to loss of both synapses and dendritic spines, changes previously connected to violent behaviors (17)(18)(19).

Cholesterol comprises 30–40% of plasma and mitochondrial membranes and, like phospholipids, is found in the lipid bilayer, where it maintains the balance between membrane fluidity and rigidity required for optimal neurotransmission (Fig. 1). In neurons, cholesterol drives the formation of dendritic spines and neurites, implicating this lipid in memory and cognition (20). For example, loss of dendritic arborizations of inhibitory parvalbumin interneurons was associated with aggression, further linking the lipidome to violence (21).

Lipophilic antipsychotic drugs, including phenothiazines, enter the lipid bilayer and oppose lipid peroxidation and neuronal membrane deformation (22)(23)(24) (see the section on lipid rehabilitation). Indeed, lipid peroxidation markers in SCZ can be detected in plasma and the cerebrospinal fluid (CSF) (25). The novel antioxidant phenothiazine derivatives, such as the tetracyclic and pentacyclic compounds, developed for heart disease and cancer, are likely beneficial for patients with SCZ (26)(27).

Phenazines are natural phenothiazines synthesized by various soil and water-residing microbes that exhibit antibiotic, anticancer, neuroprotective, and likely antipsychotic properties (28). Phenazines have never been evaluated for the treatment of SCZ. However, their biochemical similarity with phenothiazines suggests antipsychotic properties (29) (below).

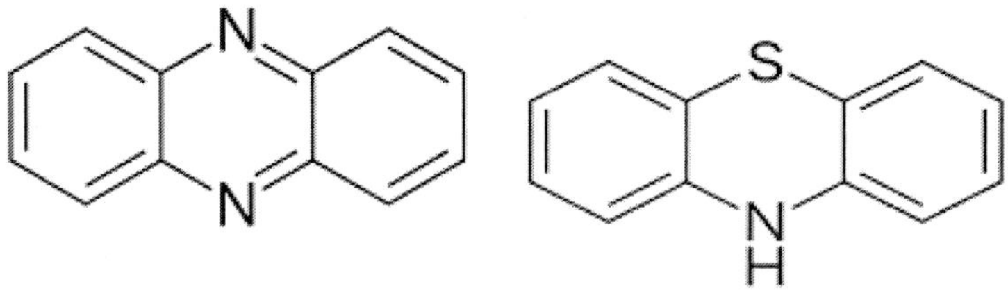


**Fig. 2 Similarities and differences between microbial phenazines and the phenothiazine antipsychotic drugs**

## Cholesterol biosynthesis

The cholesterol biosynthesis starts from acetyl-CoA and occurs in the cytoplasm and the endoplasmic reticulum (ER) of cells, including the neurons and glia. The rate-limiting enzyme in cholesterol synthesis, HMG-CoA reductase, catalyzes the conversion of HMG-CoA to mevalonate (MVA). After several reactions, 7-dehydrocholesterol (7-DHC) and desmosterol are generated (30).

Cholesterol acts via sterol regulatory element binding protein (SREBP) transcription factors 1 and 2 (SREBF-1 and SREBF-2). HMG-CoA reductase inhibitors, statins, induce the SREBP-2 pathway, increasing the transcription of the cholesterol efflux pump, ABCA1 (31). Since a subgroup of individuals with SCZ upregulates ABCA1, these patients exhibit low cholesterol levels and aggressive behavior (32)(33). Indeed, the Women's Ischemia Syndrome Evaluation (WISE) study found that statins predispose to aggression without affecting hostility or mood, suggesting that cholesterol-lowering drugs may promote violence (34)(35). In addition, statins have been known to trigger cellular senescence, an action independent of their lipid-lowering properties, further linking cholesterol dyshomeostasis to aggressive behavior (36)(37)(38)(39). Moreover, several studies found that statins can generate psychiatric adverse effects, including irritability and aggression in SCZ patients with low cholesterol levels (34)(40)(41)(42).

More studies are needed in this area as the literature regarding statin-associated neuropsychiatric changes remains limited (40).

## Gray matter loss

GMV reduction, a hallmark of SCZ, demonstrated by many neuroimaging studies, is seldom considered in this disorder's etiopathogenesis and seems refractory to most treatments. This is in line with SCZ outcome studies, which show that only a minority of patients with this disorder achieve sustained recovery, suggesting that brain volume loss may be irreversible (43). White matter is also decreased in SCZ, although at a lower rate, likely reflecting myelin damage.

GMV reduction in SCZ is associated with aggression and violence, further linking cholesterol dyshomeostasis to criminal violations (44). As GMV loss was found in unmedicated SCZ patients and the first psychotic outbreak, it likely pertains to pathology and not the antipsychotic treatment (45)(46).

## ABCA1 upregulation

Several studies have demonstrated that a subgroup of patients with SCZ exhibit low intracellular cholesterol and upregulated ABCA1 proteins that pump cholesterol out of cells, including the neurons (47)(48). This is why some individuals with SCZ may be susceptible to cholesterol-lowering agents, such as statins. Indeed, several novel studies have shown that total low cholesterol and low-density lipoproteins (LDLs) can trigger aggression, hostility, and suicidal behavior, linking the dysfunctional lipidome to these pathologies (49)(50). Along this line, reduced intraneuronal cholesterol disrupts the outgrowth of neurites as well as the density of dendritic spines, which may be responsible for the aggressive behavior (51)(52)(Fig.1). Moreover, ABCA1 upregulation in lysosomal membranes was shown to induce premature cellular senescence via cholesterol accumulation (53). Interestingly, ABCA1 is an influx pump in the lysosomes, increasing intra-lysosomal lipids (54).

## Premature cellular/neuronal senescence

Some call SCZ "segmental progeria" due to premature cellular and neuronal senescence, shortened telomeres, and upregulated senescence markers (55)(56)(57)(58). Indeed, SCZ patients exhibit both shorter lifespans and early onset of age-related diseases, including neurodegeneration, highlighting the critical role of cellular senescence in this disorder (59).

Cholesterol is a precursor of both vitamin D and 7-ketocholesterol (7KCl), a toxin known for incorporating into the lipid bilayer of neuronal membranes, disrupting neurotransmission (60)(61) (Fig, 1). In addition, 7KCh promotes premature cellular senescence via AhR activation (49). The active form of vitamin D3 (calcitriol), an AhR ligand, averts the formation of 7KCl, while low calcitriol leads to toxicity by 7KCh accumulation.

Recent studies have shown that 7KCl can increase intracellular iron and calcium, promoting AhR-mediated oxidative stress and ferroptosis, a non-apoptotic cellular/neuronal death found in SCZ and dementias (62)(63)(64). Moreover, cholesterol oxides were shown to alter the fluidity of neuronal and mitochondrial membranes, triggering neuropathology by changing the biochemical membrane conformation and disrupting neurotransmission.

Taken together, low cholesterol due to ABCA1 upregulation decreases GMV, increasing aggression and premature cellular senescence. GMV depletion was associated with violence directed at others, while white matter loss has been linked to suicide.

## Lipidome rehabilitation

Membrane Lipid Replacement (MLR) refers to oral supplementation with natural membrane glycerophospholipids, natural phenazines, and kaempferol, a plant flavonoid (66).

Oxidized membrane phospholipids and 7KCl activate AhR, inducing premature cellular, including neuronal senescence, in patients with SCZ and dementias.

Phenazines are natural or synthetic compounds produced by diverse bacteria, which possess anticancer, antibiotic, and trophic properties. Many phenazines are neuroprotective, and their similarity to phenothiazine suggests antipsychotic efficacy (67).

Phenazine derivatives have established antioxidant properties and, like phenothiazines, intercalate themselves in the lipid bilayer of cell membranes, opposing peroxidation-induced membrane deformation (68) (Fig. 3). For example, the natural phenazine derivative iodinin (1,6-dihydroxy phenazine 5,10-dioxide, 6), is a potent iron chelator, highlighting anti-ferroptosis properties of this compound (69) (See chapter on ferroptosis…).

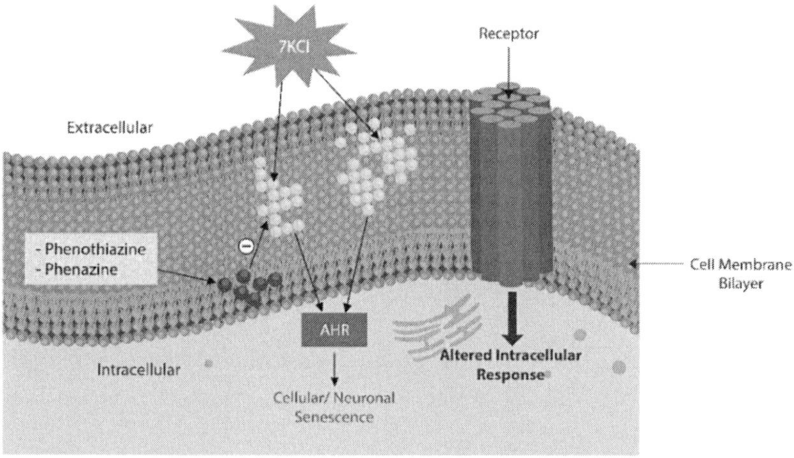


**Phospholipid and cholesterol oxides, including 7KCl, deform neuronal membranes, misaligning the cell surface receptors and disrupting neurotransmission. Phenothiazines and natural phenazines are antioxidants that intercalate into the lipid bilayer, reversing oxidation and membrane changes. This mechanism may reflect a novel antipsychotic mechanism of action of these compounds.**

MLR combined with phenazines may be more advantageous than each component alone as they can replace or repair the lipidomes of cell and organelle membranes. In addition, phenazines likely exert antipsychotic properties without the adverse effects of conventional antipsychotics.

# Article for Chapter 9: Neurolipidomics in Schizophrenia: Oiling Violent Behavior

Adonis Sfera[1], Ioana Ciuperca[2], Jacob J. Anton[3] and Dragos Turturica[4]

*1. Department of Psychiatry, Patton State Hospital, Patton, CA, USA*
*2. Paton State Hospital, CA, USA*
*3. California Baptist University, Riverside, CA, USA*
*4. College Medical Center, Long Beach, CA, USA*

## Abstract

Most patients with schizophrenia (SCZ) do not exhibit violent behaviors and are more likely to be victims rather than perpetrators of violent acts. However, a subgroup of forensic detainees with SCZ exhibit tendencies to engage in criminal violations. Although numerous models have been proposed, ranging from substance use, serotonin transporter gene, and cognitive dysfunction, the molecular underpinnings of violence in SCZ patients remain elusive.

Lithium and clozapine have established anti-aggression properties, and recent studies have linked low cholesterol levels and ultraviolet (UV) radiation with human aggression, while vitamin D3 reduces violent behaviors. A recent study found that vitamin D3, omega-3 fatty acids, magnesium, and zinc lower aggression in the forensic population.

In this review article, we look closer at the aryl hydrocarbon receptor (AhR) and the dysfunctional lipidome in neuronal membranes, emphasizing cholesterol and vitamin D3 depletion as sources of aggressive behavior. We also discuss modalities to increase the fluidity of neuronal membranes via lipid replacement therapy and natural or synthetic polyphenols.

## Introduction

For the past 70 years, psychiatry has been preoccupied with developing dopamine (DA) blocking drugs and paid much less attention to the measurable characteristics of schizophrenia (SCZ), such as gray matter loss, premature cellular senescence, gamma oscillations, and impaired insight or anosognosia. Novel SCZ studies have implicated GABAergic interneurons in these pathologies, especially the altered plasma membrane lipid bilayer. The therapeutic strategies derived from this model may, for the first time, improve SCZ outcomes. For example, low vitamin D3 and cholesterol levels were demonstrated to induce gray matter loss as well as violent behaviors.

Lithium and clozapine have well-established anti-aggression properties, and recent studies have associated low cholesterol and ultraviolet (UV) radiation with violent behavior. Conversely, vitamin D3 was reported to reduce violence in forensic institutions (1). In this regard, a recent study found that vitamin D3, omega-3 fatty acids, magnesium, and zinc lower aggression in the forensic population (2-3).

Decreasing gray matter loss, associated with criminal behavior, can be accomplished by protecting and repairing neuronal and mitochondrial membranes and the cholesterol/calciferol axis.

AHR, an essential regulator of cellular senescence, is a ligand-activated transcription factor that binds cholesterol and vitamin D3. Several neurotransmitters, including DA and serotonin (5-HT), tryptophan metabolites, and the environmental toxin dioxin, are AhR ligands. AhR activation induces premature senescence in many cell types, including lymphocytes, endothelial cells, and neurons (4)(5). For example, AhR agonists were shown to trigger thymic involution and premature brain aging (6)(7)(8). Interestingly, decreased low-density lipoprotein (LDLs) and low cholesterol were shown to activate AhR, linking this receptor to neurolipidomics (9)(10). Several neurotransmitters and psychotropic drugs, including DA, clozapine, and carbidopa, are AhR ligands, bringing this transcription factor into the psychiatric arena (11). This is significant as clozapine is known for lowering aggressive and violent behaviors, while low LDL and cholesterol augment this behavior (12)(13).

AhR resides in the cytosol and is stabilized by two heat shock protein 90 (HSP90) molecules. When uncoupled from its chaperone, AhR undergoes heterodimerization with an aryl hydrocarbon receptor nuclear translocator (ARNT) and enters the nucleus. AhR influences the transcription of many genes in the genome, probably including the SCZ vulnerability genes (14)(15).

Under physiological circumstances, adequate levels of vitamin D3, an AhR ligand, lower aggression, while suboptimal levels have the opposite effect (16)(17)(18). Vitamin D3/AhR interaction likely explains the higher incidence of SCZ in the Nordic areas of the globe with less sunshine. As vitamin D3 is generated from cholesterol, low cholesterol may deplete this vitamin.

## AhR, cholesterol, and aggression

AhR is activated by several environmental pollutants, including plasticizers and toxins generated within the body. These toxic compounds were associated with SCZ, violent behaviors, and homicide (19). AhR chaperone, heat shock protein 90 (HSP90), responds to the ambient temperature and, under pathological circumstances, can trigger chronic pain and behavioral disturbances (20)(21)(22).

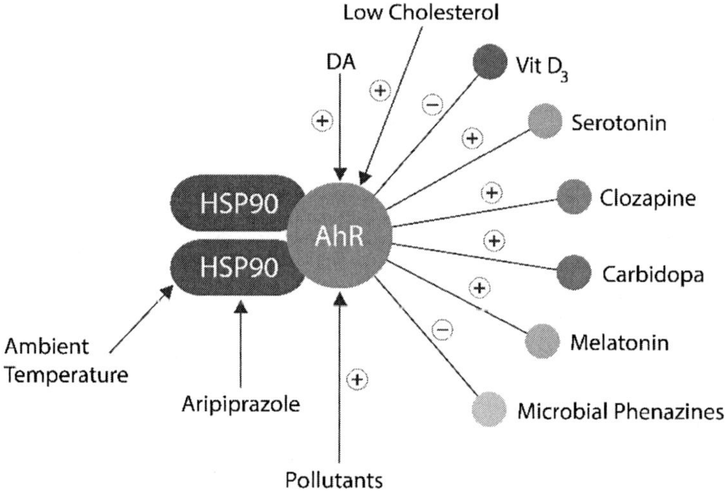


**Fig. 1 AhR and HSP90 ligands. AhR is stabilized in the cytosol by two molecules of HSP90. AhR activation separates this protein from its chaperone. Active AhR enters the nucleus and acts as a transcription factor. Several neurotransmitters, including dopamine (DA) and serotonin (5-HT2), activate AhR. Clozapine and carbidopa are also AhR ligands. Pollutants can activate AhR, explaining their link with SCZ. Low cholesterol and vitamin D3 are AhR activators. Environmental temperature and aripiprazole bind HSP90, strengthening its bond with AhR.**

AhR ligands relevant for psychiatry include ultraviolet (UV) radiation-generated 6-formylindolo(3,2-b) carbazole, neurotransmitters, metabolites, psychotropic drugs, and pollutants. Aripiprazole binds HSP90, enhancing the AhR bond. Taken together, aside from the postsynaptic dopaminergic blockade, antipsychotic drugs may "work" by AhR antagonism. Microbial phenazines are endogenous antipsychotic compounds produced by the gut microbiota. Low cholesterol levels activate AhR, while natural or synthetic phenols antagonize this receptor (23) (Table 1).

**Table 1 Exogenous and endogenous AhR agonists and antagonists**

| Exogenous agonists | Endogenous agonists | Dietary antagonists | Synthetic antagonists |
|---|---|---|---|
| Benzotriazole UV stabilizer | Tryptophan photo metabolites and FICZ | Quercetin | Salicylamide |
| Plasticizers (Bisphenol) | Indoles | Apigenin | 1,3-diketone |
| Clozapine | D3 hydroxyderivatives | Luteolin | IK-175 |
| Carbidopa | DA | Alstonine | HBU651 |

Low systemic and cell membrane cholesterol has been associated with criminal or suicidal behavior (24)(25)(26)(27)(28). Indeed, cholesterol is believed to comprise a biological marker of aggression in psychiatric patients (29).

The inverse correlation between aggression and cholesterol may be mediated by serotonergic signaling, which depends on cell membranes' integrity (29)(30). Cholesterol is transported across the cell membranes coupled with other lipids, including phosphoinositides, phosphatidylserine (PS), and sphingolipids (31). Low cholesterol in neuronal membranes disrupts dendritic growth, a pathology previously associated with violent behaviors (23)(24)(25). Indeed, SCZ patients with lower high-density lipoproteins (HDL) and cholesterol were found to exhibit three times higher aggression compared to those with normal cholesterol (13).

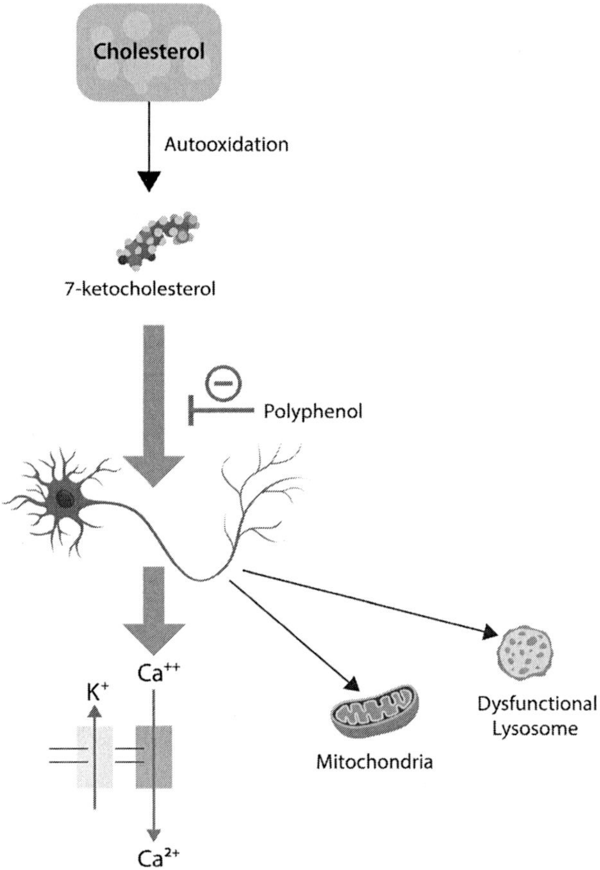


**Fig. 2 Cholesterol oxidation leads to the formation of 7-ketocholesterol, a toxic compound known for disrupting neuronal membranes, upregulating intracellular calcium (Ca++), and lowering potassium (K+). These changes can also disrupt mitochondria and the lysosomes. Polyphenols oppose the action of 7-ketocholesterol, protecting neuronal membranes.**

Cholesterol, a precursor of both vitamin D and 7-ketocholesterol, is processed by 7-dehydrocholesterol reductase, the rate-limiting enzyme in charge of this metabolic step (32)(33) (Fig. 2). Oxidized cholesterol is converted into various oxysterols, out of which 7-dehydrocholesterol is the most common one. This toxic compound is incorporated into the neuronal membranes' lipid bilayer, disrupting neurotransmission (34)(35). In addition, by facilitating calcium (Ca2+) entry and potassium (K+) exit from neuronal cells, 7-dehydrocholesterol disrupts the lysosomes and autophagy (36). Normal levels of vitamin D3 inhibit 7-dehydrocholesterol reductase, averting the conversion of cholesterol into the toxic 7-ketocholesterol. Conversely, low vitamin D3 may contribute to toxicity by accumulating this toxin.

Recent studies connected 7-ketocholesterol to iron overload and ferroptosis (37)(38). Moreover, cholesterol oxides decrease the fluidity of neuronal and mitochondrial membranes, disrupting neurotransmission as well as the Ca++ and K+ transport (39)(40)(Fig. 2). Indeed, 7-ketocholesterol induces premature senescence in many cell types, including neurons, lymphocytes, and pancreatic β-cells (41). This is significant because SCZ is characterized by premature cellular senescence and dysfunctional neurolipidome. For this reason, lipid replacement therapy (LRT) may be indicated for aggression and enhancing immunity and pancreatic function (42).

Taken together, SCZ has been associated with premature cellular senescence and early brain aging. Senescence contributes to gray matter loss, depletion of GABAergic interneurons, and likely poor insight or anosognosia.

## Vitamin D physiology and pathology

Vitamin D3 is synthesized in the outer layers of the cutaneous tissue via ultraviolet B (UVB) radiation, which converts 7-dehydrocholesterol into pre-vitamin D3, a compound that rapidly isomerizes into the pro-vitamin D3. Subsequently, the pro-vitamin is metabolized in the liver to 25-hydroxyvitamin D, which is then released into the systemic circulation, comprising the plasma vitamin D marker. To become biologically active, the 25-hydroxyvitamin D requires another hydroxylation, turning into the 1,25-dihydroxyvitamin D, or calcitriol. The final hydroxylation and activation occur in the kidney and some other tissues, including the prostate, breast, colon, lung, and immune cells, via one alpha-hydroxylase (43)(44)(45).

In the brain, microglia contain 1 alpha-hydroxylase, suggesting that calcitriol may play a key role in deactivating these cells (46-47). Aside from microglia, several neuronal networks, including substantia nigra, contain one alpha-hydroxylase and vitamin D receptor (VDR)(48).

Aside from vitamin D3, humans may utilize diet-derived ergocalciferol or vitamin D2. However, this is a compound that the body cannot synthesize. Vitamin D3 can also be obtained through the diet, especially from animal-based foods, including fish and milk (49) (Fig.3). Whether vitamin D2 and D3 have equivalent potency is a controversial but significant issue, especially since many preparations and food supplements in the US contain vitamin D2. Novel studies report a better vitamin D3 bio-efficacy in humans compared to D2, pointing to the need for vitamin D3 supplementation and fortification (50). Although calcitriol is the end-product of both vitamin D forms, serum 25(OH)D level is believed to be raised more effectively by vitamin D3 (50).

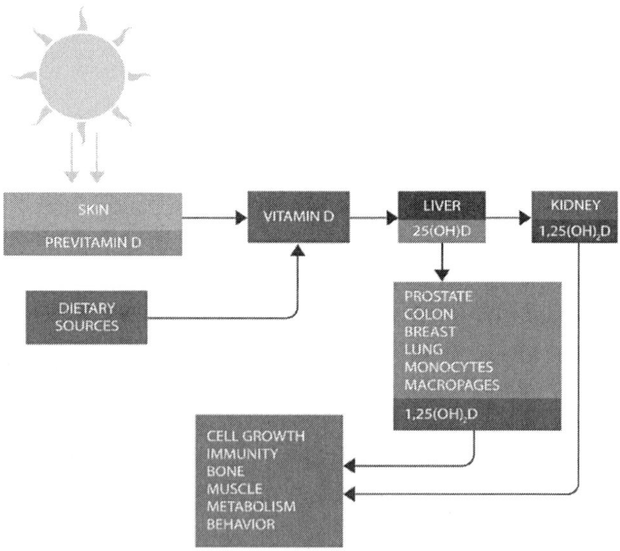


**Figure 3 adapted from Holick. Vitamin D3 is generated in the skin by UVB radiation. Vitamin D requires hydroxylation in the liver and kidney to become biologically active. Diet-derived vitamins D2 and D3 require similar activation. The tissues containing one alpha-hydroxylase activate 25(OH) vitamin D into calcitriol. In the brain, this enzyme is found in microglia and some neuronal groups, including the dopaminergic neurons in the substantia nigra.**

Aside from the well-established role in calcium homeostasis, vitamin D3 is involved in a multitude of biological functions, including immune regulation, cell cycle, apoptosis, metabolism, neuronal maturation, and homeostasis (51). At the molecular level, after entering the cells, vitamin D3 binds to vitamin D receptors (VDRs), forming dimers with the retinoic acid X-receptors (RXRs). Subsequently, the entire complex, calcitriol, VDRs, and RXRs enter the nucleus and modulate the target genes by binding to the vitamin D–D-responsive elements (VDREs) on their promoters (51)(52).

Recent studies have reported that unliganded VDRs and unbound RXRs may promote pathology, including cancer and metabolic dysfunction (53)(54). Other studies reported that unoccupied VDRs are tagged for degradation, a mechanism linked to premature aging (52-53). This is significant as SCZ is characterized by early brain aging. Moreover, genetic studies have associated VDR polymorphisms with aggression, obesity, and substance use disorders (55)(56)(57)(58).

In the CNS, vitamin D3 functions as a neurohormone/transcription factor that controls the expression of several genes, including tyrosine hydroxylase (TyrH) and tryptophan hydroxylase 2 (TPH2), facilitating DA and 5-HT. For example, the dopaminergic neurons in the substantia nigra, nucleus basalis of Meynert, and Purkinje cells in the cerebellum were reported to contain VDRs, demonstrating modulation by calcitriol (59)(60).

Active microglia, the CNS immune cells, are well-known for promoting neuroinflammation, and several studies have linked activation of these cells with aggression encountered in suicide, bipolar disorder, schizophrenia, and autism (61). Moreover, activated microglia were shown to selectively attack the substantia nigra dopaminergic neurons, contributing to Parkinson's disease (PD) (62)(63). Interestingly, vitamin D3 was found to play a major role in PD by preventing both DA depletion and microglial activation (64-65). Furthermore, activated microglia were associated with alcohol and drug addictions, suggesting a role for inflammation in pathological impulsivity related to substance abuse (66-67).

## Forensic detainees and vitamin D3

Several studies reported that more than 50% of forensic psychiatric patients exhibited low vitamin D3 levels (68)(69).

Aggression and violence have reached epidemic proportions worldwide; thus, understanding the molecular underpinnings of these behaviors is of utmost importance. Over the past decade, several studies have reported a high prevalence of hypovitaminosis D in the general population, pointing to a potentially more significant deficit in psychiatric patients. Pathological impulsivity is an overlapping domain, stretching across several disorders, ranging from SCZ, mania, attention deficit hyperactivity disorder (ADHD), and drug addictions, as well as neurodegenerative and personality disorders (70)(71)(72).

After more than four decades of neurotransmitter research, the consensus was reached that dysregulated serotonergic and dopaminergic signaling comprise the root cause of pathological impulsivity (73). However, despite the evidence of excessive cross-talk between vitamin D and monoaminergic pathways, the relationship between calcitriol and aggression remains poorly defined. Recent studies have reported beneficial effects of calcitriol in several neuropsychiatric syndromes marked by pathological impulsivity, including SCZ, bipolar disorder, ADHD, autism, suicide, and drug addictions (72)(73).

A novel line of research has associated calcitriol with increased DA and 5-HT signaling by augmenting TyrH and TPH2 gene expression. Aside from explaining the beneficial effect of vitamin D3 in depression and anxiety, this mechanism highlights a potential anti-impulsivity action (74)(75). - Indeed, TPH2 genetic polymorphisms were associated with pathological impulsivity encountered in oppositional defiant and borderline personality disorder (BPD), ADHD, anxiety, and possibly bipolar disorder and SCZ (76)(77)(78). Furthermore, calcitriol may augment melatonin, explaining its beneficial effect for insomnia (79). Interestingly, one study reported that the melatonergic drug ramelteon showed beneficial effects in autism-related impulsivity, further linking this disorder to 5-HT (80). Another novel study showed decreased tolerance for unfairness or reactive aggression in individuals on melatonin therapy (81).

Aside from its role in augmenting the brain 5-HT and DA signaling, calcitriol was demonstrated to function as an antioxidant, counteracting the adverse effects of reactive oxygen and nitrogen species (ROS)(RNS)(82). Like calcitriol, lithium, and selective serotonin uptake inhibitors (SSRIs) are reported to possess antioxidant effects (83)(84). The resemblance between vitamin D3 and psychotropic drugs does not stop here. Recent studies have reported that vitamin D3 is an Akt pathway activator, a mechanism of action shared with the established anti-impulsivity drugs lithium and clozapine (85)(86).

At the molecular level, activation of the Akt pathway by phosphoinositide-3 kinase (Pi3K) phosphorylation inhibits the downstream glycogen synthase kinase three beta (GSK3 beta), a well-known target of lithium, clozapine, and possibly SSRIs (87)(88). Moreover, Akt dysfunction is considered SCZ risk, equal to disruption in schizophrenia 1 (DISC1) and neuregulin (89)(90). Furthermore, it was recently reported that Akt phosphorylation is required for clozapine to block PCP-induced psychosis (91) successfully.

## Clinical case

MT (initials modified) is a 49 years old Caucasian female in forensic custody since 2001 due to second-degree robbery and multiple probation violations.

The patient's psychiatric history started with a suicide attempt at the age of 19 when she was first hospitalized and diagnosed with bipolar disorder. She was hospitalized again at the age of 22, treated with lithium carbonate, and remained stable until the birth of her first child at age 24. Postpartum, she experienced a prolonged depressive episode with psychotic features. MT was first arrested at the age of 26 for robbery. While incarcerated, she engaged in at least five serious suicide attempts and several self-injurious behaviors, such as cutting her arms and wrists. When she was not detained, MT was using cocaine and opioids daily.

In 2001, MT was admitted to a forensic institution where, over the years, she had multiple episodes of assaultive and self-injurious behaviors along with auditory hallucinations, paranoia, disorganized thoughts, and manic episodes manifested by pressured speech, racing thoughts, flight of ideas, low frustration tolerance, irritability, impulsivity, and psychomotor agitation.

She was diagnosed with schizoaffective disorder, bipolar type, borderline personality disorder, cocaine and opioid use disorder, severe. MT's medical history was significant for hypothyroidism, hepatitis C, and obesity, which were addressed with medications and diet. She was partially stabilized on clozapine 250 mg per day and mirtazapine 45 mg daily. However, she continued to present with intermittent assaultive behaviors and received rescue medications on multiple occasions. MT had four serious aggressive acts in 2015 and two in 2016.

In March 2017, MT presented with a 25 [OH] vitamin D level of 11 ng/ml. She was started on vitamin D3 2400 units a day, and the vitamin D level reached 77 ng/ml by August 2017. During this time, the use of rescue medications decreased considerably, and MT requested less diphenhydramine for sleep. She had no assaultive behaviors and became actively involved in her treatment.

## Vitamin D3 and schizophrenia

Multiple studies have associated vitamin D with SCZ over the past four decades due to lower levels in patients with this condition. This link is substantiated further by vitamin D receptors (VDRs) in the brain regions relevant for SCZ (92). In addition, vitamin D has been associated with dopaminergic neurogenesis during development (93). Along this line, the CASPIAN-III study found a direct correlation between VDR loss and violent behaviors in patients with SCZ (94). Indeed, vitamin D not only regulates DA during development but is also involved in the dopamine dysregulation syndrome (DDS) (95)(96). DDS is a recently defined iatrogenic entity manifested by impulsive acts triggered by DA replacement therapy in PD patients (97). Moreover, a case for vitamin D supplementation in neuropsychiatric syndromes was made by several researchers over the past two decades (vitamin D hypothesis of SCZ) (98)(99)(!00)(101)(102).

We have observed amelioration of metabolic markers in several patients on clozapine and olanzapine treatment supplemented with vitamin D3. Our observations are in line with several studies showing the beneficial effect of calcitriol in metabolic disorders (103)(104)(105)(106)(107)(108).

In a previous review, we hypothesized that correcting metabolic dysregulation may improve the efficacy of antipsychotic drugs in SCZ patients. We indicated that glucagon-like peptide-1 agonists (GLP-1), such as liraglutide, may lower impulsivity via dopamine/GLP-1 cross-talk (109)(110).

A related issue of increasing popularity lately is the combined supplementation of omega-3 fatty acids and vitamin D3, linking calcitriol to the cell membrane phospholipids. This combination was found beneficial in ADHD, bipolar disorder, and SCZ, conditions associated with impulsive aggression (111). It appears that this combined supplementation affects the ratio of omega-6/omega-3, an emerging marker of neuropathology associated with several pathologies, including SCZ (112)(113)(114). Omega-3 fatty acids were associated with vitamin D activation, indirectly augmenting monoaminergic and Akt signaling (115). Indeed, VITAL is a current study attempting to evaluate the omega-3/Vitamin D3 combination in cancer and cardiovascular disease (CVD) (116)(117).

Vitamin D receptor (VDRs) is the master regulator of tryptophan metabolism and enhances 5-HT transcription. VDRs have been implicated in autism spectrum disorder (ASD), linking this developmental disorder to vitamin D3. The link between 5-HT and impulsivity is further highlighted by the tryptophan depletion studies, which have reported aggressive behaviors in individuals on a low tryptophan diet (118)(119). As it is the sole precursor of human serotonin, deficient dietary tryptophan leads to low brain serotonin, generating pathology (120). Moreover, genetic studies provide additional evidence on the serotonin-impulsivity link as the TPH2 polymorphisms were associated with suicide, SCZ, bipolar, oppositional defiant, and borderline personality disorder, conditions marked by pathological impulsivity (121)(122). On the other hand, a low aggression phenotype was associated with the TPH2 allele -703G/T (rs4570625), further emphasizing the role of 5-HT in preventing aggression (123). Furthermore, serotonin 5-HT1B, and to a lesser extent 5-HT1A receptors, were connected to impulsivity by several studies, pointing to potential biomarkers (124). For example, a recent study associated the absence of 5-HT1B receptors with aggressive behavior later in life. Others have linked 5-HT-1B receptor polymorphisms with pathological impulsivity related to drug addictions (125)(126). Novel studies have presented evidence of direct 5-HT1B/GSK3 interaction, linking 5-HT signaling to the Akt pathway (127)(128).

Vitamin D-mediated serotonergic and dopaminergic augmentation (via TyrH and TPH2) may account for the beneficial effects in ADHD, PD, SCZ, mania, drug addictions, and suicide (129)(130)(131)(132)(133)(134).

Taken together, four mechanisms were identified for vitamin D3-mediated deterrence of violent and aggressive behaviors:

1. calcitriol-induced TyrH and TPH2 gene expression,
2. modulation of 5-HT1B receptors.
3. optimization of omega6/omega-3 ratio,
4. AhR antagonism.

In addition, calcitriol exhibits a favorable metabolic profile as it improves insulin sensitivity and lowers the risk of obesity. Therefore, adding calcitriol to SCZ treatment could ameliorate neuropsychiatric and metabolic symptoms.

## Is the AKT-GSK3 axis the driver of violent behavior?

Protein kinase B or Akt is a serine-threonine kinase involved in multiple cellular processes, including proliferation, apoptosis, chronobiology, and glycogenesis. Akt pathway is activated by phosphoinositide 3-kinases (Pi3K) in response to ligands occupying various cell membrane receptors. For example, growth factors, including the brain-derived neurotrophic factor (BDNF), binding to receptor tyrosine kinases (RTKs), activate the Akt pathway via Pi3K phosphorylation (135) (Fig.2).

Glycogen synthase kinase 3 (GSK3) is a downstream kinase negatively regulated by Akt. GSK3 comprises two isoforms, GSK3 alpha, and GSK3 beta, both suppressed by Akt via phosphorylation of serine residues. For example, phosphorylation of serine 21 inactivates GSK alpha, while GSK beta is shut off by serine nine phosphorylation (136). GSK3 alpha and beta were involved in multiple biological processes, including immunity, cancer, and SCZ (137).

The association of GSK3 with aggressive behavior originated with the realization that mood stabilizers, lithium, and valproic acid suppress GSK3 by phosphorylation (38). Subsequent studies linked the Akt-GSK3 axis to dopaminergic and serotonergic signaling and the action mechanism of psychotropic drugs (138)(139). For example, clozapine blocks PCP-induced psychosis by activating Akt and suppressing GSK3 (135). Lithium inhibits GSK3 beta both directly and indirectly by activating Akt. However, the therapeutic significance of direct lithium-GSK3 inactivation is uncertain as higher than therapeutic doses are required for this effect (140). Moreover, lithium does not inhibit GSK3 in the absence of Akt, indicating that the indirect Akt activation is the actual mechanism of GSK3 inhibition (141)(142).

Calcitriol was demonstrated to augment the expression of monoamine oxidase A (MAOA) gene (via Akt) (143). Under-expression of MAOA, nicknamed the "warrior gene," was shown to drive aggression and violence (144)(145). For example, a recent study from Finland found dysfunctional MAOA gene expression in violent offenders with antisocial personality disorder (146). Interestingly, valproic acid was reported to augment MAOA expression by activating Akt (147). Aside from antisocial personality disorder, the MAOA gene was associated with inducing impulsive behavior, including borderline personality disorder, ADHD, bipolar disorder, and SCZ (148)(149). Lipid replacement therapy (LRT) (see below) inhibits 3-phosphoinositide-dependent kinase 1 (PDK1), a molecule connecting cell membrane phosphoinositides with Akt, enhancing GSK3 inhibition.

Several studies over the past decade have linked pathological impulsivity to the Akt-GSK3 axis. These serine-threonine kinases appear to bridge the gap between the observed clinical efficacy of psychotropic drugs and the genes associated with this pathology. Like lithium and clozapine, calcitriol activates the Akt pathway, blocking GSK3 and augmenting the expression of the MAOA gene (150). More studies are needed to clarify the role of vitamin D3 in aggression and violence, an epidemic that has been comorbid with hypovitaminosis D.

## AhR antagonists as antipsychotics

The antipsychotic properties of AhR antagonists comprise the proof of concept that excessive AhR activation triggers psychosis. The following natural and synthetic AhR inhibitors were found therapeutic in SCZ (table 1):

**Quercetin** is a natural flavonoid, a plant pigment found in many fruits that exhibits anti-inflammatory, antioxidant, and anticancer activities. In the CNS, quercetin is a negative allosteric modulator of gamma-aminobutyric A (GABA-A) receptors; it lowers the inhibition of the prefrontal cortex, potentiating glutamatergic transmission, deficient in SCZ with negative symptoms (151)(152). In addition, quercetin inhibits the apoptosis of cortical neurons, likely preventing gray matter loss.

**Alstonine** is an indole alkaloid with antipsychotic properties that does not affect dopaminergic pathways but increases serotonergic transmission instead (153).

**Apigenin** is a plant-based remedy extract from Elsholtzia rugulosa used by traditional African psychiatrists to treat mental illnesses. Aside from antagonizing AhR, apigenin exhibits vasorelaxant and antioxidant properties (154).

**Luteolin,** a natural antipsychotic that reduces microglial inflammation, is currently in clinical trials for SCZ (NCT05204407) (155).

### Synthetic AhR antagonists

**Salicylamide,** an analgesic drug, induces a potent and long-lasting inhibition of AhR-induced Cyp1a enzyme activity. Salicylamide has shown antipsychotic properties in preclinical studies (156).

**1,3-diketone** reacts with arginine-containing peptides and proteins, protecting against lipid peroxidation and ferroptosis (157)

**IK-175,** structure undisclosed, was shown by preclinical studies to block ligand-stimulated AHR activation of Cyp1a (158)

**HBU651** are novel synthetic AhR antagonists developed primarily for cancer but appear to have a favorable profile for SCZ (159) (Table 1).

**Lipid replacement therapy**

LRT refers to the oral intake of natural glycerophospholipids to which we added kaempferol (3,4′,5,7-tetrahydroxyflavone), a natural flavonoid. LRT+ kaempferol aims to gradually replace the damaged lipids in neuronal cell membranes with natural glycerides containing phosphatidylserine (PS) and plant-derived kaempferol.

LRT interacts with a pathway previously implicated in SCZ: PDK1/AKT/GSK3β. PDK1, found upstream of AKT and GSK3β, contains a pleckstrin homology (PH) domain that binds PS in the cytoplasmic leaflet of cell membranes. PS/PDK1 attachment has two beneficial effects: 1) recruitment of PDK1 at the cell membrane, and 2) maintaining PDK1 in an inactive conformation (160)(161). This modulates the downstream phosphorylome, inhibiting GSK3β. In contrast, unrestrained GSK3β promotes psychosis, while several antipsychotic drugs and lithium are inhibitors of this enzyme (162).

## Conclusions

While aggression and violence have become public health problems, low vitamin D levels have been detected in populations worldwide. Is it possible that the two recent epidemics have a common denominator?

Cholesterol-lowering drugs and low-cholesterol diets to reduce the incidence of CVD may have had the undesired consequence of increasing violence not only in the forensic population but also in society at large.

Calcitriol is a positive regulator of TyrH and TFH2, rate-limiting enzymes for synthesizing DA and 5-HT. In the forensic psychiatric population, lithium and clozapine have been utilized extensively to avert aggression and impulsivity. These drugs activate the Akt pathway, augmenting MAOA expression.

## References

1. Fuller Torrey E. Deinstitutionalization and the rise of violence. CNS Spectr. 2015 Jun;20(3):207-14. doi: 10.1017/S1092852914000753.
2. Bonta J, Law M, Hanson K.The prediction of criminal and violent recidivism among mentally disordered offenders: a meta-analysis Psychological Bull. 1998123123–142
3. Every-Palmer S, Souter V. Low vitamin D levels found in 95 % of psychiatric inpatients within a forensic service. Aust N Z J Psychiatry. 2015 Apr;49(4):391-2. doi: 10.1177/0004867414562047
4. Sankaranarayanan A, Pratt R, Anoop A, Smith A, Espinoza D, Ramachandran P, Tirupati S. Serum lipids and suicidal risk among schizophrenia spectrum disorders: Systematic review and meta-analysis. Acta Psychiatr Scand. 2021 Aug;144(2):125-152. doi: 10.1111/acps.13305.
5. Roaldset, J.O., Linaker, O.M. & Bjørkly, S. Triglycerides as a biological marker of repeated re-hospitalization resulting from deliberate self-harm in acute psychiatry patients: a prospective observational study. BMC Psychiatry 14, 54 (2014). https://doi.org/10.1186/1471-244X-14-54
6. Sen P, Adewusi D, Blakemore AI, Kumari V. How do lipids influence the risk of violence, self-harm, and suicidality in people with psychosis? A systematic review. Aust N Z J Psychiatry. 2022 May;56(5):451-488. Doi: 10.1177/00048674211025608.
7. Pereira H. The Importance of Cholesterol in Psychopathology: A Review of Recent Contributions. Indian J Psychol Med. 2017 Mar-Apr;39(2):109-113. doi: 10.4103/0253-7176.203117
8. Björkhem I, Meaney S. Brain cholesterol: long secret life behind a barrier. Arterioscler Thromb Vasc Biol. 2004 May;24(5):806-15. doi: 10.1161/01.ATV.0000120374.59826.1b. Epub 2004 Feb 5. PMID: 14764421.

9. Snipes GJ, Suter U. Cholesterol and myelin. Subcell Biochem. 1997;28:173-204. doi: 10.1007/978-1-4615-5901-6_7. PMID: 9090 295.

10. Ward MA, Bendlin BB, McLaren DG, Hess TM, Gallagher CL, Kastman EK, Rowley HA, Asthana S, Carlsson CM, Sager MA, Johnson SC. Low HDL Cholesterol is Associated with Lower Gray Matter Volume in Cognitively Healthy Adults. Front Aging Neurosci. 2010 Jul 15;2:29. Doi: 10.3389/fnagi.2010.00029.

11. Vita A, De Peri L, Deste G, Sacchetti E. Progressive loss of cortical gray matter in schizophrenia: a meta-analysis and meta-regression of longitudinal MRI studies. Transl Psychiatry. 2012 Nov 20;2(11): e190. doi: 10.1038/tp.2012.116. Erratum in: Transl Psychiatry. 2013;3:e275.

12. Wright IC, Rabe-Hesketh S, Woodruff PWR, David AS, Murray RM, Bullmore ET. Meta-analysis of regional brain volumes in schizophrenia. Am J Psychiatry. 2000;157:16–25.

13. Chester DS, Lynam DR, Milich R, DeWall CN. Physical aggressiveness and gray matter deficits in the ventromedial prefrontal cortex. Cortex. 2017 Dec;97:17-22. doi: 10.1016/j.cortex.2017.09.024.

14. Hofhansel, L., Weidler, C., Votinov, M. et al. Morphology of the criminal brain: Gray matter reductions are linked to antisocial behavior in offenders. Brain Struct Funct 225, 2017–2028 (2020). https://doi.org/10.1007/s00429-020-02106-6

15. Seok JW, Cheong C. Gray Matter Deficits and Dysfunction in the Insula Among Individuals With Intermittent Explosive Disorder. Front Psychiatry. 2020 May 20;11:439. doi: 10.3389/fpsyt.2020.00439.

16. Kim B, Oh J, Kim MK, Lee S, Tae WS, Kim CM, Choi TK, Lee SH. White matter alterations are associated with suicide attempts in patients with panic disorder. J Affect Disord. 2015 Apr 1;175:139-46. doi: 10.1016/j.jad.2015.01.001.

17. Yonezawa K, Tani H, Nakajima S, Nagai N, Koizumi T, Miyazaki T, Mimura M, Takahashi T, Uchida H. AMPA receptors in schizophrenia: A systematic review of postmortem studies on

receptor subunit expression and binding. Schizophr Res. 2022 May;243:98-109. doi: 10.1016/j.schres.2022.02.033.

18. Hering H, Lin CC, Sheng M. Lipid rafts in maintaining synapses, dendritic spines, and surface AMPA receptor stability. J Neurosci. 2003 Apr 15;23(8):3262-71. doi: 10.1523/JNEUROSCI.23-08-03262.2003.
19. Moyer CE, Shelton MA, Sweet RA. Dendritic spine alterations in schizophrenia. Neurosci Lett. 2015 Aug 5;601:46-53. doi: 10.1016/j.neulet.2014.11.042.
20. Jose M, Sivanand A, Channakeshava C. Membrane Cholesterol Is a Critical Determinant for Hippocampal Neuronal Polarity. Front Mol Neurosci. 2021 Oct 21;14:746211. doi: 10.3389/fnmol.2021.746211.
21. Li X, Sun H, Zhu Y, Wang F, Wang X, Han L, Cui D, Luo D, Zhai Y, Zhuo L, Xu X, Yang J, Li Y. Dysregulation of prefrontal parvalbumin interneurons leads to adult aggression induced by social isolation stress during adolescence. Front Mol Neurosci. 2022 Oct 4;15:1010152. doi: 10.3389/fnmol.2022.1010152.
22. Dalla Tiezza M., Hamlin T.A., Bickelhaupt F.M., Orian L. Radical Scavenging Potential of the Phenothiazine Scaffold: A Computational Analysis. ChemMedChem. 2021;16:3763–3771. doi: 10.1002/cmdc.202100546.
23. Yu MJ, McCowan JR, Thrasher KJ, Keith PT, Luttman CA, Ho PP, Towner RD, Bertsch B, Horng JS, Um SL, et al. Phenothiazines as lipid peroxidation inhibitors and cytoprotective agents. J Med Chem. 1992 Feb 21;35(4):716-24. doi: 10.1021/jm00082a012. PMID: 1542098.
24. Keynes RG, Karchevskaya A, Riddall D, Griffiths CH, Bellamy TC, Chan AWE, Selwood DL, Garthwaite J. N10 -carbonyl-substituted phenothiazines inhibiting lipid peroxidation and associated nitric oxide consumption powerfully protect brain tissue against oxidative stress. Chem Biol Drug Des. 2019 Sep;94(3):1680-1693. doi: 10.1111/cbdd.13572
25. Dietrich-Muszalska A, Kontek B. Lipid peroxidation in patients with schizophrenia. Psychiatry Clin Neurosci. 2010 Oct;64(5):469-75. doi: 10.1111/j.1440-1819.2010.02132.x. PMID: 20923426.

26. Voronova O, Zhuravkov S, Korotkova E, Artamonov A, Plotnikov E. Antioxidant Properties of New Phenothiazine Derivatives. Antioxidants (Basel). 2022 Jul 14;11(7):1371. doi: 10.3390/antiox11071371.
27. Engwa GA, Ayuk EL, Igbojekwe BU, Unaegbu M. Potential Antioxidant Activity of New Tetracyclic and Pentacyclic Nonlinear Phenothiazine Derivatives. Biochem Res Int. 2016;2016:9896575. doi: 10.1155/2016/9896575.
28. Serafim B, Bernardino AR, Freitas F, Torres CAV. Recent Developments in the Biological Activities, Bioproduction, and Applications of Pseudomonas spp. Phenazines. Molecules. 2023 Feb 1;28(3):1368. doi: 10.3390/molecules28031368.
29. Sfera, Adonis. 2023. "Six Decades of Dopamine Hypothesis: Is Aryl Hydrocarbon Receptor the New D2?" Reports 6, no. 3: 36. https://doi.org/10.3390/reports6030036
30. Singh P, Saxena R, Srinivas G, Pande G, Chattopadhyay A. Cholesterol biosynthesis and homeostasis in regulation of the cell cycle. PLoS One. 2013;8(3):e58833. doi: 10.1371/journal.pone.0058833.
31. Wong J, Quinn CM, Brown AJ. SREBP-2 positively regulates the cholesterol efflux gene ABCA1 transcription by generating oxysterol ligands for LXR. Biochem J. 2006 Dec 15;400(3):485-91. doi: 10.1042/BJ20060914.
32. Cheng W, Frei O, van der Meer D, et al. Genetic Association Between Schizophrenia and Cortical Brain Surface Area and Thickness. JAMA Psychiatry. 2021;78(9):1020–1030. doi:10.1001/jamapsychiatry.2021.1435
33. Zhou X, Shin S, He C, Zhang Q, Rasband MN, Ren J, Dai C, Zorrilla-Veloz RI, Shingu T, Yuan L, Wang Y, Chen Y, Lan F, Hu J. Qki regulates myelinogenesis through Srebp2-dependent cholesterol biosynthesis. Elife. 2021 May 4;10:e60467. doi: 10.7554/eLife.60467.
34. Leppien E, Mulcahy K, Demler TL, Trigoboff E, Opler L. Effects of Statins and Cholesterol on Patient Aggression: Is There a Connection? Innov Clin Neurosci. 2018 Apr 1;15(3-4):24-27. PMID: 29707423; PMCID: PMC5906086.

35. Olson MB, Kelsey SF, Matthews KA, Bairey Merz CN, Eteiba W, McGorray SP, Cornell CE, Vido DA, Muldoon MF. Lipid-lowering medication use and aggression scores in women: a report from the NHLBI-sponsored WISE study. J Womens Health (Larchmt). 2008 Mar;17(2):187-94. doi: 10.1089/jwh.2007.0379.
36. Wang ST, Huang SW, Liu KT, Lee TY, Shieh JJ, Wu CY. Atorvastatin-induced senescence of hepatocellular carcinoma is mediated by the downregulation of hTERT by suppressing the IL-6/STAT3 pathway. Cell Death Discov. 2020 Mar 30;6:17. Doi: 10.1038/s41420-020-0252-9.
37. Shu X, Wu J, Zhang T, Ma X, Du Z, Xu J, You J, Wang L, Chen N, Luo M, Wu J. Statin-Induced Geranylgeranyl Pyrophosphate Depletion Promotes Ferroptosis-Related Senescence in Adipose Tissue. Nutrients. 2022 Oct 18;14(20):4365. doi: 10.3390/nu14204365.
38. Fuentes-Fayos AC, G-García ME, Pérez-Gómez JM, Montero-Hidalgo AJ, Martín-Colom J, Doval-Rosa C, Blanco-Acevedo C, Torres E, Toledano-Delgado Á, Sánchez-Sánchez R, Peralbo-Santaella E, Ortega-Salas RM, Jiménez-Vacas JM, Tena-Sempere M, López M, Castaño JP, Gahete MD, Solivera J, Luque RM. Metformin and simvastatin exert additive antitumor effects in glioblastoma via senescence-state: clinical and translational evidence. EBioMedicine. 2023 Apr;90:104484. doi: 10.1016/j.ebiom.2023.104484.
39. Ahmadi, Y., Fard, J.K., Ghafoor, D. et al. Paradoxical effects of statins on endothelial and cancer cells: the impact of concentrations. Cancer Cell Int 23, 43 (2023). https://doi.org/10.1186/s12935-023-02890-1
40. Cham S, Koslik HJ, Golomb BA. Mood, Personality, and Behavior Changes During Treatment with Statins: A Case Series. Drug Saf Case Rep. 2016 Dec;3(1):1. Doi: 10.1007/s40800-015-0024-2.
41. Golomb BA, Dimsdale JE, Koslik HJ, Evans MA, Lu X, Rossi S, Mills PJ, White HL, Criqui MH. Statin Effects on Aggression: Results from the UCSD Statin Study, a Randomized Control Trial. PLoS One. 2015 Jul 1;10(7):e0124451. doi: 10.1371/journal.pone.0124451.

42. Tatley M, Savage R. Psychiatric adverse reactions with statins, fibrates, and ezetimibe: implications for lipid-lowering agents. Drug Saf. 2007;30(3):195-201.
doi: 10.2165/00002018-200730030-00003. PMID: 17343428.
43. Lappin JM, Heslin M, Lomas B, Jones PB, Doody GA, Reininghaus UA, Croudace T, Craig T, Fearon P, Murray RM, Dazzan P, Morgan C. Early sustained recovery following first-episode psychosis: Evidence from the AESOP10 follow-up study. Schizophr Res. 2018 Sep;199:341-345. doi: 10.1016/j.schres.2018.03.014.
44. Soyka M. Neurobiology of aggression and violence in schizophrenia. Schizophr Bull. 2011 Sep;37(5):913-20. doi: 10.1093/schbul/sbr103. PMID: 21860037; PMCID: PMC3160223
45. Liu, N., Xiao, Y., Zhang, W. et al. Characteristics of gray matter alterations in never-treated and treated chronic schizophrenia patients. Transl Psychiatry 10, 136 (2020).
https://doi.org/10.1038/s41398-020-0828-4
46. Gur RE, Turetsky BI, Bilker WB, Gur RC. Reduced Gray Matter Volume in Schizophrenia. Arch Gen Psychiatry. 1999;56(10):905–911. doi:10.1001/archpsyc.56.10.905
47. Luquain-Costaz C, Kockx M, Anastasius M, Chow V, Kontush A, Jessup W, Kritharides L. Increased ABCA1 (ATP-Binding Cassette Transporter A1)-Specific Cholesterol Efflux Capacity in Schizophrenia. Arterioscler Thromb Vasc Biol. 2020 Nov;40(11): 2728-2737. Doi: 10.1161/ATVBAHA.120.314847.
48. Ota M, Fujii T, Nemoto K, Tatsumi M, Moriguchi Y, Hashimoto R, Sato N, Iwata N, Kunugi H. A polymorphism of the ABCA1 gene confers susceptibility to schizophrenia and related brain changes. Prog Neuropsychopharmacol Biol Psychiatry. 2011 Dec 1;35(8): 1877-83. doi: 10.1016/j.pnpbp.2011.07.012.
49. Suneson K, Asp M, Träskman-Bendz L, Westrin Å, Ambrus L, Lindqvist D. Low total cholesterol and low-density lipoprotein are associated with aggression and hostility in recent suicide attempters. Psychiatry Res. 2019 Mar;273:430-434.
doi: 10.1016/j.psychres.2019.01.056.

50. Buydens-Branchey L, Branchey M, Hudson J, Fergeson P. Low HDL cholesterol, aggression and altered central serotonergic activity. Psychiatry Res. 2000 Mar 6;93(2):93-102. doi: 10.1016/s0165-1781(99)00126-2.
51. Dotti CG, Esteban JA, Ledesma MD. Lipid dynamics at dendritic spines. Front Neuroanat. 2014 Aug 8;8:76. doi: 10.3389/fnana.2014.00076. PMID: 25152717; PMCID: PMC4126552.
52. Anilkumar S, Patel D, de Boer SF, Chattarji S, Buwalda B. Decreased dendritic spine density in posterodorsal medial amygdala neurons of proactive coping rats. Behavioural Brain Research. 2021 Jan;397:112940. doi: 10.1016/j.bbr.2020.112940. PMID: 33126115.
53. Roh K, Noh J, Kim Y, Jang Y, Kim J, Choi H, Lee Y, Ji M, Kang D, Kim MS, Paik MJ, Chung J, Kim JH, Kang C. Lysosomal control of senescence and inflammation through cholesterol partitioning. Nat Metab. 2023 Mar;5(3):398-413. doi: 10.1038/s42255-023-00747-5.
54. Boadu E, Nelson RC, Francis GA. ABCA1-dependent mobilization of lysosomal cholesterol requires functional Niemann-Pick C2 but not Niemann-Pick C1 protein. Biochim Biophys Acta. 2012 Mar;1821(3):396-404. doi: 10.1016/j.bbalip.2011.11.013.
55. Papanastasiou E, Gaughran F, Smith S. Schizophrenia as segmental progeria. J R Soc Med. 2011 Nov;104(11):475-84. doi: 10.1258/jrsm.2011.110051. PMID: 22048679; PMCID: PMC3206717.
56. Feng Y, Shen J, He J, Lu M. Schizophrenia and cell senescence candidate genes screening, machine learning, diagnostic models, and drug prediction. Front Psychiatry. 2023 Apr 11;14:1105987. doi: 10.3389/fpsyt.2023.1105987.
57. Tanya T Nguyen, Lisa T Eyler, Dilip V Jeste, Systemic Biomarkers of Accelerated Aging in Schizophrenia: A Critical Review and Future Directions, Schizophrenia Bulletin, Volume 44, Issue 2, March 2018, Pages 398–408, https://doi.org/10.1093/schbul/sbx069
58. Solana, Corona, Diana Pereira, and Raquel Tarazona. 2018. "Early Senescence and Leukocyte Telomere Shortening in SCHIZOPHRENIA: A Role for Cytomegalovirus Infection?" Brain Sciences 8, no. 10: 188. https://doi.org/10.3390/brainsci8100188

59. Adamowicz DH, Lee EE. Dementia among older people with schizophrenia: an update on recent studies. Curr Opin Psychiatry. 2023 May 1;36(3):150-155. doi: 10.1097/YCO.0000000000000861.
60. Wilson KA, Wang L, O'Mara ML. Site of Cholesterol Oxidation Impacts Its Localization and Domain Formation in the Neuronal Plasma Membrane. ACS Chem Neurosci. 2021 Oct 20;12(20):3873-3884. doi: 10.1021/acschemneuro.1c00395.
61. Anderson A, Campo A, Fulton E, Corwin A, Jerome WG 3rd, O'Connor MS. 7-Ketocholesterol in disease and aging. Redox Biol. 2020 Jan;29:101380. doi: 10.1016/j.redox.2019.101380.
62. Hamsanathan S, Gurkar AU. Lipids as Regulators of Cellular Senescence. Front Physiol. 2022 Mar 4;13:796850. doi: 10.3389/fphys.2022.796850. PMID: 35370799; PMCID: PMC 8965560.
63. Zhao T, Guo X, Sun Y. Iron Accumulation and Lipid Peroxidation in the Aging Retina: Implication of Ferroptosis in Age-Related Macular Degeneration. Aging Dis. 2021 Apr 1;12(2):529-551. doi: 10.14336/AD.2020.0912. PMID: 33815881; PMCID: PMC7990 372.
64. Reichert, C.O.; de Freitas, F.A.; Sampaio-Silva, J.; Rokita-Rosa, L.; Barros, P.d.L.; Levy, D.; Bydlowski, S.P. Ferroptosis Mechanisms Involved in Neurodegenerative Diseases. Int. J. Mol. Sci. 2020; 21: 8765. https://doi.org/10.3390/ijms21228765
65. Feng S, Chen J, Qu C, Yang L, Wu X, Wang S, Yang T, Liu H, Fang Y, Sun P. Identification of Ferroptosis-Related Genes in Schizophrenia Based on Bioinformatic Analysis. Genes (Basel). 2022 Nov 20;13(11):2168. doi: 10.3390/genes13112168
66. Nicolson GL, Ferreira de Mattos G, Ash M, Settineri R, Escribá PV. Fundamentals of Membrane Lipid Replacement: A Natural Medicine Approach to Repairing Cellular Membranes and Reducing Fatigue, Pain, and Other Symptoms While Restoring Function in Chronic Illnesses and Aging. Membranes (Basel). 2021 Nov 29;11(12):944. Doi: 10.3390/membranes11120944.
67. Cha JW, Lee SI, Kim MC, Thida M, Lee JW, Park JS, Kwon HC. Pontemazines A and B, phenazine derivatives containing a methylamine linkage from Streptomyces sp. UT1123 and their

protective effect on HT-22 neuronal cells. Bioorg Med Chem Lett. 2015 Nov 15;25(22):5083-6. Doi: 10.1016/j.bmcl.2015.10.019.

68. Chen JJ, Chen W, He H, Li DB, Li WW, Xiong L, Yu HQ. Manipulation of microbial extracellular electron transfer by changing molecular structure of phenazine-type redox mediators. Environ Sci Technol. 2013 Jan 15;47(2):1033-9. doi: 10.1021/es304189t.

69. Alatawneh, Nadeem and Meijler, Michael M. Unraveling the Antibacterial and Iron Chelating Activity of N-Oxide Hydroxy-Phenazine Natural Products and Synthetic Analogs against Staphylococcus aureus (2023) Israel Journal of Chemistry, volume 63, number 5-6.

# CHAPTER 10

# IRON, SENESCENT MICROGLIA, AND GRAY MATTER REDUCTION

Reduced gray matter volume (GMV) in the brain has been directly correlated with aggressive behavior, suggesting that neuronal elimination by ferroptosis or aberrant phagocytosis by iron-activated microglia may drive criminal violations (1)(2).

There is a growing body of evidence that iron accumulation in senescent microglia activates these cells, converting them to neurotoxicity, a phenotype known for eliminating viable neurons and synapses (3)(4) (5). Indeed, neurotoxic microglia not only engage in the phagocytosis of live neurons, but also convert astrocytes into neurotoxic cells, further contributing to GMV reduction.

Lysine lactylation (Kla) in histone proteins is a posttranslational modification of lactate which plays a key role in behavior regulation (6)(7). Lactate modulates iron metabolism via hepcidin, a liver hormone in charge of iron egress from cells, including neurons (8). In addition, a novel iron-histone pathway was recently described, further linking this biometal to lactate and lactylation (9). Lactylation appears to play a major role in disseminating neurotoxicity from senescent microglia to astrocytes (10)(11). For example, iron as well as lactylation of histone 3 lysine 18 (H3K18) can trigger astrocytic neurotoxicity and subsequent reduction in GMV (12)(13).

Microglia are resident brain macrophages, hypervigilant cells which surveil the microenvironment for debris and pathogens and at the same time facilitate synaptic transmission and neurogenesis. Novel studies have shown that several microglial phenotypes may become neurotoxic, engaging not only in the elimination of synapses and intact neurons but can also drive neurotoxicity in astrocytes (14).

Cellular senescence is a phenotype adopted by cells in distress to avoid apoptosis, malignant transformation, or irreversible DNA damage. Cellular senescence averts cancer, however, inflammation promoted by the toxic secretome known as senescence associated secretory phenotype (SASP) can paradoxically facilitate tumorigenesis (15). In addition, SASP has been shown to reduce GMV and to promote cortical thinning, linking senescence to behavioral disturbances, including aggression (16).

In the brain, senescent neurons can undergo ferroptosis, if astrocytes are damaged, or ferrosenescence if astrocytes are viable and capable of supplying the neurons with the necessary antioxidants, such as GPX-4 and ferritin as well as "fresh" organelles, such as mitochondria and lysosomes (Fig.1). The transfer of protective biomolecules from astrocytes to neuron occurs via tunneling nanotubules or extracellular vesicles. Antidepressant drugs, selective serotonin reuptake inhibitors (SSRIs) facilitate this process, suggesting a non-serotonergic mechanism for combating depression, in other words, a paradigm shift (17).

Cellular senescence was believed to be irreversible however, newer studies have demonstrated that aging cells can be rejuvenated via phosphatidylinositol dependent kinase 1 (PDK1) inhibitors, including the BBB-crossing OSU-03012 (18)(Fig.1). Aside from PDK1 inhibitors, inhibiting the downstream protein kinase B (Akt)/ glycogen synthase kinase 3 β (GSK3 β) pathway may accomplish the same effect (19). Indeed, many drugs, including some antipsychotics and lithium, inhibit GSK3 β, suggesting that natural compounds exerting this effect may be beneficial against affective and psychotic disorders. For example, kaempferol, a polyphenol, and berberine as well as membrane lipid replacement (MLR) may exhibit antipsychotic properties (20)(21).

In this chapter we take a closer look at MLR, and some natural or synthetic compounds that may prevent GMV depletion and aggression.

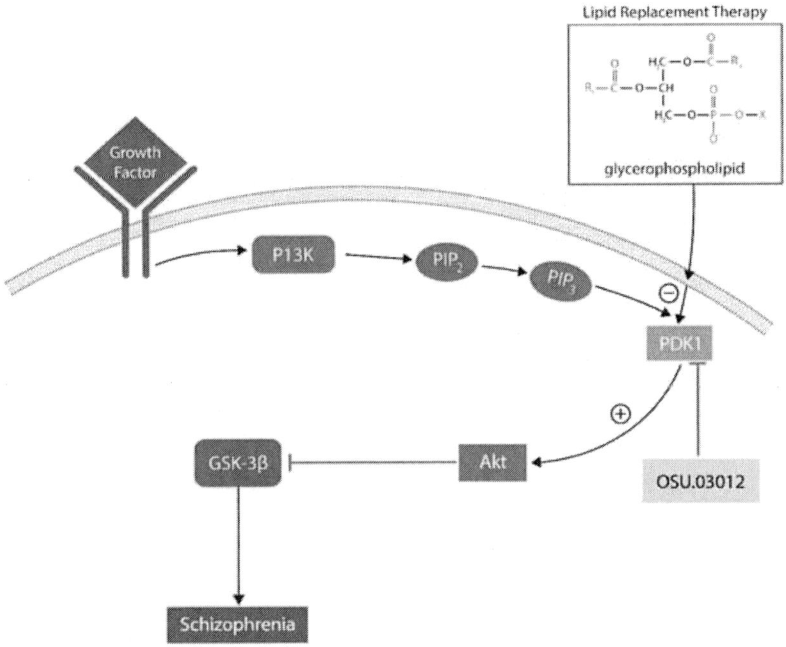


**Fig, 1. MLR inhibits PDK1 as exogenous phosphatidylserine (PS) binds PDK1, inactivating the downstream kinases, protein kinase B (Akt), and glycogen synthase kinase 3 beta (GSK-3β). MLR and PDK1 inhibitors act as natural antipsychotic agents. The novel PDK1 inhibitor OSU 03012 readily crosses the BBB, enhancing the antipsychotic properties of MLR.**

# References

1. Liu S, Gao X, Zhou S. New Target for Prevention and Treatment of Neuroinflammation: Microglia Iron Accumulation and Ferroptosis. ASN Neuro. 2022;14. doi:10.1177/17590914221133236
2. Zhang YD, Zhou JS, Lu FM, Wang XP. Reduced gray matter volume in male adolescent violent offenders. PeerJ. 2019 Sep 3;7:e7349. doi: 10.7717/peerj.7349. PMID: 31534834; PMCID: PMC6730529.
3. Hu Y, Fryatt GL, Ghorbani M, Obst J, Menassa DA, Martin-Estebane M, Muntslag TAO, Olmos-Alonso A, Guerrero-Carrasco M, Thomas D, Cragg MS, Gomez-Nicola D. Replicative senescence dictates the emergence of disease-associated microglia and

contributes to Aβ pathology. Cell Rep. 2021 Jun 8;35(10):109228. doi: 10.1016/j.celrep.2021.109228.
4. Ng PY, McNeely TL, Baker DJ. Untangling senescent and damage-associated microglia in the aging and diseased brain. FEBS J. 2023 Mar;290(5):1326-1339. doi: 10.1111/febs.16315.
5. Donley DW, Realing M, Gigley JP, Fox JH. Iron activates microglia and directly stimulates indoleamine-2,3-dioxygenase activity in the N171-82Q mouse model of Huntington's disease. PLoS One. 2021 May 14;16(5):e0250606. doi: 10.1371/journal.pone.0250606.
6. Hagihara H, Shoji H, Otabi H, Toyoda A, Katoh K, Namihira M, Miyakawa T. Protein lactylation induced by neural excitation. Cell Rep. 2021 Oct 12;37(2):109820. doi: 10.1016/j.celrep.2021.109820. PMID: 34644564.
7. Zhang D, Tang Z, Huang H, Zhou G, Cui C, Weng Y, et al. Metabolic regulation of gene expression by histone lactylation. Nature. 2019;574(7779):575–80.
8. Gregory J Anderson, David M Frazer, Lactate as a regulator of iron homeostasis, Life Metabolism, Volume 2, Issue 5, October 2023, load033, https://doi.org/10.1093/lifemeta/load033
9. Shapiro, J. S. et al. Iron drives anabolic metabolism through active histone demethylation and mTORC1. Nat. Cell Biol. 25, 1478–1494 (2023)
10. Wei L, Yang X, Wang J, Wang Z, Wang Q, Ding Y, Yu A. H3K18 lactylation of senescent microglia potentiates brain aging and Alzheimer's disease through the NFκB signaling pathway. J Neuroinflammation. 2023 Sep 11;20(1):208. doi: 10.1186/s12974-023-02879-7
11. Galle, E., Wong, CW., Ghosh, A. et al. H3K18 lactylation marks tissue-specific active enhancers. Genome Biol 23, 207 (2022). https://doi.org/10.1186/s13059-022-02775-y
12. Chen A-N, Luo Y, Yang Y-H, Fu J-T, Geng X-M, Shi J-P and Yang J (2021) Lactylation, a Novel Metabolic Reprogramming Code: Current Status and Prospects. Front. Immunol. 12:688910. doi: 10.3389/fimmu.2021.688910

13. Li B, Xia M, Zorec R, Parpura V, Verkhratsky A. Astrocytes in heavy metal neurotoxicity and neurodegeneration. Brain Res. 2021 Feb 1;1752:147234. doi: 10.1016/j.brainres.2020.147234.
14. Gao, C., Jiang, J., Tan, Y. et al. Microglia in neurodegenerative diseases: mechanism and potential therapeutic targets. Sig Transduct Target Ther 8, 359 (2023). https://doi.org/10.1038/s41392-023-01588-0
15. Coppé JP, Desprez PY, Krtolica A, Campisi J. The senescence-associated secretory phenotype: the dark side of tumor suppression. Annu Rev Pathol. 2010;5:99-118. doi: 10.1146/annurev-pathol-121808-102144.
16. Blinkouskaya Y, Caçoilo A, Gollamudi T, Jalalian S, Weickenmeier J. Brain aging mechanisms with mechanical manifestations. Mech Ageing Dev. 2021 Dec;200:111575. doi: 10.1016/j.mad.2021.111575.
17. Wang Y, Ni J, Gao T, Gao C, Guo L, Yin X. Activation of astrocytic sigma-1 receptor exerts antidepressant-like effect via facilitating CD38-driven mitochondria transfer. Glia. 2020 Nov;68(11):2415-2426. doi: 10.1002/glia.23850.
18. An S, Cho SY, Kang J, Lee S, Kim HS, Min DJ, Son E, Cho KH. Inhibition of 3-phosphoinositide-dependent protein kinase 1 (PDK1) can revert cellular senescence in human dermal fibroblasts. Proc Natl Acad Sci U S A. 2020 Dec 8;117(49):31535-31546. doi: 10.1073/pnas.1920338117.
19. Emamian ES. AKT/GSK3 signaling pathway and schizophrenia. Front Mol Neurosci. 2012 Mar 15;5:33. doi: 10.3389/fnmol.2012.00033.
20. Ren J, Lu Y, Qian Y, Chen B, Wu T, Ji G. Recent progress regarding kaempferol for the treatment of various diseases. Exp Ther Med. 2019 Oct;18(4):2759-2776. doi: 10.3892/etm.2019.7886.
21. Shri SR, Manandhar S, Nayak Y, Pai KSR. Role of GSK-3β Inhibitors: New Promises and Opportunities for Alzheimer's Disease. Adv Pharm Bull. 2023 Nov;13(4):688-700. doi: 10.34172/apb.2023.071.

## Highlights

- Dysfunctional lipids in neuronal and mitochondrial membranes drive cellular senescence.
- Oxidized phospholipids and cholesterol in plasma and mitochondrial membranes activate AhR, inhibiting Akt and disinhibiting GSK-3β.
- Overactive GSK-3β was associated with SCZ, while several antipsychotic drugs and lithium inhibit this enzyme.
- Like phenothiazines, MLR and Kaempferol inhibit GSK-3β, likely exerting antipsychotic effects.
- MLR and Kaempferol are natural compounds that may alleviate psychotic symptoms with fewer or no adverse effects.

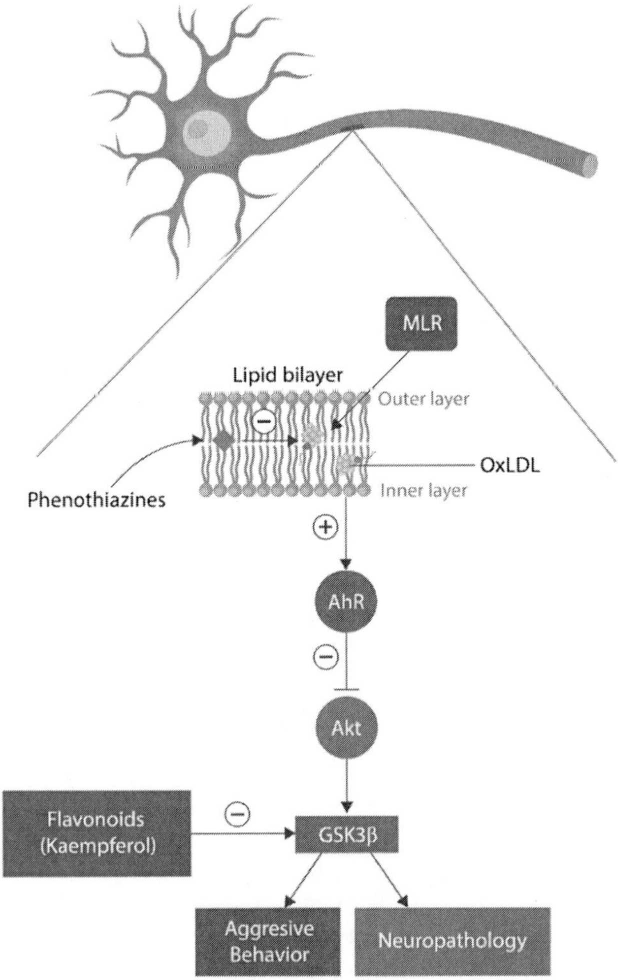


## Visual Abstract

**Oxidized low-density lipoproteins (OxLDL), including phospholipids, in neuronal membranes, activate AhR, inhibiting Akt, which in return disinhibits the Downstream GSK-3β, an enzyme implicated in aggressive behavior, SCZ, and dementias. Phenothiazine antipsychotics can insert themselves into the lipid bilayer, reversing the effects of OxLDLs by averting lipid peroxidation. MLR accomplishes the same result by substituting oxidized lipids. Flavonoids, including kaempferol, inhibit GSK-3β, complementing the action of MLR.**

For the past 70 years, psychiatry has been preoccupied with the development of more and more dopamine (DA) blocking drugs. It has paid less attention to the quantifiable characteristics of SCZ, such as gray matter volume (GMV) loss, premature cellular senescence, attenuation of gamma oscillations on electroencephalogram (EEG), alteration of cell membrane lipids, and metabolic abnormalities.

Therapeutic strategies derived from this model, membrane lipid replacement (MLR) and polyphenol therapeutics, could alleviate the symptoms of SCZ, including aggressive behavior. Low vitamin D3 and decreased cholesterol levels were found to promote GMV loss in the central nervous system (CNS), a pathology previously associated with SCZ and aggressive behavior (1)(2)(3). In addition, progressive depletion of GMV, a consistent neuroimaging marker, was found even in unmedicated patients with the first psychotic episode, suggesting a primary lipidome defect (4)(5)(6)(7). Continuous GMV reduction in SCZ is in line with the poor outcome of this disorder.

Several antipsychotic drugs, including phenothiazines, were shown to interact directly with the neuronal membrane of the lipid bilayer, correcting the lipid pathology. Due to their antioxidant properties, phenothiazines oppose lipid peroxidation, emphasizing the role of redox dysfunction in this condition (8)(9)(10). In contrast, excessive lipid oxides, markers of poor treatment response, have been associated with SCZ, childhood trauma, as well as various comorbidities encountered in forensic patients (11)(12)(13).

Several studies found that oxidative stress and lipid peroxidation trigger premature cellular/neuronal senescence, an established characteristic of SCZ. Previous studies have documented other hallmarks of this disorder, including shortened telomeres, upregulation of senescence markers, and early development of age-related diseases (14)(15). MLR likely lowers phospholipid and cholesterol oxides by replacing them with healthy glycerophospholipids and antioxidants, such as flavonoids.

MLR may also carry therapeutic agents directly to the plasma membranes. For example, treating SCZ with MLR carrying natural phenazines could be beneficial, antioxidant, and likely well tolerated (16).

A subgroup of patients with SCZ exhibit low intracellular cholesterol due to upregulated ATP-binding cassette transporter A1 (ABCA1), an efflux pump that ejects intracellular cholesterol into the extracellular space (ECS) (17). This SCZ characteristic may render patients more susceptible to cholesterol-lowering strategies, including statins, a phenomenon noted by many researchers and clinicians.

Vitamin D deficiency was demonstrated in over 95% of forensic patients with SCZ, connecting this hypovitaminosis to neuropsychiatric pathology (18). Moreover, since cholesterol is a precursor of vitamin D, low cholesterol may enhance an existing D3 deficit, explaining the high prevalence of this condition in SCZ (19). Along this line, a recent study has shown that supplementation with omega-3 fatty acids, vitamin D3, magnesium, and zinc decreased aggression and violence in forensic psychiatric patients, further emphasizing the critical role of these nutrients in SCZ (20).

Premature brain aging, a cellular senescence-mediated characteristic of SCZ, led some researchers and clinicians to conceptualize this disorder as a "segmental progeria" (21).

AhR, the master regulator of cellular senescence, is a ligand-activated transcription factor that binds both cholesterol and vitamin D3 while at the same time inhibiting protein kinase B (Akt), linking it to the pathogenesis of SCZ. Moreover, several neurotransmitters, including dopamine (DA), serotonin (5-HT), melatonin, tryptophan metabolites, and environmental toxins, are AhR ligands, further linking this receptor to SCZ. Furthermore, the AhR connection to psychosis is also supported by the premature cellular senescence induced by ligand-overactivated AhR (20)(22). For example, AhR agonists were shown to induce thymic involution, immune senescence, and premature brain aging (22)(23)(24). Interestingly, decreased levels of low-density lipoprotein (LDLs) were shown to activate AhR, connecting this receptor to aggressive behavior (25)(26)(27). Moreover, as AhR is activated by oxidized lipids, including 7-ketocholesterol (7KCl), a dysfunction of this transcription factor connects premature brain aging to SCZ (28).

Most patients with SCZ do not exhibit violent behaviors and are more likely to be victims of aggressive acts perpetrated by others. However, a subgroup of forensic detainees with hypocholesterolemia and hypovitaminosis D3 engage in criminal violations, linking the dysfunctional membrane lipidome to aggression and violence (29)(30)(31)(32).

In this mini-view, we examine potential therapeutic interventions to correct the cell membrane lipidome, alleviate the symptoms of SCZ, and lower aggressive behaviors. In addition to vitamin D3 supplementation, we discuss polyphenols and MLR treatment of cell /mitochondrial membranes.

## Behavioral lubrication: cholesterol averts aggression

Several studies have demonstrated that low systemic and neuronal membrane cholesterol increases the prevalence of criminal or suicidal behavior (33)(34)(35)(36)(37). Indeed, cholesterol level is considered a biological marker of psychiatric aggression as it likely reflects dysfunctional serotonergic signaling secondary to defective plasma and mitochondrial membranes (38)(39)(40).

Cholesterol is transported across the cell membranes with other lipids, including phosphoinositides, phosphatidylserine (PS), and sphingolipids (41). Impaired cholesterol transport was demonstrated to disrupt dendritic spines, inducing GMV loss with subsequent violent behavior (42). For example, patients with psychosis and decreased cholesterol exhibit three times higher aggression than controls (40). A recent systematic review of patients with SCZ found a correlation between low cholesterol serum levels and aggression toward self or others (43). Another study in women with SCZ found an inverse correlation between decreased cholesterol HDL levels and aggressive behavior (44).

Cholesterol is a precursor of both vitamin D and 7KCl. The latter, generated via 7-dehydrocholesterol reductase, is highly toxic and disrupts neurotransmission when incorporated into neuronal membranes (47)(48). In addition, 7KCl promotes premature cellular senescence, a phenotypic marker of SCZ (49). Vitamin D3 (calcitriol) inhibits 7-dehydrocholesterol reductase, averting the formation of 7KCh. In contrast, low vitamin D3 leads to 7KCh accumulation and activation of AhR, a key driver of cellular senescence.

Recent studies have shown that 7KCl can increase intracellular iron ($Fe^{2+}$), promoting AhR-mediated oxidative stress and ferroptosis, a non-apoptotic cell death demonstrated in SCZ and dementias (50)(51)(52). Moreover, cholesterol oxides were shown to decrease the fluidity of neuronal and mitochondrial membranes, disrupting neurotransmission. Furthermore, accumulation of intracellular $Ca^{2+}$ enhances neuronal senescence, promoting SCZ (53) (Fig. 1). Aside from neurons, 7KCl was shown to induce premature senescence in pancreatic β-cells, linking this toxin to SCZ-associated metabolic syndrome (54). In contrast, treatment with MLR may avert not only aggression but also pancreatic pathology (55). Taken together, SCZ has been associated with dysmetabolism, premature cellular senescence, and early brain aging. Senescence contributes to gray matter loss, predisposing to aggressive behaviors. 7KCl promotes brain aging via AhR overactivation, $Fe^{2+}$, and $Ca^{2+}$ accumulation.

## Vitamin D3 physiology and pathology, a quick reminder

Vitamin D3, or calcitriol, is synthesized in the outer layers of the cutaneous tissue via ultraviolet B (UVB) radiation, which converts 7-dehydrocholesterol into pre-vitamin D3. This compound rapidly isomerizes into the pro-vitamin D3. Subsequently, the pro-vitamin is metabolized in the liver to 25-hydroxyvitamin D (25[OH]D), which is then released into the systemic circulation and measured as plasma vitamin D level (Fig.2). However, to become biologically active 25[OH]D requires another hydroxylation, turning it into 1,25-dihydroxyvitamin D, or calcitriol. The final hydroxylation by one alpha-hydroxylase occurs in the kidney and some other tissues, including prostate, breast, colon, lung, and immune cells (56)(57). In the brain, microglia contain one alpha-hydroxylase, suggesting that calcitriol may play a vital role in the activation/deactivation of these cells (58). Aside from microglia, several neuronal networks, including those in the *Substantia nigra*, express one alpha-hydroxylase and vitamin D receptors (VDRs), linking calcitriol to dopaminergic signaling (59)(60) (Fig. 2).

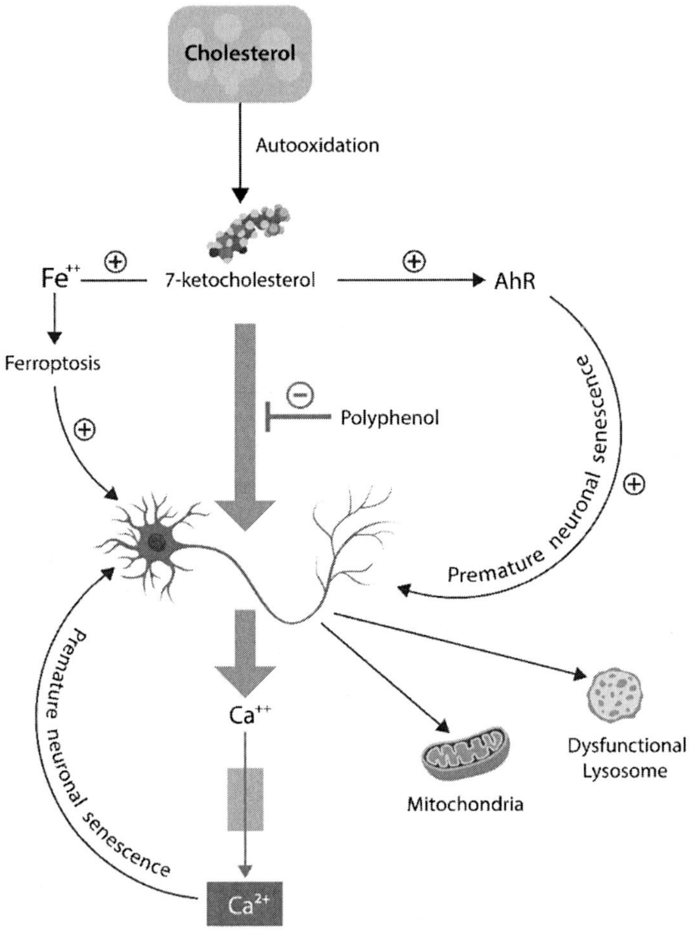


**Fig. 1 7KCl-induced damage to neuronal and organelles' membrane. Cholesterol oxidation leads to forming 7KCl, a toxic compound known for disrupting. Neuronal membranes upregulate intracellular calcium (Ca2+) and promote premature brain aging. 7KCl also activates AhR, inducing further senescence. 7KCl upregulates intracellular iron, promoting neuronal ferroptosis. Membrane biophysical changes can also disrupt the organelles, including mitochondria and lysosomes. In contrast, MLR and polyphenols, including kaempferol, oppose the action of 7KCl, protecting neuronal membranes.**

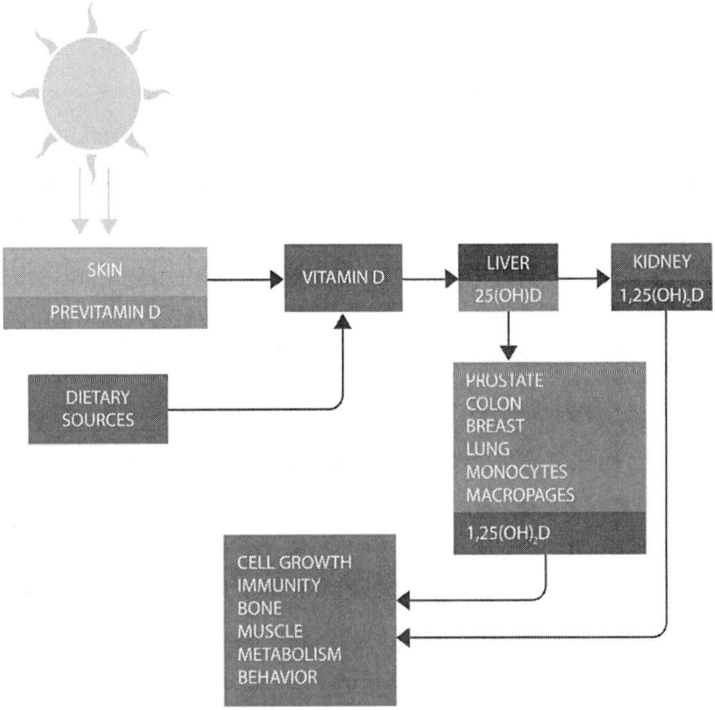


**Figure 2 adapted from Holick. Vitamin D3 is generated in the skin by UVB radiation. Vitamin D requires hydroxylation in the liver and kidney to become biologically active. Diet-derived vitamin D2 requires similar activation. Tissues containing one alpha hydroxylase activate i25[OH]D into calcitriol (vitamin D3). In the brain, this enzyme is found in microglia and some neuronal groups, including the dopaminergic neurons in the *Substantia nigra*.**

Aside from vitamin D3, humans can utilize the diet-derived ergocalciferol or vitamin D2, a compound not synthesized by the body. Vitamin D3 can also be obtained through the diet, especially from animal-based foods, including fish and milk (61) (Fig.2). Whether vitamin D2 and D3 have equivalent potency is currently unclear, but this is a significant issue, as many preparations and food supplements in the US contain only vitamin D2. Novel studies have reported a better bio-efficacy of vitamin D3 than D2, indicating the need for vitamin D3 supplementation and fortification

(62). Although calcitriol is the end-product of both vitamin D forms, it is believed that serum 25(OH)vitamin D levels are raised more effectively by vitamin D3 (62).

Aside from the well-established role in calcium homeostasis, vitamin D3 is involved in many biological functions, including immune regulation, cell cycle, apoptosis, metabolism, and neuronal homeostasis (63). After crossing the cell membrane, vitamin D3 binds to vitamin D receptors (VDRs), forming dimers with the retinoic acid X-receptors (RXRs). Subsequently, the entire complex, calcitriol, VDRs, and RXRs enter the nucleus and modulate target genes by binding to the vitamin D–D-responsive elements (VDREs) on the promoters of these genes (63)(64).

Recent studies have reported that unliganded VDRs and unbound RXRs may trigger metabolic dysfunction and certain cancers (65). Other studies found that unoccupied VDRs are tagged for degradation, leading to premature aging (64). This is significant, as SCZ is characterized by early brain aging and subsequent GMV loss. Moreover, genetic studies have associated VDR polymorphisms with aggression, obesity, and substance use disorders, linking this receptor to impulsivity (66)(67)(68).

In the CNS, vitamin D3 functions as a neurohormone/transcription factor that controls the expression of several genes, including tyrosine hydroxylase (TyrH) and tryptophan hydroxylase 2 (TPH2), known for participating in DA and 5-HT biosynthesis. For example, dopaminergic neurons in the *Substantia nigra*, nucleus basalis of Meynert, and Purkinje cells in the cerebellum express VDRs, highlighting the role of calcitriol in maintaining the integrity of DA signaling (69)(70).

Under pathological circumstances, microglia, the CNS-resident macrophages, were shown to promote neuroinflammation, contributing to aggression associated with several disorders, including suicide, bipolar disorder, SCZ, and autism spectrum disorders (ASD)(71). Moreover, activated microglia were shown to selectively target the dopaminergic neurons *insubstantial nigra*, contributing to Parkinson's disease (PD) (72)(73). Interestingly, vitamin D3 was therapeutic for PD as it averts DA depletion and microglial activation (74). Furthermore, aberrantly activated microglia may engage in the phagocytosis of healthy neurons and synapses, likely explaining SCZ-related GMV loss (75).

## The role of AhR-calcitriol crosstalk

AhR is becoming a receptor of interest in psychiatry as its ligands, including vitamin D3, DA, 5-HT, cholesterol, microbial molecules, several psychotropic drugs, SCZ-associated pollutants and neuropsychiatric toxins, bisphenol A (BPA), and phthalates (Fig.3). In addition, AhR regulates the expression of human cytochrome P450 1A1 (CYP1A1), an enzyme involved in the metabolism of cholesterol. In contrast, low cholesterol activates AhR via a feedback mechanism (76).

Polyphenols, both natural and synthetic, are AhR inhibitors that can reverse the effects of oxidized lipids on this receptor, ameliorating neuropathology (76)(77)(78)(79) (Table 1) (Fig.3). Indeed, AhR overactivation was strongly associated with cardiovascular diseases (CVD), including atherosclerosis, myocarditis, coronary heart disease, and pulmonary arterial hypertension, highlighting a link between heart disease and neuropsychiatric disorders (23).

Multiple studies over the past four decades have associated low levels of vitamin D3 with SCZ, while VDRs were found in the brain areas relevant to this psychotic disorder (80). In addition, during early development, vitamin D3 participates in the neurogenesis of DA neurons, suggesting that aberrant activation of this process later in life may lead to the development of PD (81). For example, vitamin D has been implicated in the dopamine dysregulation syndrome (DDS), an iatrogenic condition occurring in PD patients treated with DA replacement therapy (82)(83).

The CASPIAN-III study of SCZ found a direct correlation between violent behaviors and decreased expression of VDRs, while calcitriol supplementation enhanced the expression of these proteins (84)(85)(86). Along the same line, we have observed amelioration of metabolic markers.

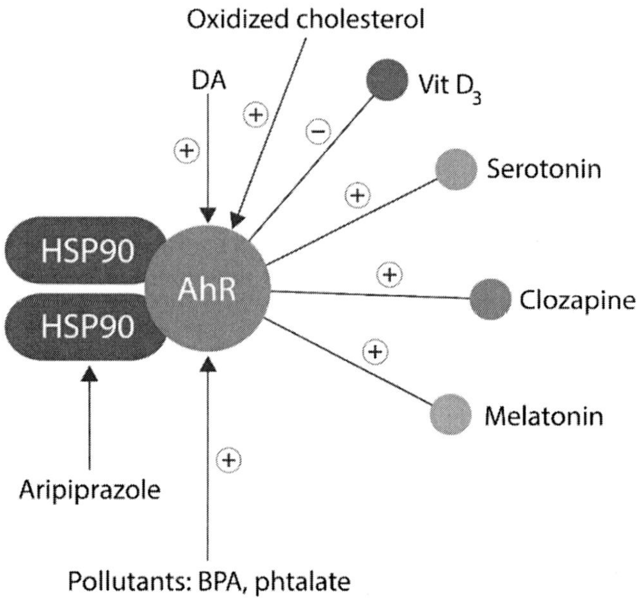


**Fig. 3 AhR and HSP90 ligands. AhR is stabilized in the cytosol by two molecules of HSP90. AhR activation separates this protein from its chaperones. Active AhR enters the nucleus and acts as a transcription factor. Several neurotransmitters, including dopamine (DA) and serotonin (5-HT), activate AhR. Clozapine and carbidopa are also AhR ligands. Pollutants can activate AhR, explaining their link to SCZ. Low cholesterol and vitamin D3 are AhR activators. Aripiprazole binds HSP90, strengthening its bond with AhR and keeping this transcription factor in the cytosol.**

| Exogenous agonists | Endogenous agonists | Dietary antagonists | Synthetic antagonists |
|---|---|---|---|
| Benzotriazole UV stabilizer | Tryptophan photo metabolites and FICZ | Quercetin | Salicylamide |
| Plasticizers (Bisphenol) | Indoles | Apigenin | 1,3-diketone |
| Clozapine | D3 hydroxyderivatives | Luteolin | IK-175 |
| Carbidopa | DA | Alstonine | HBU651 |

**Table 1 AhR agonists and antagonists**

In SCZ, patients are treated with clozapine or olanzapine and supplemented with vitamin D3 (unpublished data). Our observations are in line with several other studies showing the beneficial effects of calcitriol in metabolic disorders, regardless of etiology (87)(88)(89)(90)(91). Along this line, we have hypothesized previously that correcting dyslipidemia could lower aggressive behavior and other SCZ symptoms. For example, treatment with glucagon-like peptide-1 (GLP-1) agonists, such as liraglutide, was found to reduce the impulsivity associated with neuropsychiatric pathology (92)(93).

## Does the Akt-GSK3 axis drive violent behavior?

Protein kinase B or Akt is a serine-threonine kinase involved in multiple cellular processes, including the homeostasis of cell membrane lipids. The Akt pathway is activated by phosphoinositide 3-kinases (Pi3K) in response to receptor occupancy on the cell membrane. For example, brain-derived neurotrophic factor (BDNF) binding to its receptor tyrosine kinases (RTKs) can activate the Akt pathway via Pi3K phosphorylation at serine 473 and threonine 308 (94). GSK3 beta (GSK-3β) is a downstream kinase negatively regulated by Akt via phosphorylation at serine 9 (95) (visual abstract). This kinase is implicated in numerous physiological and pathological processes, including SCZ and aggressive behavior (96).

The link between GSK-3β and aggression originated with the realization that mood stabilizers, such as lithium and valproic acid, suppress this kinase, modulating dopaminergic and serotonergic signaling (97)(98)(99). In addition, the reserve antipsychotic drug, clozapine, an AhR ligand, blocks phencyclidine-induced psychosis by activating Akt, which, in turn, suppresses GSK-3β (100). Like clozapine, calcitriol activates Akt, inhibiting GSK-3β and, at the same time, augmenting the expression of monoamine oxidase A (MAOA), a gene previously implicated in aggressive behavior (101)(102)(103)(104). For example, a recent study from Finland has found decreased expression of the MAOA gene in violent offenders with antisocial personality disorder (APD), suggesting that enhancing MAOA expression may lower aggression (105). Interestingly, valproic acid has been reported to lower aggression by augmenting MAOA, suggesting novel targets (106). MAOA gene was also involved in other neuropsychiatric syndromes, including borderline personality disorder (BPD), bipolar, attention deficit hyperactivity disorder (ADHD), and SCZ (107).

Novel studies have found that the Akt/GSK-3β pathway interacts with the lipidome when Akt is recruited to the cell membrane, where it binds to cell membrane lipids, assuming an inactive conformation (108). For example, oxidized membrane low-density lipoproteins (oxLDL), including phospholipids, inactivate Akt, disinhibiting GSK-3β.

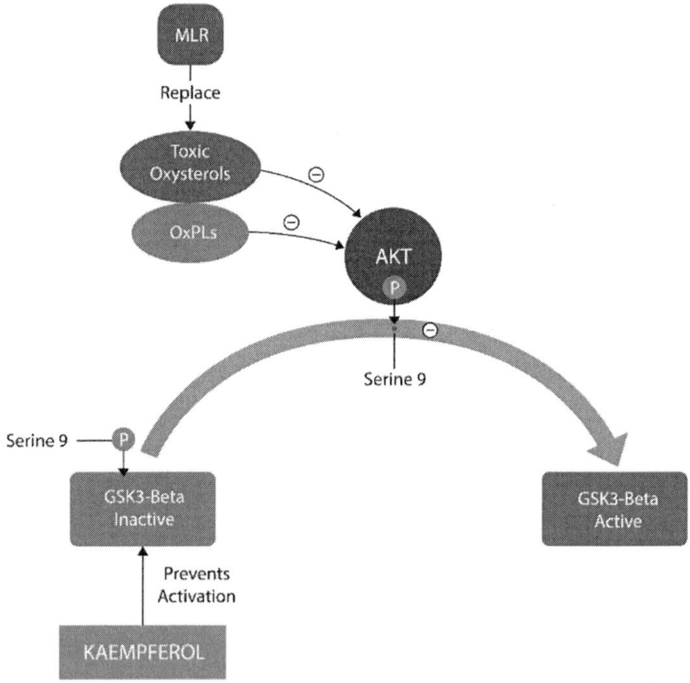


**Fig. 4 Oxidized phospholipids (OxPLs) and cholesterol (oxysterols) in neuronal membranes alter neurotransmission by modifying the biophysical properties of cell membranes, which anchor the receptors for central brain signaling pathways. In addition, oxidized lipids inhibit Akt, disinhibiting GSK-3β (by phosphorylation at serine 9). GSK-3β activation was associated with several pathologies, including premature cellular senescence and SCZ. Membrane lipid replacement (MLR) substitutes the oxidized with healthy lipids, reactivating Akt and inhibiting GSK-3β. Kaempferol inhibits GSK-3β thus, combining MLR with kaempferol enhances GSK-3β inhibition.**

MLR substitutes the oxidized with healthy lipids, likely reactivating Akt and inhibiting GSK-3β (108). Kaempferol is a natural GSK-3β inhibitor that can increase the efficacy of MLR by synergistic actions (109).

Taken together, the dysfunctional Akt-GSK3 axis promotes neuropathology, impulsivity, and aggression, potentially linking criminal behaviors to dysfunctional lipidome. Like lithium and clozapine, vitamin D3 augments the expression of the MAOA gene, activating Akt and suppressing GSK-3β.

## AhR antagonists as antipsychotics

The antipsychotic properties of AhR antagonists comprise the proof of concept that excessive AhR activation can trigger psychosis (Fig.4). The following natural and synthetic AhR inhibitors were found therapeutic in SCZ (table 1):

**Quercetin** is a natural flavonoid and plant pigment with anti-inflammatory, antioxidant, and anticancer properties. Quercetin is a negative allosteric modulator of the CNS gamma-aminobutyric A (GABA-A) receptor. As such, it lowers the inhibition of the prefrontal cortex, potentiating glutamatergic neurotransmission, known for being hypofunctional in SCZ (110)(111). In addition, quercetin inhibits apoptosis of cortical neurons, likely preventing GMV loss and subsequent aggression.

**Alstonine** is an indole alkaloid with antipsychotic properties that does not affect dopaminergic pathways but increases serotonergic transmission (112).

**Apigenin** is a plant-based remedy extract from *Elsholtzia rugulosa* used by traditional African psychiatrists to treat mental illness. Aside from antagonizing AhR, apigenin exhibits vasorelaxant and antioxidant properties (113).

**Luteolin** is a natural antipsychotic that reduces microglial inflammation and is currently in clinical trials for SCZ (NCT05204407) (114).

**Synthetic AhR antagonists**

**Salicylamide,** an analgesic drug, is a potent and long-lasting inhibitor of the AhR-induced CYP1A enzyme. In preclinical studies, salicylamide has shown antipsychotic properties (115).

**1,3-diketone** reacts with arginine-containing peptides and proteins, protecting against lipid peroxidation and ferroptosis, pathologies documented in SCZ (116).

**IK-175**, structure undisclosed, was shown to block ligand-mediated AhR activation in preclinical studies (117).

**HBU651** is a novel synthetic AhR antagonist developed primarily for cancer, and it appears to be a suitable candidate for SCZ (118) (Table 1).

## Membrane Lipid Replacement (MLR) therapy

MLR refers to the oral supplementation with natural membrane glycerophospholipids and Kaempferol (3,4′,5,7-tetrahydroxyflavone), a natural plant flavonoid (55). The aim of MLR + kaempferol is to gradually replace the damaged phospholipids in neuronal cell membranes with inulin-protected natural glycerophospholipids and plant-derived kaempferol. The MLR/kaempferol combination interacts with Akt/ GSK-3β, a pathway previously implicated in SCZ and aggressive behavior (119)(120)(Fig.4).

Oxidized membrane phospholipids and oxysterols induce premature cellular senescence, a marker SCZ. For example, a novel study found that lowered cholesterol precursor, mevalonate (MVA), plays a pivotal role in cellular senescence, suggesting that MLR supplementation with this lipid or the downstream coenzyme Q10 may avert premature brain aging (121)(122). Since statins inhibit MVA and are associated with aggressive behavior, forensic detainees with SCZ may be more susceptible to these agents (due to ABCA1 upregulation), a phenomenon in need of closer scrutiny (123)(124). This is significant as several non-statin lipid-lowering drugs are currently available, including Ezetimibe, Inclisiran, Lomatipide, and Pelacarsen, agents which could substitute statins in forensic psychiatric patients with CVD (125)(126).

MLR aims to replace oxLDL with healthy lipids, avoiding AhR activation and Akt inhibition (Fig.4). MLR also reverses cell membrane curvature induced by oxidized lipids, which alters receptor alignment and neurotransmission. This action is not very different from phenothiazine antipsychotics, which intercalate themselves into the lipid bilayer, inhibiting the ability of annexins to curve the cell membrane (127). In contrast, oxidized lipids form looped structures, generating membrane curvatures and pores, which lead to cell death (128). In addition, phenothiazines exert anti-peroxidation properties and protect against lipid pathology (129)(130). Indeed, a novel category of antioxidant phenothiazine derivatives has recently been developed with potential use in neuropsychiatry and CVD (131).

## Conclusions

Aggression and violence have reached epidemic proportions worldwide, as well as in forensic psychiatric institutions. Hypovitaminosis D3, a widespread pathology affecting worldwide populations, may be more problematic in forensic institutions compared to other settings, probably due to excessive GMV loss, a hallmark of both SCZ and psychopathy.

It has been established that even unmedicated patients with SCZ exhibit low intracellular cholesterol, indicating a phenotypic trait. In addition, patients with SCZ exhibit premature cellular senescence, which may reflect hypocholesterolemia and hypovitaminosis D3, associated with premature aging by previous studies.

According to this model, cholesterol-lowering strategies may increase violence and aggression in forensic detainees, a phenomenon that requires more studies.

Drugs, such as lithium and clozapine, have been utilized in psychiatry to lower aggressive behavior and injuries to self or others. Like vitamin D3, lithium, and clozapine activate Akt, inhibiting GSK-3β, suggesting a common mechanism of action with MLR and kaempferol. MLR, like phenothiazines, exerts antioxidant properties and prevents cell membrane alteration and receptor misalignment.

Taken together, a better understanding of cell membrane lipidome has opened new therapeutic opportunities for chronic mental illness. MLR can be used as an intramembrane delivery system for other therapeutics and for correcting lipid pathology in cellular and mitochondrial membranes. MLR provides a safe and natural alternative to the synthetic, canonical therapeutics.

# ARTICLE FOR CHAPTER 10: RUSTY MICROGLIA: TRAINERS OF INNATE IMMUNITY IN ALZHEIMER'S DISEASE

ADONIS SFERA[1,2], ROBERTO GRADINI[3], MICHAEL CUMMINGS[2], EDDIE DIAZ[2], AMY I. PRICE[4] AND CAROLINA OSORIO[1]

*1. Psychiatry, Loma Linda University, Loma Linda, CA, United States,*
*2. Patton State Hospital, San Bernardino, CA, United States,*
*3. Department of Pathology, La Sapienza University of Rome, Rome, Italy,*
*4. Evidence Based Medicine, University of Oxford, Oxford, United Kingdom.*

## Abstract

Alzheimer's disease, the most common form of dementia, is marked by progressive cognitive and functional impairment believed to reflect synaptic and neuronal loss. Recent preclinical data suggests that lipopolysaccharide (LPS)-activated microglia may contribute to the elimination of viable neurons and synapses by promoting a neurotoxic astrocytic phenotype, defined as A1. The innate immune cells, including microglia and astrocytes, can either facilitate or inhibit neuroinflammation in response to peripherally applied inflammatory stimuli, such as LPS. Depending on previous antigen encounters, these cells can assume activated (trained) or silenced (tolerized) phenotypes, augmenting or lowering inflammation. Iron, reactive oxygen species (ROS), and LPS, the cell wall component of gram-negative bacteria, are microglial activators, but only the latter can trigger immune tolerization. In Alzheimer's disease, tolerization may be impaired as elevated LPS levels, reported in this condition, fail to lower neuroinflammation. Iron is closely linked to immunity as it plays a key role in immune cells proliferation and maturation, but it is also indispensable to pathogens and malignancies which compete for its capture. Danger signals, including LPS, induce intracellular iron sequestration in innate immune cells to withhold it from pathogens. However, excess cytosolic iron increases the risk of inflammasomes' activation, microglial training and neuroinflammation. Moreover, it was suggested that free iron can awaken the dormant central nervous system (CNS) LPS-shedding microbes, engendering prolonged neuroinflammation that may override immune tolerization, triggering autoimmunity. In this review, we focus on iron-related innate immune pathology in Alzheimer's disease and discuss potential immunotherapeutic agents for microglial de-escalation along with possible delivery vehicles for these compounds.

**Keywords:** inflammasomes, astrocytes, microglia, exosomes, trained immunity, tolerized immunity.

## Highlights

- LPS activates microglial TLRs, training these cells excessively and triggering the release of C1q, TNF-alpha, and IL-1 alpha, biomolecules associated with autoimmunity.
- A1 astrocytes, likely autoimmune, eliminate viable neurons and oligodendrocytes, contributing to Alzheimer's disease neuronal and synaptic loss.
- LPS, a danger signal, promotes intracellular iron sequestration, increasing the risk of ROS. LPS also promotes ferritinophagy, increasing the free intracellular iron levels.
- ROS and iron activate NLRP3 inflammasomes, generating prolonged inflammation which may override microglial tolerization, engendering autoimmune A1 astrocytes.
- Promoting tolerization and lowering training may de-escalate microglia, lowering the risk of neuronal loss and Alzheimer's disease.

## Introduction

Alzheimer's disease (AD), the most common form of dementia, is marked by progressive memory impairment and functional decline believed to reflect synaptic and neuronal loss. Elimination of these structures may be carried out by an aggressive astrocytic phenotype, defined as A1. Preclinical studies show that LPS-activated microglia enable the conversion of trophic to A1 astrocytes by releasing several cytokines, including tumor necrosis factor alpha (TNF-alpha), interlukin-1 alpha (IL-1 alpha), and complement component C1q. These molecules alter astrocytic transcriptomes, promoting the neurotoxic A1 cells observed to engage in the phagocytosis of healthy neurons and oligodendrocytes, contributing to their loss (1). In this article we take the position that A1 astrocytes are autoimmune in nature, resulting from the prolonged microglial activation that overrides LPS tolerization.

LPS tolerization refers to the absence of an inflammatory response after repeated or prolonged exposure to this microbial endotoxin as re-challenged "tolerant" innate immune cells are incapable of immunological activation. This is relevant to AD because the constantly elevated brain LPS levels, detected in this disorder, fail to trigger microglial tolerization and lower neuroinflammation (2, 3).

Excess LPS in the brain microenvironment, a danger signal, is detected by microglial TLRs which activate the pathogenmediated iron sequestration via hepcidin-ferroportin axis (4) (Figure 1). Indeed, recent neuroimaging studies detected ironcontaining microglia in the hippocampi of AD patients, likely reflecting LPS-triggered iron sequestration (5).

The source of brain LPS is unclear at this time, but it has been hypothesized that it may derive from the gastrointestinal (GI) tract microbial community. These bacteria were found to lie dormant in various tissues, possibly including the brain, for prolonged periods of time restrained by the lack of free iron (3, 6). Later in life, impaired iron homeostasis caused by aging and/or defective ferritinophagy may provide these microbes with enough metal to resume their growth and LPS shedding, engendering inflammatory neuropathology (6).

Iron is closely linked to immunity as it plays a key role in immune cells proliferation and maturation, but it is also indispensable to pathogens and malignancies which compete for its capture (discussed in The Trained Arm of Innate Immunity section). To safeguard iron, innate immune cells, including microglia and astrocytes, sequestrate it intracellularly bound to cytosolic and mitochondrial ferritin, an arrangement which can generate excessive ROS and inflammation when disrupted (4). Indeed, iron-ferritin dissociation was demonstrated in AD animal models in which LPS-induced ferritinophagy increased intracellular free iron, engendering neuroinflammation (7, 8). Moreover, iron-damaged mitochondria were shown to act as danger signals, activating the inflammatory cascade by igniting inflammasomes, including NLRP3 (9). LPS-activated microglia release cytokines, including TNFalpha, IL-1 alpha, and C1q, that have been associated with autoimmune inflammation, an association that led to the development of vaccines, including anti-TNF-alpha antibodies (for the treatment of autoimmune disorders) and anti-C1q antibody, currently in phase I trials for both AD and autoimmunity (10, 11).

In contrast to immune tolerization which may be an adaptive mechanism to prevent autoimmune inflammation, allowing the clearance of damaged self-components, immune training may serve the purpose of overriding immune anergy encountered in various pathologies, including sepsis and cancer (12, 13). Indeed, the peripheral and central innate immune cells are engaged in a balancing act as they must be sufficiently trained to effectively defend the host against pathogens and malignancies, while at the same time tolerant enough to accept self-components, food, the fetus and commensal microbes. Disruption of this fine equilibrium may either cause unchecked inflammation or excessive tolerance (12). Iron interferes with this balance by promoting activation and inflammation, a property exploited in oncology to train tumor-associated macrophages (TAMs) in fighting malignant cells (14). On the other hand, iron chelators oppose training, providing therapeutic benefit in AD. Indeed, deferiprone, currently in phase 2 clinical trials, may soon become the first FDA approved iron chelator indicated for AD (15). Along these lines, a recent preclinical study demonstrated that in response to peripherally applied inflammatory stimuli, microglia can undergo either activation (training) or tolerization, the former augmenting, the latter lowering neuroinflammation (13). This is important for AD because this study also found that training increases while tolerization decreases β-amyloid accumulation, suggesting that central tolerance can be promoted by peripheral stimulation, comprising a novel therapeutic strategy (13). Previous AD studies are in line with this model as it was demonstrated that immune trained subjects (positive for TNF-alpha) presented with memory loss, while the tolerized patients (TNF-alpha negative) lacked cognitive deterioration (16). Moreover, trained microglia and astrocytes were found able to undergo transcriptomic alterations, morphing into antigen presenting cells (APCs) that can establish immunologic synapses with infiltrating peripheral lymphocytes, further perpetuating neuroinflammation (17).

Traditionally, immunological memory has been associated with adaptive immunity, however novel studies indicate that innate immune cells, including microglia and astrocytes can "recall" prior vaccinations or infections (13). For example, β-glucan, a cell wall component of Candida Albicans and bacillus Calmette-Guerin (BCG), was shown to train monocytes, improving the outcome of sepsis-induced immune paralysis (18). Indeed, the development of treatments based on innate immune memory manipulation has been encouraged by the recent FDA approval of immune training-inducers, the BCG vaccine for the treatment and prophylaxis of urinary bladder carcinoma in situ (CIS) and muramyl tripeptide for osteosarcoma (19). Along these lines, innate immune memory manipulation may improve AD outcome by de-escalating microglia via peripherallyapplied tolerizing stimuli (13). Since tolerized immunity, unlike immunosuppression, is antigen specific and natural, harnessing it may not only benefit AD but also cancer and autoimmune disorders (20, 21). The recent finding that altered endogenous molecules, including dysfunctional mitochondria, can trigger microglial training will likely result in novel AD strategies, including mitophagy-activating therapeutics (22).

In this article we look beyond iron chelators, focusing on lowering the consequences of iron pathology, especially microglial training and defective tolerization.

The immunotherapeutic agents discussed here include inflammasome inhibitors, histone deacetylase inhibitors, activators of co-inhibitory receptors, acetylcholinesterase inhibitors and selective serotonin reuptake inhibitors.

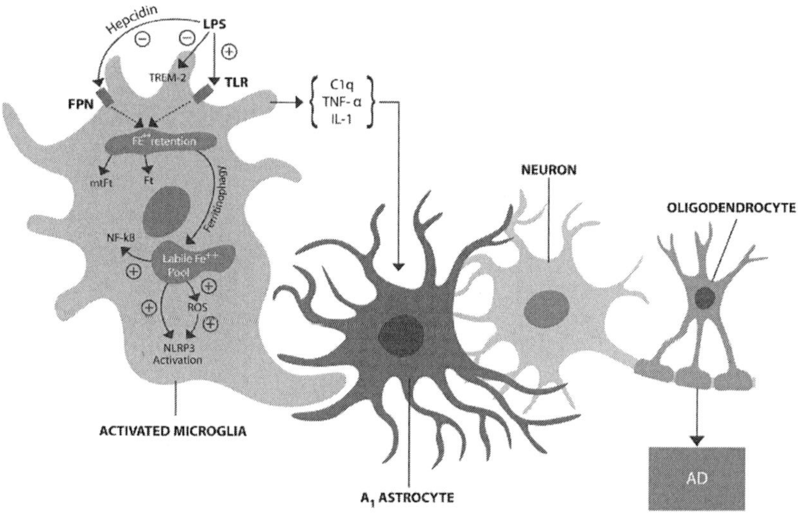


**Figure 1 | LPS, a danger signal, binds to TLRs of microglia, inducing pathogen-mediated intracellular iron sequestration. LPS also promotes astrocytic hepcidin synthesis which via FPN prevents iron egress. In addition, LPS inhibits TREM-2 expressed on microglial cells. Intracellular iron is stored in Ft and mtFt. Iron can dissociate from ferritins via ferritinophagy, augmenting the free iron (labile iron pool). Unbound iron directly and indirectly (via ROS) activates NLRP3 and NF-kB, inducing microglial activation (training). Microglial release of cytokines, including TNF-alpha, IL-1, and C1q induces A1 astrocytes shown to engage in the phagocytosis of viable neurons and oligodendrocytes, contributing to neuronal loss and possibly AD.**

## Iron Homeostasis and the Innate Immune System

Iron is an indispensable but potentially toxic trace element and for this reason it has to be circulated throughout the body attached to its carrier protein, transferrin (Tf). Dietary iron is absorbed in the gut by crossing the enterocyte brush border membrane via divalent metal-ion transporter 1 (DMT-1). After conversion from ferrous to ferric iron by hephaestin and/or ceruloplasmin it is exported through the basolateral membrane via ferroportin (FPN) channels (23).

Novel studies have demonstrated that gram-negative commensal gut microbes are able to generate more than one type of LPS, thus activating or inhibiting innate immune responses (24). For example, Escherichia coli LPS was found to be an activator of innate immunity, while LPS derived from Bacteroides dorei was linked to immune tolerance (25).

Interestingly, Bacteroides fragilis LPS (BF-LPS) was shown to contribute to autoimmune pathology by selectively inhibiting innate immune tolerization (26). Since the host and microbes share a common iron pool, its availability is directly linked to the survival and growth of the LPS-shedding bacteria.

Iron enters the CNS together with Tf (iron-Tf complex) by binding to transferrin receptor-1 (TFR-1) expressed by the endothelial cells of brain capillaries. After crossing into the cytosol of these cells and satisfying their metabolic needs, excess iron is stored in the cytosolic and mitochondrial ferritin. The remaining iron is exported via FPN into the extracellular space (27).

One of the key roles of the innate immune system is pathogen-mediated intracellular iron sequestration to deny it to bacteria and malignancies which are dependent on this biometal for growth (discussed in The Trained Arm of Innate Immunity section). Iron sequestration is initiated in response to exogenous and endogenous danger signals, consisting of pathogen-associated molecular patterns (PAMPs) or, damage-associated molecular patterns (DAMPs), respectively. For example, LPS, the cell wall component of gram-negative bacteria, is a PAMP that activates microglial TLR-4. In contrast, the endogenously produced ROS is a DAMP that activates the cytosolic inflammasome NOD-like receptor pyrin domaincontaining-3 (NLRP3) (28). Iron, itself and/or iron-induced ROS were shown to activate NLRP3 inflammasomes, engendering neuroinflammation (9) (Figure 1).

Iron enters neurons via DMT-1 and TFR-1 receptors but can only exit these cells through FPN, a receptor controlled by hepcidin, the master regulator of iron metabolism. Hepcidin is biosynthesized in the liver, but since only a small fraction of this this peptide hormone crosses the brain-blood barrier (BBB), the brain produces its own hepcidin. High hepcidin levels are associated with intracellular iron accumulation, as this biomolecule binds to FPN, internalizing this receptor (29). LPS and pro-inflammatory cytokines stimulate hepcidin production, inducing hypoferremia, a mechanism involved in the anemia of chronic inflammation pathogenesis (30). Interestingly, astrocytes were shown to induce neuronal death in response to LPS-activated microglia and to synthesize hepcidin via the IL-6/STAT3 pathway, likely linking hepcidin to A1 astrocytes (31). In addition, iron activates nuclear factor kappa-light-chainenhancer of activated B cells (NF-kB), a transcription factor involved in innate immune training and inflammation (27).

Microglia are yolk-sac-derived myeloid cells, comprising up to 20% of the total brain glial cell population (32). Their main function consists of brain parenchyma surveillance, searching for endogenous or exogenous danger signals to which they respond by activation (33). Another major function of microglia, assisted by astrocytes, consists of tolerization or acceptance of self-molecules, food, commensal microbes, and the fetus. This task is accomplished by phagocytosis via prompt clearance of molecular debris, including dead or dying cells that were shown to trigger inflammation and autoimmunity when allowed to accumulate (34). Taken together, disruption of phagocytosis can lead to unchecked inflammation, impaired immune tolerance and autoantibodies against self-components. Indeed, increased levels of autoantibodies were documented in AD, suggesting that autoimmunity may play a role in this disorder (35).

## The Trained Arm of Innate Immunity

Pathogen-mediated iron sequestration is an effective mechanism that protects the host against bacteria and malignancies at the risk of inflammation and ROS triggered by increased intracellular iron (36). To lower this risk, iron must be properly stored into the cytosolic and mitochondrial ferritin, a process that may be disrupted by inflammation and age-related pathology. In the CNS, pathogen-mediated iron sequestration is initiated upon detection of PAMPs and/or DAMPs by microglia and astrocyte, followed by the release acute phase proteins, including hepcidin and lipocalin-2 (LCN-2), to internalize iron (29, 37).

Aging augments the expression of hepcidin and LCN-2, which along with impaired ferritinophagy, increases the risk of free intracellular iron and prolonged inflammation via NLRP3 inflammasomes activation (16, 38). Both hepcidin and LCN-2 have been associated with neurotoxicity and AD, despite some studies describing them as neuroprotective (39–42). These findings are contradictory in appearance only because hepcidin and LCN-2 may have both beneficial and detrimental effects, depending on the phase of inflammation. For example, during the acute phase, iron sequestration may be adaptive as it is denied to pathogens, limiting infection and inflammation. On the other hand, with chronic inflammation and increasing age, intracellular iron may become detrimental as it activates NLRP3 likely overwhelming immune tolerization and triggering neuronal loss. In addition, iron also activates NF-kB implicated in tolerization disruption and autoimmunity when in excess or inappropriately activated (43) (Figure 1). Iron may impair immune tolerance directly by altering microglial secretome, enhancing the release of TNF-alpha, IL-1, and C1q, cytokines that promote A1 astrocytes (1). Indeed, the pathological phagocytosis that A1 cells engage in may reflect the loss of neuronal and oligodendrocytic tolerization. Interestingly, a different study reported A1 astrocytes' upregulation in healthy elderly individuals, linking these cells to the chronic inflammation of aging or inflammaging, considered by some an AD prodrome (44, 45). Moreover, a novel study found that glucagon-like peptide-1 receptor (GLP1R) agonists can block the conversion of trophic to A1 astrocytes, suggesting that Diabetes mellitus type 2 treatments, including liraglutide, may benefit inflammaging and AD (46). Interestingly, liraglutide was documented to lower inflammatory responses by decreasing the expression of NLRP3, suggesting that this drug may function as an inflammasome inhibitor (47).

Inflammasomes are cytosolic multiprotein complexes activated in innate immune cells in response to PAMPs or DAMPs (16, 48). Inflammation is ignited by the inflammasome assembly with caspase1-induced maturation of interleukin-1β and IL-18 which in turn activate multiple inflammatory pathways (49) (Figure 2). NLRP3 inflammasomes, abundantly expressed by microglia and astrocytes, may play a major role in AD as they can be activated by beta amyloid, iron and ROS, maintaining chronic inflammation (48, 50, 51). Indeed, continuous immune training in inflammaging and AD was associated with perpetually elevated NLRP1 and NLRP3 mRNA levels (52–54). Similarly, chronic NLRP3 activation was associated with atherosclerosis and Western diets, linking metabolism and chronic inflammation (55, 56).

Recently the mitochondrion was identified as the interface connecting immunity and metabolism as this organelle contains the mammalian target of rapamycin (mTOR), a protein involved in shifting the metabolic gears from oxidative phosphorylation (OXPHOS), characterizing tolerized immunity, to aerobic glycolysis, marking immune training (11). Iron has been demonstrated to induce mitochondrial damage, probably lowering OXPHOS and prompting NLRP3 inflammasome assembly and microglial training (57, 58) (Figure 2). In fact, iron-disrupted OXPHOS may leave aerobic glycolysis as the only metabolic option for microglia and a possible source of neuroinflammation in AD. Along these lines, a recent study described a direct cross-talk between mTOR and iron metabolism, suggesting a connection between this biometal and aerobic glycolysis (59, 60). Mitophagy or elimination of damaged mitochondria (including that which is iron-induced) was reported to inhibit NLRP3 and lower immune training in AD models, pointing to mitophagy as a potential AD treatment (61–64). Interestingly, liraglutide, a GLP-1R agonist, was shown to promote mitophagy in addition to, or because of NLRP3 inhibition, indicating a potential "off label" use of this drug (65). A recent preclinical study linked the NLRP3 component, apoptosis-associated speck-like protein containing a caspase recruitment domain (ASC), with the prion-like seeding of beta amyloid (66). Similarly, in a previous study, ASC was reported as capable of migrating through the extracellular space (67). Another novel study found a link between NLRP3 inflammasomes and prion disease (68). Furthermore, multiple studies over the past decade established a close connection between various forms of prion diseases and autoimmunity, suggesting a common denominator (69, 70). Interestingly, iron was associated with both prion disease and autoimmunity, and chelation was found therapeutic in CNS autoimmune disorders, including MS and experimental autoimmune encephalomyelitis (EAE) (71–74). For example, brain iron dyshomeostasis was demonstrated in prion disease patients, while another study found a higher incidence of autoimmune disorders in individuals with hemochromatosis (71, 74). A preliminary study found that deferiprone, a BBB-crossing iron chelator, was therapeutic in MS patients

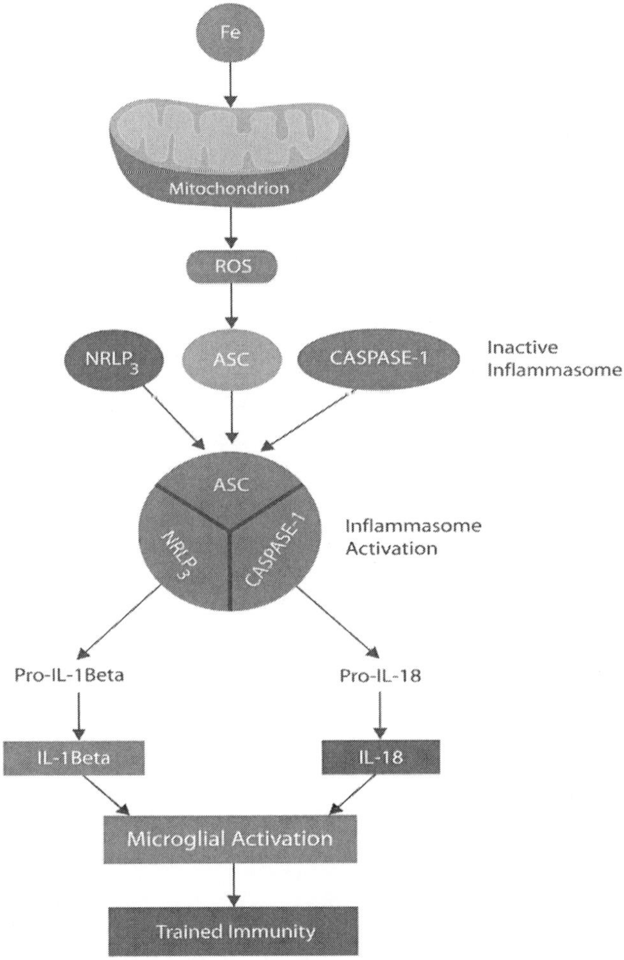


**Figure 2 | NLRP3 inflammasomes activation: iron-damaged mitochondria, acting as a DAMP, directly or via ROS triggers inflammation by activating NLRP3 inflammasomes. Inflammasomes are comprised of a sensor, the nucleotide-binding oligomerization domain (NOD), in this case the (NOD)-like receptor protein 3 (NLRP3), apoptosis-associated speck-like protein containing a caspase recruitment domain (ASC) and caspase-1 which, upon stimulation, assemble and cleave premature IL-1 beta and IL-18 into their biologically active forms, activating microglia (trained immunity).**

(73). Moreover, some iron chelators were found beneficial in AD and Parkinson's disease (PD), possibly pointing to the role of autoimmune inflammation in these disorders (75– 77). Indeed, over the past decade, several studies have associated autoimmunity with AD as serum and CSF autoantibodies against β-amyloid, tau, ceramide and adenosine triphosphate (ATP) synthase were detected in this disorder (35, 78–82). Interestingly, these molecules were also associated with iron and NLRP3, making it worthwhile to search for ASC autoantibodies in AD (83–87).

## The Tolerized Arm of Innate Immunity

Effective protection from pathogens and malignant cells is an important function of the innate immune system, but an equally important task is protection against autoimmune inflammation by maintaining immunologic tolerance to self-structures, food, the fetus, and commensal bacteria. Tolerized immunity or absence of immune responses to repeated or prolonged LPS stimulation was originally described in rodents which survived the administration of a lethal endotoxin dose after previous exposure to sublethal concentrations (88). The adaptive role of this mechanism in the CNS may include "tolerating" elevated levels of LPS demonstrated in the brains of aging individuals and AD patients (2). Indeed, aging and AD have been associated with increased gram-negative bacteria titers in the GI tract and gums (89). For example, individuals with AD were found to have three times higher LPS blood levels compared to controls (90). Interestingly, novel studies have shown that B. fragilis generates a structurally different LPS (BF-LPS), that selectively inhibits immune tolerization, possibly contributing to the pathogenesis of both autoimmune disorders and AD (25, 26).

Aside from the LPS response, brain tolerized immunity may serve the purpose of inhibiting inflammation during phagocytosis of apoptotic cells, synapses, or damaged endogenous molecules, a process we define as tolerant phagocytosis (91, 92). Preclinical studies have shown that disruption of this pathway and accumulation of molecular debris activates autoimmune inflammation, inflicting neuronal damage (93, 94). A novel study has reported that LPS downregulates the expression of the triggering receptor expressed on myeloid cells 2 (TREM2), the microglial receptor associated with immune tolerance (95) (Figure 1). Apolipoprotein E (ApoE) is a TREM2 ligand and their interaction may be necessary for tolerant phagocytosis (96–98). Indeed, TREM-2 blockade was demonstrated to exacerbate EAE and MS, linking this receptor to the CNS autoimmune disorders (99, 100).

A recent pivotal study established the existence of an ApoETREM-2 axis which under normal circumstances engenders tolerized or homeostatic microglial phenotypes (101). In contrast, a dysfunctional ApoE-TREM-2 axis was associated with deficient tolerization and unopposed inflammation. For example, ApoE4 isoform, linked to late onset AD, presents with poor TREM-2 binding, leading to the activation of NLRP3 and immune training instead of tolerization (102, 103).

In AD, the tolerized arm of innate immunity appears to be impaired as persistently elevated LPS brain levels fail to induce tolerance, probably triggering the autoimmune elimination of neurons and oligodendrocytes via A1 astrocytes (1, 2, 98, 104). Moreover, LPS elevation in AD was linked to iron as dormant microbes, including B. fragilis, may survive in the CNS in an inactive state limited by the lack of free iron (6). During aging, impaired iron homeostasis provides these microbes with enough metal to resume their growth and LPS shedding, possibly explaining the LPS upregulation observed in AD (105). Indeed, iron may facilitate B. fragilis resuscitation in the brain as this microbe was shown to require iron or heme for surviving outside of the GI tract (106). In addition, iron-induced endothelial cells' damage may open the BBB (a property exploited in the treatment of gliomas), allowing microbial passage (107, 108). On the other hand, iron chelators were demonstrated to inhibit B. fragilis growth, lowering LPS brain levels, perhaps explaining some of the beneficial effects of these compounds in AD (109). In addition, LPS, not only promotes ferritinophagy, but also the astrocytic expression of hepcidin via IL6/STAT3, further augmenting the cellular free iron pool along with the chances of dormant bacterial resuscitation (31).

At the molecular level, tolerized immunity was shown to be associated with microglial TREM-2 receptors, interacting with anti-inflammatory molecules, including ApoE, and complement components C1q/C3 (110–112) (Figure 3). In addition, tolerized immunity was shown to be modulated by iron-dependent hypoxia-inducible factor 1α (HIF-1α), suggesting another tolerization target (113).

Under physiological circumstances C1q and C3 facilitate phagocytosis by tagging dysfunctional synapses for engulfment by microglia and astrocytes (114, 115). In addition, C1q enhances immune tolerance and inhibits NLRP3-induced immune activation (116). Pathologically, deficient C1q was found in over 90% of systemic lupus erythematosus (SLE) patients, linking this protein to autoimmune inflammation (117). In contrast, ApoE4-induced C1q upregulation was associated with inappropriate elimination of healthy synapses by astrocytes, connecting this phenomenon to autoimmunity and the A1 cells (118). Indeed, the development of anti-C1q antibodies may comprise a novel therapeutic strategy for both AD and autoimmunity (10).

Iron disrupts tolerized immunity by lowering ApoE expression in microglia, impairing the ApoE-TREM-2 axis and amyloid plaque phagocytosis (119–121). Indeed, ApoEimmunoreactive microglia were found closely associated with senile plaques, suggesting a key role in AD pathology (122). In addition, iron disrupts tolerized immunity by upregulating C3 and altering the C1q expression, likely preventing their ApoE binding (123, 124). Indeed, C3 upregulation was linked to increased beta amyloid and phosphorylated tau, linking once more iron to AD pathogenesis (110, 125) (Figure 3). Other recent studies connected iron-upregulated C3 with the A1 astrocytes by demonstrating high complement levels in astrocyte-derived exosomes obtained from AD patients (114, 126).

Aside from ApoE and C1q/C3, iron inhibits α-secretase or ADAM-10, the enzyme involved in the generation of soluble TREM-2 (sTREM-2), linking again this biometal to autoimmunity (102, 123, 124, 127–129) (Figure 4).

Adenosine-triphosphate (ATP) synthase, the mitochondrial enzyme involved in ATP biosynthesis, is a newly identified AD target, especially because extracellular ATP (eATP) is a potent NLRP3 activator associated with autoimmune disorders (81– 85). This is relevant as preclinical studies show iron-associated augmentation of F1 and F0 components of ATP synthase with loss of mitochondrial ATP, possibly suggesting ATP displacement to the extracellular compartment (130). In addition, ironbinding protein, lactoferrin clears eATP, presenting with a beneficial role in AD (see the section on exosomes and Inflammasomes). Furthermore, blockade of purinergic receptors P2Y1 was associated with improved cognition in AD models, while P2X7 inhibition was found beneficial in autoimmune disorders, linking eATP and iron to impaired immune tolerance (87, 130, 131).

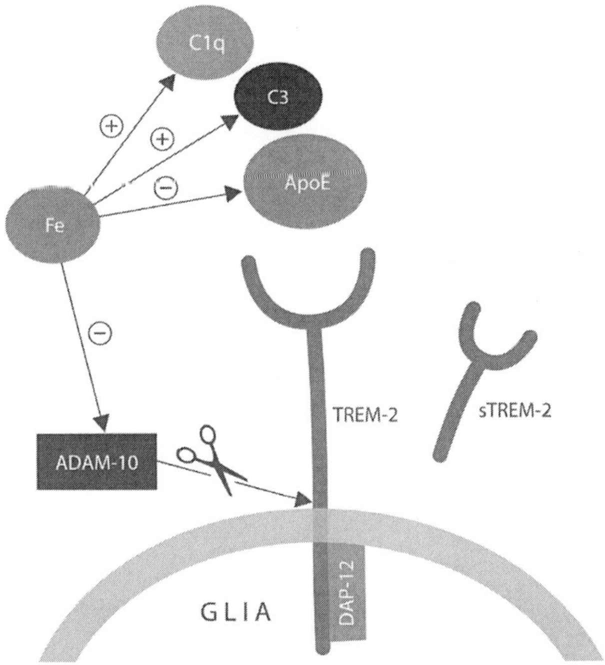


**Figure 4 | A closer view of microglial ApoE-TREM-2 axis: ApoE, C1q, and C3 engender tolerant phagocytosis (lack of inflammatory response during the clearance of damaged self-components). Iron disrupts this process by promoting prolonged inflammation that overrides immune tolerization. In addition, iron impairs tolerization by altering C1q and ApoE along with C3 upregulation. Iron also inhibits alpha secretase (ADAM-10) which cleaves tolerant TREM-2 receptor into sTREM-2, likely impairing phagocytosis. DAP-12 is a TREM-2 adapter, anchoring this receptor into the cell membrane. ADAM-10 is the same enzyme that cleaves amyloid precursor protein (APP), preventing the formation of amyloid-beta peptide.**

## The Innate-Adaptive Continuum

Novel preclinical studies indicate a close cooperation between the innate and adaptive immune systems via NLRP3 inflammasomes and IL-1β (132, 133). Microglia and astrocytes communicate extensively with peripheral lymphocytes, inducing their activation and CNS migration (10, 134). IL-1β is known for increasing BBB permeability, facilitating the infiltration of peripheral cytotoxic T-cells (CTCs) into the CNS (135). In addition, iron is known for altering the BBB by inflicting endothelial cells damage, facilitating peripheral cells access to the CNS (107). In addition, peripheral lymphocytes may access the brain via the newly discovered CNS-draining lymphatics (17).

The newly arrived cells were shown to activate NLRP3, attracting more blood-borne immune cells into the brain (136). On the other hand, tolerized glia may orchestrate the CNS import of T-regs or the newly identified regulatory B1a cells which in turn lower microglial training (137–140). In addition, B-cells have been known to facilitate the recruitment of T-regs to the CNS, augmenting their immunosuppressive activities (141).

T-regs, the preservers of immune tolerance, were found to delay AD progression, linking this condition to autoimmune inflammation (142, 143). The anti-inflammatory IL-10 released by tolerized microglia and T-regs was demonstrated to negatively regulate iron metabolism, possibly explaining the beneficial role of Tregs in AD (144). In addition, IL-4 also regulates iron metabolism and promotes immune tolerance (145). Indeed, iron has been shown to facilitate the CNS infiltration of peripheral CTCs, while iron chelation produces the opposite effect (146). Furthermore, IL-10 was demonstrated to inhibit aerobic glycolysis, the metabolic driver of trained immunity, promoting the tolerant OXPHOS (144, 147, 148). Interestingly, a recent preclinical study discovered a CNS population of cerebral T-regs, documenting that aside from blood borne, the brain maintains its own tolerogenic lymphocyte population (139). Other novel studies demonstrated the existence of various T-regs subpopulations, expressing different co-inhibitory Tcell receptors, including the T-cell immunoglobulin and ITIM Domain (TIGIT) that regulates immunity exclusively via ironlowering IL-10, linking this receptor to iron downregulation (149, 150).

Co-inhibitory receptors, including cytotoxic T-lymphocyte associated protein 4 (CTLA-4), programmed cell death protein 1 (PD-1), lymphocyte-activation protein 3 (Lag-3), and TIGIT play an essential role in the prevention of autoimmune disorders by promoting tolerized responses (151, 152). A growing body of evidence reveals that dysfunctional co-inhibitory receptors may contribute to AD neuroinflammation as under normal circumstances they function to inhibit inflammation-generating co-stimulatory signals (153). For example, upregulation of PD1 expressed on both microglia and T-regs, was found beneficial in AD animal models (154). Another study demonstrated that non-PD-1 expressing T-regs were upregulated in mild cognitive impairment (MCI), demonstrating the beneficial role of PD-1 receptors in preventing the development of full-blown AD (155). Indeed, tolerized microglia also express PD-1, activating T-regs and probably facilitating their CNS import (156, 157).

These findings suggest that other co-inhibitory receptors, including TIGIT, may activate T-regs. Interestingly, a recent study found elevated TIGIT in the peripheral blood of healthy elderly individuals (158). As upregulated A1 astrocytes were also found in normal aging, TIGIT and A1 may comprise novel AD risk markers (45). In addition, as TIGIT modulates immunity via the iron-lowering IL-10, this receptor may be elevated in normal aging in a compensatory manner in response to iron overload (149). TIGIT is yet to be demonstrated on glial cells, however like PD-1, it may be a coordinator of adaptive and immune responses.

Taken together, this data suggests that innate and adaptive immunity operate on a continuum as trained immunity may activate CTCs, while tolerized immunity the T-regs, therefore targeting trained and tolerized immunity may lower the CNS infiltration of peripheral lymphocytes.

## Microglial Reprograming: Trained and Tolerized Therapies

The recent FDA approval of immune training-inducers prompted research for similar therapies for cancer and neurodegeneration (18). Immune stimulatory vaccines, comprised of antigen and pro-inflammatory molecules, activate TLRs or NLRP3, inducing immune activation. These therapeutics have been utilized to train APCs and reverse cancer or sepsisinduced T cell anergy. Iron as an inducer of trained immunity has been utilized to activate TAMs and several nanoparticles are currently being designed for its delivery (14). On the other hand, the development of specific tolerized therapies, including "inverse vaccines," capable of improving pathology without causing generalized immunosuppression, has been vexing (20). The same is true regarding the first-generation AD vaccines, like AN1793, based on anti-Aβ1-42 antibodies which was abandoned due to adverse effects (159). However, despite these draw backs, a new generation of AD vaccines, including anti-C1q mentioned above, are currently being developed. Since neuroinflammation represents the predominant pathology in many neurodegenerative and even psychiatric disorders, de-escalating iron-trained microglia may comprise an effective treatment strategy. Indeed, the anti-inflammatory iron chelator deferiprone is currently in phase 2 trials for AD (15, 160). Deferiprone may have a dual mechanism of action, lowering trained immunity and augmenting tolerization, suggesting that simultaneously targeting both arms of innate immunity may yield better therapeutic outcomes than addressing each one in isolation. Another dual-mechanism-of-action compound, hydroxamic acid, is a promising histone deacetylase-6 inhibitor (HDAC6i) which presents with the added benefit of being an iron chelator (161, 162). Histone deacetylases are enzymes involved in the removal of acetyl groups from histone proteins, altering the chromatin landscape and gene expression. HDACs have been associated with AD pathogenesis, while some HDACis were found to improve cognition (163, 164). In addition, selective HDAC inhibitors were shown to suppress LPS-trained microglia via IL-6 and TNF-α, suggesting a therapeutic potential in AD neuroinflammation (165). Moreover, HDACs 1 and 2 inhibitors are augmenters of microglial β amyloid phagocytosis, linking these compounds to the immuno-metabolic reprograming via OXPHOS augmentation (165, 166).

## Inflammasome Inhibitors

NLRP3 inhibition to lower immune training and the subsequent neuroinflammation is an emerging therapeutic strategy in AD and traumatic brain injury (TBI) (167–169).

Purinergic receptor blockers, ASC inhibitors, diarylsulphonylurea inhibitors, β-sulfonyl nitrile compounds, and caspase-1 blockers are the broad categories of recently developed NLRP3 inhibitors (170, 171). The most studied compound, MCC950 is a diarylsulphonylurea inhibitor, a potent anti-inflammatory drug and a facilitator of β amyloid clearance in AD animal models (172). Another recently developed molecule, OLT1177, is a β-sulfonyl nitrile which inhibits NLRP3 by limiting ROS generation after LPS challenge. This compound is currently in phase I clinical trials.

Suppressing NLRP3 by ASC inhibition is an attractive AD strategy as ASC was recently found to disseminate β amyloid throughout the CNS (66, 172). Interestingly, saxagliptin, a dipeptidyl peptidase-4 (DPP-4) inhibitor, which increases plasma GLP-1 concentration, appears to selectively inhibit ASC, suggesting a role in preventing the spread of AD pathology (173). This is significant since GLP-1R agonists were found to inhibit the conversion of trophic into A1 astrocytes, probably linking ASC to this neurotoxic phenotype (1, 46). Moreover, Tranilast, an anti-allergic drug derived from tryptophan, was also reported to selectively inhibit ASC, suggesting a preventive potential in AD (174).

## Of Exosomes and Inflammasomes

Exosomes are (50–150 nm) extracellular nanovesicles released by most cell types, including neurons and glia, which can carry molecular cargos and trigger functional changes in target cells. Exosomes cross the BBB, facilitating the transfer of inflammation as they can carry a variety of peripheral molecules, including inflammasome-derived proteins (175, 176).

Exosomes, involved in innate immune cells' cross talk, participate in microglial training or tolerization by augmenting or lowering neuroinflammation, depending on their cells of origin (17, 177, 178). Novel studies have found that neuronal exosomes have beneficial effects, while astrocytesderived exosomes (ADE) are mostly detrimental, inducing neurodegeneration. Neuronal exosomes present with the adaptive function of clearing β amyloid by delivering it to microglia for phagocytosis. For this reason, pharmacological facilitation of neuronal exosomes' synthesis could be developed into an AD therapy (176). For example, designer neuronal exosomes were recently developed and utilized in animal models of Parkinson's disease (170). Interestingly, microglial cells were shown to release exosomes that were previously reported to originate from B cells and dendritic cells, suggesting pro-inflammatory roles (179). CNS autoimmune disorders have been associated with exosomes transporting histocompatibility complex (MHC) class II proteins released by interferon-γ activated microglia (180).

ADE were shown to promote the conversion of trophic to A1 astrocytes by releasing exosomes containing complement components C1q and C3 (126, 181–183). Preventing ADE release may comprise another potential AD strategy. Moreover, a novel study has demonstrated that excessive interstitial ATP can facilitate the generation of A1 astrocytes, suggesting clearance of ATP from the extracellular space (ECS) as a potential AD treatment modality (174). Interestingly, the natural iron chelator, lactoferrin, was found to facilitate the ECS removal of ATP, indicating a novel therapeutic application (184). Indeed, a recent study suggested that engineered lactoferrin-containing exosomes could accomplish this goal (185).

## Histone Deacetylases Inhibitors (Hdaci)

Innate immune cells are endowed with an epigenetically regulated memory of previous antigen encounters, suggesting that epigenome manipulation may comprise an efficient reprograming strategy in these cells (17). Acetylation and deacetylation of DNA and histone proteins are the most studied epigenetic mechanisms regulating innate immune cells. Indeed, HDACi were shown to lower the LPS-induced microglial training, promoting tolerization (165). For example, valproic acid, a HDACi utilized in the treatment of bipolar disorder and epilepsy, was shown to downregulate the mammalian target of rapamycin (mTOR), restoring OXPHOS, the driver of immune tolerance (11, 186–188). Furthermore, HDACi were recently shown to augment astrocytic ApoE secretion (189). Since ApoE inhibits NLRP3 activation, HDAC inhibition may have a potential therapeutic value in the fight against AD neuroinflammation (Figure 3).

HDACi are facilitators of ferritin storage, lowering intracellular free iron and the risk of NLRP3 activation (161, 190). In addition, HDACi reverse the iron-induced augmentation of glycogen synthase kinase-3β (GSK3β), a proinflammatory enzyme implicated in AD (191, 192). GSK-3β inhibitors, including lithium, were shown to promote immune tolerance, suggesting a therapeutic role in lowering iron levels (193–195). Interestingly, the tolerizing receptor TREM-2 is a negative regulator of GSK-3β, further associating this protein with decreasing iron-induced neuroinflammation (191, 196).

## Co-Inhibitory T-Cell Receptors in Ad

Dysfunctional co-inhibitory receptors may contribute to AD neuroinflammation as under normal circumstances, they block co-stimulatory signals, lowering inflammation (153). For example, stimulation of PD-1 receptors, expressed on both microglia and T-regs, was found beneficial in AD animal models (154). On the other hand, increased number of nonPD-1 expressing T-regs in MCI, shows the importance of this co-inhibitory receptor in AD prevention (155).

T cell activation by APCs is crucial for mounting adequate adaptive immune responses. In the CNS, microglia and astrocytes can become APCs, engendering immunologic synapses with peripheral T cells (10). The proliferation, differentiation, and migration of these cells is triggered by the interplay between co-stimulatory and co-inhibitory signals which fine tune T cell responses (197). For example, the co-stimulatory receptors promote effector T-cells function, while co-inhibitory receptors function to inhibit co-stimulatory signals, promoting T-regs (6). Activation of co-inhibitory receptors, including CTLA-4, PD-1, LAG-3, TIM-3, and TIGIT, induce immune tolerance, therefore their stimulation would be beneficial in autoimmune disorders (198). On the other hand, their blockade was shown to train TAMs in a manner similar to iron and eliminate cancer cells (199). Interestingly, TIGIT competes with the co-stimulatory signal CD226 for a common ligand CD155, suggesting that promoting the TIGIT-CD155 axis may lower intracellular iron as TIGIT operates exclusively via the iron-lowering IL-10 (200). Indeed, IL-10 or CD-155 loaded exosomes may enhance the co-inhibitory receptor TIGIT, lowering microglial intracellular iron. In addition, the CD226 genetic variant, Gly307Ser, was associated with several autoimmune disorders, suggesting that CD 226 inhibition may facilitate tolerized immunity and benefit the treatment of these conditions as well (201, 202).

## Tolerized Immunity and Acetylcholinesterase Inhibitors

Acetylcholinesterase inhibitors (AChEIs) are cholinergic compounds widely utilized in AD. AChEIs, including donepezil, rivastigmine, and galantamine function by inhibiting cholinesterase, the acetylcholine-degrading enzyme, increasing its synaptic availability in the cholinergic tracts. Some of these drugs may be modulators of trained or tolerized immunity as they oppose iron-induced NLRP3 activation and the inhibition of ADAM-10, the protective α-secretase, in charge of cleaving both TREM-2 and APP (203–205) (Figure 4). In addition, α7and α9 nicotinic acetylcholine receptor (nAChR) agonists were found to lower autoimmune inflammation, by augmenting tolerization (206, 207). Moreover, activation of α7nAChRs was found to reverse post-surgical cognitive impairment, suggesting that AChEIs-linked cognitive enhancement may be due to their anti-inflammatory actions (208). On the other hand, a recent study demonstrated that iron and ROS can inhibit α7nAChRs signaling, likely disrupting tolerized immunity (209, 210). Interestingly, conjugation of an AChEI, such as galantamine, with the natural iron chelator, lactoferrin, was recently proposed as an AD therapy (211).

## Tolerized Immunity and Selective Serotonin Reuptake Inhibitors (SSRIs)

Serotonin reuptake inhibitors (SSRIs) are widely prescribed antidepressant drugs that block 5-hydroxytryptamine reuptake in the presynaptic neurons of brain serotonergic tracts, augmenting the synaptic availability of this neurotransmitter. However, these compounds were found to also lower trained immune responses. For example, a recent study indicated that the SSRI, fluoxetine reduces the central and peripheral levels of IL-1β by inhibiting NLRP3 (212, 213).

Another group demonstrated the existence of a cross talk between the brain innate immunity and serotonin signaling, possibly linking major depressive disorder with NLRP3 activation (214). Along the same lines, it was recently shown that indoleamine 2,3-dioxygenase-1 (IDO-1), an enzyme associated with tryptophan catabolism, is abundantly expressed by microglia and astrocytes, connecting serotonergic signaling with tolerized immunity (215). IDO-1 induces immune tolerance by processing tryptophan to L-kynurenine, an inhibitor of immune cells' proliferation and maturation (216). IDO-1 is known for orchestrating mother's immune acceptance of the fetus, however some bacteria and cancers were found to exploit this pathway (217, 218). Indeed, an IDO vaccine to block cancer-induced immune tolerance is currently under development (219). Moreover, IDO-1 contributes to the biosynthesis of quinolinic acid (QUIN), a neurotoxic tryptophan catabolite that was linked to AD pathogenesis (220). Interestingly, iron-QUIN complexes were demonstrated in this neurodegenerative disorder, indicating that QUIN toxicity may be iron-related (221, 222). QUIN was demonstrated to activate microglia and astrocytes, resulting in neuronal death, possibly by inducing A1 cells (223–225).

## Conclusions

The healthy immune system must keep trained and tolerized immunity in balance to ensure effective defenses against pathogens and malignancies, while at the same time accepting the self-components, food, the fetus, and commensal microbes. Iron interferes with this process as it triggers a competition between the host and pathogens. Both biological systems have developed mechanisms to capture iron and deny it to the opposing side. The innate immune cells sequestrate iron to restrict its availability to pathogens, but elevated intracellular iron increases the risk of mitochondrial damage, ROS generation, and autoimmune inflammation.

Aging and iron are associated with increased permeability of both GI and brain microvessels, allowing gut microbes, including B. fragilis, to migrate into the CNS and shed LPS, disrupting immune tolerization. Manipulation of trained and tolerized immunity, especially via exosomes and nanoparticles loaded with iron chelators could represent future AD strategies (76). Indeed, iron-oxide loaded exosomes for magnetic hyperthermia have been successfully used in oncology (226).

Tolerogenic immunization also known as "inverse vaccines," can for example, utilize CD-155 loaded exosomes to enhance the co-inhibitory receptor TIGIT and lower AD neuroinflammation (227). In addition, nanoparticles containing NLRP3-inhibitors, HDACi or ASC blockers may soon become parts of the AD armamentarium.

**Author Contributions:** All authors listed have made a substantial, direct and intellectual contribution to the work, and approved it for publication.

**Conflict of Interest Statement:** The authors declare that the research was conducted in the absence of any commercial or financial relationships that could be construed as a potential conflict of interest.



## References

1. Chester DS, Lynam DR, Milich R, DeWall CN. Physical aggressiveness and gray matter deficits in the ventromedial prefrontal cortex. Cortex. 2017 Dec;97:17-22. doi: 10.1016/j.cortex.2017.09.024.
2. Zhang YD, Zhou JS, Lu FM, Wang XP. Reduced gray matter volume in male adolescent violent offenders. PeerJ. 2019 Sep 3;7:e7349. doi: 10.7717/peerj.7349. PMID: 31534834; PMCID: PMC6730529.
3. Hofhansel L, Weidler C, Votinov M, Clemens B, Raine A, Habel U. Morphology of the criminal brain: gray matter reductions are linked to antisocial behavior in offenders. Brain Struct Funct. 2020 Sep;225(7):2017-2028. doi: 10.1007/s00429-020-02106
4. Vita A, De Peri L, Deste G, Sacchetti E. Progressive loss of cortical gray matter in schizophrenia: a meta-analysis and meta-regression of longitudinal MRI studies. Transl Psychiatry. 2012 Nov 20;2(11):

e190. Doi: 10.1038/tp.2012.116. Erratum in: Transl Psychiatry. 2013;3:e275.

5. Sun, D., Stuart, G., Jenkinson, M. et al. Brain surface contraction mapped in first-episode schizophrenia: a longitudinal magnetic resonance imaging study. Mol Psychiatry 14, 976–986 (2009). https://doi.org/10.1038/mp.2008.34
6. Thompson PM, Vidal C, Giedd JN, Gochman P, Blumenthal J, Nicolson R, Toga AW, Rapoport JL. Mapping adolescent brain change reveals a dynamic wave of accelerated gray matter loss in very early-onset schizophrenia. Proc Natl Acad Sci U S A. 2001 Sep 25; 98(20):11650-5. doi: 10.1073/pnas.201243998. PMID: 11573002
7. Li M, Gao Y, Wang D, Hu X, Jiang J, Qing Y, Yang X, Cui G, Wang P, Zhang J, Sun L, Wan C. Impaired Membrane Lipid Homeostasis in Schizophrenia. Schizophr Bull. 2022 Sep 1;48(5):1125-1135. doi: 10.1093/schbul/sbac011.
8. Alves I, Staneva G, Tessier C, Salgado GF, Nuss P. The interaction of antipsychotic drugs with lipids and subsequent lipid reorganization was investigated using biophysical methods. Biochim Biophys Acta. 2011 Aug;1808(8):2009-18.
doi: 10.1016/j.bbamem.2011.02.021
9. Murphy C.M., Ravner H., Smith N.L. Mode of Action of Phenothiazine-Type Antioxidants. Ind. Eng. Chem. 1950;42:2479–2489. doi: 10.1021/ie50492a027
10. Ohlow MJ, Moosmann B. Phenothiazine: the seven lives of pharmacology's first lead structure. Drug Discov Today. 2011 Feb;16(3-4):119-31. doi: 10.1016/j.drudis.2011.01.001. Epub 2011 Jan 13. PMID: 21237283.
11. Medina-Hernández V, Ramos-Loyo J, Luquin S, Sánchez LF, García-Estrada J, Navarro-Ruiz A. Increased lipid peroxidation and neuron specific enolase in treatment refractory schizophrenics. J Psychiatr Res. 2007 Oct;41(8):652-8.
doi: 10.1016/j.jpsychires.2006.02.010
12. Shu X, Wu J, Zhang T, Ma X, Du Z, Xu J, You J, Wang L, Chen N, Luo M, Wu J. Statin-Induced Geranylgeranyl Pyrophosphate Depletion Promotes Ferroptosis-Related Senescence in Adipose Tissue. Nutrients. 2022 Oct 18;14(20):4365.

doi: 10.3390/nu14204365.

13. Shichiri M. The role of lipid peroxidation in neurological disorders. J Clin Biochem Nutr. 2014 May;54(3):151-60. doi: 10.3164/jcbn.14-10. Epub 2014 Apr 9. PMID: 24895477; PMCID: PMC4042144.
14. Nousis, Lambros, Panagiotis Kanavaros, and Alexandra Barbouti. 2023. "Oxidative Stress-Induced Cellular Senescence: Is Labile Iron the Connecting Link?" Antioxidants 12, no. 6: 1250. https://doi.org/10.3390/antiox12061250
15. Ren JG, Xia HL, Just T, Dai YR. Hydroxyl radical-induced apoptosis in human tumor cells is associated with telomere shortening but not telomerase inhibition and caspase activation. FEBS Lett. 2001 Jan 19;488(3):123-32. doi: 10.1016/s0014-5793(00)02377-2.
16. Sfera A, Andronescu L, Britt WG, Himsl K, Klein C, Rahman L, Kozlakidis Z. Receptor-Independent Therapies for Forensic Detainees with Schizophrenia-Dementia Comorbidity. Int J Mol Sci. 2023 Oct 31;24(21):15797. doi: 10.3390/ijms242115797.
17. Luquain-Costaz C, Kockx M, Anastasius M, Chow V, Kontush A, Jessup W, Kritharides L. Increased ABCA1 (ATP-Binding Cassette Transporter A1)-Specific Cholesterol Efflux Capacity in Schizophrenia. Arterioscler Thromb Vasc Biol. 2020 Nov;40(11): 2728-2737. Doi: 10.1161/ATVBAHA.120.314847.
18. Every-Palmer S, Souter V. Low vitamin D levels found in 95 % of psychiatric inpatients within a forensic service. Aust N Z J Psychiatry. 2015 Apr;49(4):391-2. doi: 10.1177/0004867414562047
19. Pillinger T, Beck K, Stubbs B, Howes OD. Cholesterol and triglyceride levels in first-episode psychosis: systematic review and meta-analysis. Br J Psychiatry. 2017 Dec;211(6):339-349. Doi 10.1192/bjp.bp.117.200907.
20. Choy O. Nutritional factors associated with aggression. Front Psychiatry. 2023 Jun 21;14:1176061. doi: 10.3389/fpsyt.2023.1176061. PMID: 37415691; PMCID: PMC10320003.
21. Papanastasiou E, Gaughran F, Smith S. Schizophrenia as segmental progeria. J R Soc Med. 2011 Nov;104(11):475-84. doi: 10.1258/jrsm.2011.110051.

22. Ojo ES, Tischkau SA. The Role of AhR in the Hallmarks of Brain Aging: Friend and Foe. Cells. 2021 Oct 13;10(10):2729. doi: 10.3390/cells10102729. PMID: 34685709; PMCID: PMC8534784.
23. Yi T, Wang J, Zhu K, Tang Y, Huang S, Shui X, Ding Y, Chen C, Lei W. Aryl Hydrocarbon Receptor: A New Player of Pathogenesis and Therapy in Cardiovascular Diseases. Biomed Res Int. 2018 Jun 10;2018:6058784. Doi: 10.1155/2018/6058784.
24. Nagai H, Kubo M, Abe R, Yamamoto M, Nohara K. Constitutive activation of the aryl hydrocarbon receptor in T-lineage cells induces thymus involution independently of the Fas/Fas ligand signaling pathway. Int Immunopharmacol. 2006 Feb;6(2):279-86. doi: 10.1016/j.intimp.2005.08.015.
25. Bravo-Ferrer I, Cuartero MI, Medina V, Ahedo-Quero D, Peña-Martínez C, Pérez-Ruíz A, Fernández-Valle ME, Hernández-Sánchez C, Fernández-Salguero PM, Lizasoain I, Moro MA. Lack of the aryl hydrocarbon receptor accelerates aging in mice. FASEB J. 2019 Nov;33(11):12644-12654. doi: 10.1096/fj.201901333R.
26. Ash PEA, Stanford EA, Al Abdulatif A, Ramirez-Cardenas A, Ballance HI, Boudeau S, Jeh A, Murithi JM, Tripodis Y, Murphy GJ, Sherr DH, Wolozin B. Dioxins and related environmental contaminants increase TDP-43 levels. Mol Neurodegener. 2017 May 5;12(1):35. doi: 10.1186/s13024-017-0177-9. PMID: 28476168; PMCID: PMC5420162.
27. McMillan BJ, Bradfield CA. The aryl hydrocarbon receptor is activated by modified low-density lipoprotein. Proc Natl Acad Sci U S A. 2007 Jan 23;104(4):1412-7. doi: 10.1073/pnas.0607296104.
28. Wang BL, Zhang CW, Wang L, Tang KL, Tanaka N, Gonzalez FJ, Xu Y, Fang ZZ. Lipidomics reveal aryl hydrocarbon receptor (Ahr)-regulated lipid metabolic pathway in alpha-naphthyl isothiocyanate (ANIT)-induced intrahepatic cholestasis. Xenobiotica. 2019 May; 49(5):591-601. doi: 10.1080/00498254.2018.1467065.
29. Sankaranarayanan A, Pratt R, Anoop A, Smith A, Espinoza D, Ramachandran P, Tirupati S. Serum lipids and suicidal risk among schizophrenia spectrum disorders: Systematic review and meta-analysis. Acta Psychiatr Scand. 2021 Aug;144(2):125-152. doi: 10.1111/acps.13305.

30. Roaldset, J.O., Linaker, O.M. & Bjørkly, S. Triglycerides as a biological marker of repeated re-hospitalization resulting from deliberate self-harm in acute psychiatry patients: a prospective observational study. BMC Psychiatry 14, 54 (2014). https://doi.org/10.1186/1471-244X-14-54
31. Sen P, Adewusi D, Blakemore AI, Kumari V. How do lipids influence the risk of violence, self-harm, and suicidality in people with psychosis? A systematic review. Aust N Z J Psychiatry. 2022 May;56(5):451-488. Doi: 10.1177/00048674211025608.
32. Pereira H. The Importance of Cholesterol in Psychopathology: A Review of Recent Contributions. Indian J Psychol Med. 2017 Mar-Apr;39(2):109-113. doi: 10.4103/0253-7176.203117
33. Hung HC, Kay SA, Weber F. HSP90, a capacitor of behavioral variation. J Biol Rhythms. 2009 Jun;24(3):183-92. doi: 10.1177/0748730409333171. PMID: 19465695.
34. Tanos R, Patel RD, Murray IA, Smith PB, Patterson AD, Perdew GH. Aryl hydrocarbon receptor regulates the cholesterol biosynthetic pathway in a dioxin response element-independent manner. Hepatology. 2012 Jun;55(6):1994-2004. doi: 10.1002/hep.25571.
35. Golomb BA, Stattin H, Mednick S. Low cholesterol and violent crime. J Psychiatr Res. 2000 Jul-Oct;34(4-5):301-9. doi: 10.1016/s0022-3956(00)00024-8. PMID: 11104842.
36. Virkkunen M. Serum cholesterol levels in homicidal offenders. A low cholesterol level is connected with a habitually violent tendency under the influence of alcohol. Neuropsychobiology. 1983;10(2-3):65-9. doi: 10.1159/000117987. PMID: 6674827.
37. Mascitelli L, Pezzetta F, Goldstein MR. Low cholesterol, delinquency, and suicidality. Prim Care Companion J Clin Psychiatry. 2008;10(5):413-4. doi: 10.4088/pcc.v10n0511c
38. Repo-Tiihonen E, Halonen P, Tiihonen J, Virkkunen M. Total serum cholesterol level, violent criminal offenses, suicidal behavior, mortality and the appearance of conduct disorder in Finnish male criminal offenders with an antisocial personality disorder. Eur Arch Psychiatry Clin Neurosci. 2002 Feb;252(1):8-11. doi: 10.1007/s004060200001.

39. Mufti RM, Balon R, Arfken CL. Low cholesterol and violence. Psychiatr Serv. 1998 Feb;49(2):221-4. doi: 10.1176/ps.49.2.221. PMID: 9575009.
40. Tomson-Johanson K, Harro J. Low cholesterol, impulsivity and violence revisited. Curr Opin Endocrinol Diabetes Obes. 2018 Apr;25(2):103-107. doi: 10.1097/MED.0000000000000395. PMID: 29351110.
41. Ikonen E, Zhou X. Cholesterol transport between cellular membranes: A balancing act between interconnected lipid fluxes. Dev Cell. 2021 May 17;56(10):1430-1436. doi: 10.1016/j.devcel.2021.04.025. PMID: 34004151.
42. Moyer CE, Shelton MA, Sweet RA. Dendritic spine alterations in schizophrenia. Neurosci Lett. 2015 Aug 5;601:46-53. doi: 10.1016/j.neulet.2014.11.042.
43. Sen P, Adewusi D, Blakemore AI, Kumari V. How do lipids influence the risk of violence, self-harm, and suicidality in people with psychosis? A systematic review. Aust N Z J Psychiatry. 2022 May;56(5):451-488. doi: 10.1177/00048674211025608
44. Herceg D, Mimica N, Herceg M, Puljić K. Aggression in Women with Schizophrenia Is Associated with Lower HDL Cholesterol Levels. Int J Mol Sci. 2022 Oct 6;23(19):11858. doi: 10.3390/ijms231911858. PMID: 36233163; PMCID: PMC9570159.
45. Prabhu AV, Luu W, Sharpe LJ, Brown AJ. Cholesterol-mediated Degradation of 7-Dehydrocholesterol Reductase Switches the Balance from Cholesterol to Vitamin D Synthesis. J Biol Chem. 2016 Apr 15;291(16):8363-73. doi: 10.1074/jbc.M115.699546
46. Wnętrzak A, Makyła-Juzak K, Filiczkowska A, Kulig W, Dynarowicz-Łątka P. Oxysterols Versus Cholesterol in Model Neuronal Membrane. I. The Case of 7-Ketocholesterol. The Langmuir Monolayer Study. J Membr Biol. 2017 Oct;250(5):553-564. doi: 10.1007/s00232-017-9984-8
47. Wilson KA, Wang L, O'Mara ML. Site of Cholesterol Oxidation Impacts Its Localization and Domain Formation in the Neuronal Plasma Membrane. ACS Chem Neurosci. 2021 Oct 20;12(20):3873-3884. doi: 10.1021/acschemneuro.1c00395.

48. Anderson A, Campo A, Fulton E, Corwin A, Jerome WG 3rd, O'Connor MS. 7-Ketocholesterol in disease and aging. Redox Biol. 2020 Jan;29:101380. doi: 10.1016/j.redox.2019.101380.
49. Hamsanathan S, Gurkar AU. Lipids as Regulators of Cellular Senescence. Front Physiol. 2022 Mar 4;13:796850. Doi: 10.3389/fphys.2022.796850. PMID: 35370799; PMCID: PMC8965560.
50. Zhao T, Guo X, Sun Y. Iron Accumulation and Lipid Peroxidation in the Aging Retina: Implication of Ferroptosis in Age-Related Macular Degeneration. Aging Dis. 2021 Apr 1;12(2):529-551. Doi: 10.14336/AD.2020.0912. PMID: 33815881; PMCID: PMC7990372.
51. Reichert, C.O.; de Freitas, F.A.; Sampaio-Silva, J.; Rokita-Rosa, L.; Barros, P.d.L.; Levy, D.; Bydlowski, S.P. Ferroptosis Mechanisms Involved in Neurodegenerative Diseases. Int. J. Mol. Sci. 2020; 21: 8765. https://doi.org/10.3390/ijms21228765
52. Feng S, Chen J, Qu C, Yang L, Wu X, Wang S, Yang T, Liu H, Fang Y, Sun P. Identification of Ferroptosis-Related Genes in Schizophrenia Based on Bioinformatic Analysis. Genes (Basel). 2022 Nov 20; 13(11):2168. Doi: 10.3390/genes13112168.
53. Martin N, Zhu K, Czarnecka-Herok J, Vernier M, Bernard D. Regulation and role of calcium in cellular senescence. Cell Calcium. (2023) 110:102701. doi: 10.1016/j.ceca.2023.102701.
54. Zhu Q, Wang W, Wu N, He S, Lin X, Zhang W, Zhou J. 7-Ketocholesterol accelerates pancreatic β-cell senescence by inhibiting the SIRT1/CDK4-Rb-E2F1 signaling pathway. Islets. 2023 Dec 31;15(1):2219105. doi: 10.1080/19382014.2023.2219105.
55. Nicolson GL, Ash ME. Membrane Lipid Replacement for chronic illnesses, aging, and cancer using oral glycerolphospholipid formulations with fructooligosaccharides to restore phospholipid function in cellular membranes, organelles, cells, and tissues. Biochim Biophys Acta. 2017; 1859:1704-1724. doi: 10.1016/j.bbamem.2017.04.013
56. Wacker M, Holick MF. Sunlight and Vitamin D: A global perspective for health. Dermato-endocrinology. (2013) 5(1):51-108. doi:10.4161/derm.24494.

57. Bikle DD. Vitamin D Metabolism, Mechanism of Action, and Clinical Applications. Chemistry & biology. (2014) 21(3):319-329. doi:10.1016/j.chembiol.2013.12.016.
58. Landel V, Stephan D, Cui X, Eyles D, Feron F. Differential expression of vitamin D-associated enzymes and receptors in brain cell subtypes. J Steroid Biochem Mol Biol. 2018 Mar;177:129-134. doi: 10.1016/j.jsbmb.2017.09.008
59. Pignolo A, Mastrilli S, Davì C, Arnao V, Aridon P, Dos Santos Mendes FA, Gagliardo C, D'Amelio M. Vitamin D and Parkinson's Disease. Nutrients. 2022 Mar 14;14(6):1220. doi: 10.3390/nu14061220. PMID: 35334877; PMCID: PMC8953648.
60. Hur J, Lee P, Kim MJ, Cho Y-W. Regulatory Effect of 25-hydroxyvitamin D3 on Nitric Oxide Production in Activated Microglia. The Korean Journal of Physiology & Pharmacology : Official Journal of the Korean Physiological Society and the Korean Society of Pharmacology. (2014) 18(5):397-402. doi:10.4196/kjpp.2014.18.5.397.
61. Roger Bouillon, Lieve Verlinden, Annemieke Verstuyf, Is Vitamin D2 Bioequivalent to Vitamin D3?, Endocrinology, Volume 157, Issue 9, 1 September 2016, Pages 3384–3387, https://doi.org/10.1210/en.2016-1528
62. Tripkovic L, Lambert H, Hart K, et al. Comparison of vitamin D2 and D3 supplementation in raising serum 25-hydroxyvitamin D status: a systematic review and meta-analysis. The American Journal of Clinical Nutrition. (2012) 95(6):1357-1364. doi:10.3945/ajcn.111.031070.
63. Mitri J, Pittas AG. Vitamin D and diabetes. Endocrinology and metabolism clinics of North America. (2014) 43(1):205-232. doi:10.1016/j.ecl.2013.09.010.
64. Bikle DD. Vitamin D Metabolism, Mechanism of Action, and Clinical Applications. Chemistry & biology. (2014) 21(3):319-329. doi:10.1016/j.chembiol.2013.12.016.
65. Kongsbak M, von Essen MR, Boding L, et al. Vitamin D Up-Regulates the Vitamin D Receptor by Protecting It from Proteasomal

Degradation in Human CD4+ T Cells. Bradl M, ed. PLoS ONE. (2014) 9(5):e96695. doi:10.1371/journal.pone.0096695
66. Suzuki K, Sugihara G, Ouchi Y, Nakamura K, Futatsubashi M, Takebayashi K,et al. Microglial activation in young adults with autism spectrum disorder. AMA Psychiatry. (2013) 70(1):49-58. doi: 10.1001/jamapsychiatry.2013.272.
67. Jakobsson J, Bjerke M, Sahebi S, et al. Monocyte and microglial activation in patients with mood-stabilized bipolar disorder. Journal of Psychiatry & Neuroscience : JPN. (2015) 40(4):250-258. doi:10.1503/jpn.140183.
68. Schnieder TP, Trencevska I, Rosoklija G, et al. Microglia of Prefrontal White Matter in Suicide. Journal of neuropathology and experimental neurology. (2014) 73(9):880-890. doi:10.1097/NEN.0000000000000107.
69. Kaneko I, Sabir MS, Dussik CM, Whitfield GK, Karrys A, Hsieh JC, Haussler MR, Meyer MB, Pike JW, Jurutka PW. 1,25-Dihydroxyvitamin D regulates expression of the tryptophan hydroxylase two and leptin genes: implication for behavioral influences of vitamin D. FASEB J. 2015 Sep;29(9):4023-35. doi: 10.1096/fj.14-269811.
70. Waløen K, Kleppe R, Martinez A, Haavik J. Tyrosine and tryptophan hydroxylases as therapeutic targets in human disease. Expert Opin Ther Targets. 2017 Feb;21(2):167-180. doi: 10.1080/14728222.2017.1272581.
71. Mastroeni D, Grover A, Leonard B, et al. Microglial responses to dopamine in a cell culture model of Parkinson's disease. Neurobiology of aging. (2009) 30(11):1805-1817. doi:10.1016/j.neurobiolaging.2008.01.001.
72. Knekt P, Kilkkinen A, Rissanen H, Marniemi J, Sääksjärvi K, Heliövaara M. Serum vitamin D and the risk of Parkinson's disease. Archives of neurology. (2010) 67(7):808-811. doi:10.1001/archneurol.2010.120.
73. Mastroeni D, Grover A, Leonard B, et al. Microglial responses to dopamine in a cell culture model of Parkinson's disease. Neurobiology of aging. (2009) 30(11):1805-1817. doi:10.1016/j.neurobiolaging.2008.01.001.

74. Seidl SE, Santiago JA, Bilyk H, Potashkin JA. The emerging role of nutrition in Parkinson's disease. Frontiers in Aging Neuroscience. (2014) 6:36. doi:10.3389/fnagi.2014.00036.
75. Allyson P Mallya, Ariel Y Deutch, (Micro)Glia as Effectors of Cortical Volume Loss in Schizophrenia, Schizophrenia Bulletin, Volume 44, Issue 5, September 2018, Pages 948–957, https://doi.org/10.1093/schbul/sby088
76. Lu J, Shang X, Yao B, Sun D, Liu J, Zhang Y, Wang H, Shi J, Chen H, Shi T, Liu M, Wang X. The role of CYP1A1/2 in cholesterol ester accumulation provides a new perspective for the treatment of hypercholesterolemia. Acta Pharm Sin B. 2023 Feb;13(2):648-661. doi: 10.1016/j.apsb.2022.08.005.
77. Mohseni H, Mohammadi FM, Karampour Z, Amini S, Abiri B, Sayyah M. The relationship between history of dietary nutrients intakes and incidence of aggressive behavior in adolescent girls: a case-control study. Clin Nutr ESPEN. (2021) 43:200–5. doi: 10.1016/j.clnesp.2021.04.017
78. Rahman MM, Lorenzo M, Ban-Weiss G, Hasan Z, Azzouz M, Eckel SP, Conti DV, Lurmann F, Schlaerth H, Johnston J, Ko J, Palinkas L, Hurlburt M, Silva S, Gauderman WJ, McConnell R, Garcia E. Ambient temperature and air pollution associations with suicide and homicide mortality in California: A statewide case-crossover study. Sci Total Environ. 2023 May 20;874:162462. doi: 10.1016/j.scitotenv.2023.162462.
79. Shan J, Ma XF, Wu MY, Lin YJ, Wang Y, Wang R, Li HM, Wu ZL, Xu HM. Preliminary study on the role of aryl hydrocarbon receptor in the neurotoxicity of three typical bisphenol compounds (BPA, BPS, and TBBPA) at environmentally relevant concentrations to adult zebrafish (Danio rerio). Heliyon. 2023 May 26;9(6):e16649. doi: 10.1016/j.heliyon.2023.e16649.
80. Kuroda K, Yamada S, Tanaka M, Iizuka M, Yano H, Mori D, et al. Behavioral alterations associated with targeted disruption of exons 2 and 3 of the Disc1 gene in the mouse. Hum Mol Genet. (2011) 20(23):4666-83. doi: 10.1093/hmg/ddr400.

81. Pertile RAN, Brigden R, Raman V, Cui X, Du Z, Eyles D. Vitamin D: A potent regulator of dopaminergic neuron differentiation and function. J Neurochem. 2023 Sep;166(5):779-789. doi: 10.1111/jnc.15829. Epub 2023 May 14. PMID: 37084159
82. Weintraub D. Dopamine and Impulse Control Disorders in Parkinson's Disease. Annals of neurology. (2008) 64(Suppl 2):S93-100. doi:10.1002/ana.21454.
83. O'Sullivan SS, Evans AH, Lees AJ. Dopamine dysregulation syndrome: an overview of its epidemiology, mechanisms, and management. CNS Drugs. (2009) 23(2):157-70. doi: 10.2165/00023210-200923020-00005.
84. Ataie-Jafari A, Qorbani M, Heshmat R, Ardalan G, Motlagh ME, Asayesh H, Arzaghi SM, Tajadini MH, Nejatinamini S, Poursafa P, Kelishadi R. The association of vitamin D deficiency with psychiatric distress and violence behaviors in Iranian adolescents: the CASPIAN-III study. J Diabetes Metab Disord. 2015 Jul 22;14:62. Doi: 10.1186/s40200-015-0191-9.
85. Yüksel RN, Altunsoy N, Tikir B, et al. Correlation between total vitamin D levels and psychotic psychopathology in patients with schizophrenia: therapeutic implications for add-on vitamin D augmentation. Therapeutic Advances in Psychopharmacology. (2014)4(6):268-275. doi:10.1177/2045125314553612.
86. Cui X, McGrath JJ, Burne THJ, Eyles DW. Vitamin D and schizophrenia: 20 years on. Mol Psychiatry. 2021 Jul;26(7):2708-2720. doi: 10.1038/s41380-021-01025-0.
87. Doğan Bulut S, Bulut S, Görkem Atalan D, et al. The Relationship between Symptom Severity and Low Vitamin D Levels in Patients with Schizophrenia. Hashimoto K, ed. PLoS ONE. 2016;11(10): e0165284. doi:10.1371/journal.pone.0165284.
88. McGrath JJ, Eyles DW, Pedersen CB, Anderson C, Ko P, Burne TH, et al. Neonatal vitamin D status and risk of schizophrenia: a population-based case-control study. Arch Gen Psychiatry. 2010;67:889–94.
89. Dang R, Jiang P, Cai H, Li H, Guo R, Wu Y, et al.Vitamin D deficiency exacerbates atypical antipsychotic-induced metabolic

side effects in rats: involvement of the INSIG/SREBP pathway. Eur Neuropsychopharmacol. (2015) 25(8):1239-47. doi: 10.1016/j.euroneuro.2015.04.028
90. Nwosu BU, Meltzer B, Maranda L, et al. A potential role for adjunctive vitamin D therapy in managing weight gain and metabolic side effects of second-generation antipsychotics. Journal of pediatric endocrinology & metabolism : JPEM. 2011;24(0):619-626.
91. Nagashima T, Shirakawa H, Nakagawa T, Kaneko S. Prevention of antipsychotic-induced hyperglycemia by vitamin D: a data mining prediction followed by an experimental exploration of the molecular mechanism. Scientific Reports. 2016;6:26375. doi:10.1038/srep26375.
92. Sfera A, Osorio C, Inderias LA, Parker V, Price AI, Cummings M. The Obesity-Impulsivity Axis: Potential Metabolic Interventions in Chronic Psychiatric Patients. Front Psychiatry. 2017 Feb 13;8:20. doi: 10.3389/fpsyt.2017.00020. PMID: 28243210; PMCID: PMC5303716.
93. Jamilian M, Samimi M, Ebrahimi FA, Hashemi T, Taghizadeh M, Razavi M, et al., The effects of vitamin D and omega-3 fatty acid co-supplementation on glycemic control and lipid concentrations in patients with gestational diabetes. J Clin Lipidol. (2017) 11(2):459-468. doi: 10.1016/j.jacl.2017.01.011
94. Beaulieu J-M. A role for Akt and glycogen synthase kinase-3 as integrators of dopamine and serotonin neurotransmission in mental health. Journal of Psychiatry & Neuroscience : JPN. (2012) 37(1):7-16. doi:10.1503/jpn.110011.
95. Stambolic V, Woodgett JR. Mitogen inactivation of glycogen synthase kinase-3 beta in intact cells via serine nine phosphorylation. Biochemical Journal. (1994) 303(Pt 3):701-704.
96. Ma YX, Wang XL, Chen JQ, Li B, Hur EM, Saijilafu. Differential Roles of Glycogen Synthase Kinase 3 Subtypes Alpha and Beta in Cortical Development. Front Mol Neurosci. 2017 Nov 28;10:391. doi: 10.3389/fnmol.2017.00391.
97. Freland L, Beaulieu J-M. Inhibition of GSK3 by lithium, from single molecules to signaling networks. Frontiers in Molecular Neuroscience. (2012) 5:14. doi:10.3389/fnmol.2012.00014.

98. Goksugur SB, Tufan AE, Semiz M, Gunes C, Bekdas M, Tosun M, Demircioglu F. Vitamin D status in children with attention-deficit-hyperactivity disorder. Pediatr Int. (2014) 56(4):515-9. doi: 10.1111/ped.12286
99. Lee K. Sex-specific relationships between alcohol consumption and vitamin D levels: The Korea National Health and Nutrition Examination Survey 2009. Nutrition Research and Practice. (2012) 6(1):86-90. doi:10.4162/nrp.2012.6.1.86.
100. Smith GC, McEwen H, Steinberg JD, Shepherd PR. The activation of the Akt/PKB signaling pathway in the brains of clozapine-exposed rats is linked to hyperinsulinemia and not a direct drug effect. Psychopharmacology (Berl). 2014 Dec;231(23):4553-60. doi: 10.1007/s00213-014-3608-0.
101. Zaulkffali AS, Md Razip NN, Syed Alwi SS, Abd Jalil A, Abd Mutalib MS, Gopalsamy B, Chang SK, Zainal Z, Ibrahim NN, Zakaria ZA, Khaza'ai H. Vitamins D and E Stimulate the PI3K-AKT Signalling Pathway in Insulin-Resistant SK-N-SH Neuronal Cells. Nutrients. 2019 Oct 19;11(10):2525. doi: 10.3390/nu11102525.
102. Bortolato M, Shih JC. Behavioral Outcomes of Monoamine Oxidase Deficiency: Preclinical and Clinical Evidence. International Review of Neurobiology. (2011) 100:13-42. doi:10.1016/B978-0-12-386467-3.00002-9.
103. McDermott R, Tingley D, Cowden J, Frazzetto G, Johnson DDP. Monoamine oxidase A gene (MAOA) predicts behavioral aggression following provocation. Proceedings of the National Academy of Sciences of the United States of America. (2009) 106(7):2118-2123. doi:10.1073/pnas.0808376106.
104. Sabir MS, Haussler MR, Mallick S, Kaneko I, Lucas DA, Haussler CA, Whitfield GK, Jurutka PW. Optimal vitamin D spurs serotonin: 1,25-dihydroxyvitamin D represses serotonin reuptake transport (SERT) and degradation (MAO-A) gene expression in cultured rat serotonergic neuronal cell lines. Genes Nutr. 2018 Jul 11;13:19. Doi: 10.1186/s12263-018-0605-7.
105. Kolla NJ, Patel R, Meyer JH, Chakravarty MM. Association of monoamine oxidase-A genetic variants and amygdala morphology

in violent offenders with antisocial personality disorder and high psychopathic traits. Scientific Reports. (2017) 7:9607. doi:10.1038/s41598-017-08351-w.

106. Wu JB, Shih JC. Valproic acid induces monoamine oxidase A via Akt/forkhead box O1 activation. Mol Pharmacol. 2011 Oct;80(4): 714-23. doi: 10.1124/mol.111.072744.
107. Kwon HJ, Jin HJ, Lim MH. Association between monoamine oxidase gene polymorphisms and attention deficit hyperactivity disorder in Korean children. Genet Test Mol Biomarkers. 2014 Jul;18(7):505-9. doi: 10.1089/gtmb.2014.0066.
108. Siess KM, Leonard TA. Lipid-dependent Akt-activity: where, when, and how. Biochem Soc Trans. 2019 Jun 28;47(3):897-908. doi: 10.1042/BST20190013. Epub 2019 May 30.
109. Zhou M, Ren H, Han J, Wang W, Zheng Q, Wang D. Protective Effects of Kaempferol against Myocardial Ischemia/Reperfusion Injury in Isolated Rat Heart via Antioxidant Activity and Inhibition of Glycogen Synthase Kinase-3β. Oxid Med Cell Longev. 2015;2015:481405. doi: 10.1155/2015/481405. Epub 2015 Jul 22. PMID: 26265983
110. Schwartz DL. Quercetin as an Augmentation Agent in Schizophrenia. J Clin Psychopharmacol. 2016 Jun;36(3):282-3. doi: 10.1097/JCP.0000000000000498. PMID: 27035495.
111. Fan HR, Du WF, Zhu T, Wu YJ, Liu YM, Wang Q, Wang Q, Gu X, Shan X, Deng S, Zhu T, Xu TL, Ge WH, Li WG, Li F. Quercetin Reduces Cortical GABAergic Transmission and Alleviates MK-801-Induced Hyperactivity. EBioMedicine. 2018 Aug;34:201-213. doi: 10.1016/j.ebiom.2018.07.031.
112. Elisabetsky E, Costa-Campos L. The alkaloid alstonine: a review of its pharmacological properties. Evid Based Complement Alternat Med. 2006 Mar;3(1):39-48. doi: 10.1093/ecam/nek011.
113. Cleide S. Souza, Bruna S. Paulsen, Sylvie Devalle, Silvia Lima Costa, Helena L. Borges, Stevens K. Rehen. The pro-estrogenic flavonoid apigenin induces the commitment of human pluripotent stem cells to a neural lineage. Advances in Regenerative Biology, 2015; 2 (0) DOI: 10.3402/arb.v2.29244

114. Yan T, Li L, Sun B, Liu F, Yang P, Chen T, Li T, Liu X. Luteolin inhibits behavioral sensitization by blocking methamphetamine-induced MAPK pathway activation in the caudate putamen in mice. PLoS One. 2014 Jun 5;9(6):e98981.
doi: 10.1371/journal.pone.0098981. PMID: 24901319; PMCID: PMC4047057.

115. MacDonald CJ, Ciolino HP, Yeh GC. The drug salicylamide is an antagonist of the aryl hydrocarbon receptor that inhibits signal transduction induced by 2,3,7,8 tetrachlorodibcnzo-p-dioxin. Cancer Res. 2004 Jan 1;64(1):429-34. doi: 10.1158/0008-5472.can-03-0974. PMID: 14729655.

116. Patro BS, Rele S, Chintalwar GJ, Chattopadhyay S, Adhikari S, Mukherjee T. Protective activities of some phenolic 1,3-diketones against lipid peroxidation: possible involvement of the 1,3-diketone moiety. Chembiochem. 2002 Apr 2;3(4):364-70. doi: 10.1002/1439-7633(20020402)3:4<364::AID-CBIC364>3.0.CO;2-S.
PMID: 11933238

117. McGovern K, Castro AC, Cavanaugh J, Coma S, Walsh M, Tchaicha J, Syed S, Natarajan P, Manfredi M, Zhang XM, Ecsedy J. Discovery and Characterization of a Novel Aryl Hydrocarbon Receptor Inhibitor, IK-175, and Its Inhibitory Activity on Tumor Immune Suppression. Mol Cancer Ther. 2022 Aug 2;21(8):1261-1272. doi: 10.1158/1535-7163.MCT-21-0984. PMID: 35666806.

118. Kang S, Lee AG, Im S, Oh SJ, Yoon HJ, Park JH, Pak YK. A Novel Aryl Hydrocarbon Receptor Antagonist HBU651 Ameliorates Peripheral and Hypothalamic Inflammation in High-Fat Diet-Induced Obese Mice. Int J Mol Sci. 2022 Nov 28;23(23):14871. doi: 10.3390/ijms232314871. PMID: 36499198; PMCID: PMC9736602.

119. Matsuda, Satoru, Yuka Ikeda, Mutsumi Murakami, Yukie Nakagawa, Ai Tsuji, and Yasuko Kitagishi. 2019. "Roles of PI3K/AKT/GSK3 Pathway Involved in Psychiatric Illnesses" Diseases 7, no. 1: 22.
https://doi.org/10.3390/diseases7010022

120. Emamian ES. AKT/GSK3 signaling pathway and schizophrenia. Front Mol Neurosci. 2012 Mar 15;5:33.
doi: 10.3389/fnmol.2012.00033. PMID: 22435049; PMCID: PMC3304298.

121. Ziegler, D.V., Czarnecka-Herok, J., Vernier, M. et al. The cholesterol biosynthetic pathway induces cellular senescence through ERRα. npj Aging 10, 5 (2024). https://doi.org/10.1038/s41514-023-00128-y
122. Millner A, Atilla-Gokcumen GE. Lipid Players of Cellular Senescence. Metabolites. 2020 Aug 21;10(9):339. doi: 10.3390/metabo10090339. PMID: 32839400; PMCID: PMC7570155.
123. Huo J, Xu Z, Hosoe K, Kubo H, Miyahara H, Dai J, Mori M, Sawashita J, Higuchi K. Coenzyme Q10 Prevents Senescence and Dysfunction Caused by Oxidative Stress in Vascular Endothelial Cells. Oxid Med Cell Longev. 2018 Jul 8;2018:3181759. Doi: 10.1155/2018/3181759.
124. Leppien E, Mulcahy K, Demler TL, Trigoboff E, Opler L. Effects of Statins and Cholesterol on Patient Aggression: Is There a Connection? Innov Clin Neurosci. 2018 Apr 1;15(3-4):24-27. PMID: 29707423; PMCID: PMC5906086.
125. Jain P. Traditional and novel non-statin lipid-lowering drugs. Indian Heart J. 2023 Nov 17:S0019-4832(23)00176-1. doi: 10.1016/j.ihj.2023.11.003. Epub ahead of print. PMID: 37979722.
126. Abdul-Rahman T, Bukhari SMA, Herrera EC, Awuah WA, Lawrence J, de Andrade H, Patel N, Shah R, Shaikh R, Capriles CAA, Ulusan S, Ahmad S, Corriero AC, Mares AC, Goel A, Hajra A, Bandyopadhyay D, Gupta R. Lipid-Lowering Therapy: An Era Beyond Statins. Curr Probl Cardiol. 2022 Dec;47(12):101342. doi: 10.1016/j.cpcardiol.2022.101342.
127. Heitmann ASB, Zanjani AAH, Klenow MB, Mularski A, Sønder SL, Lund FW, Boye TL, Dias C, Bendix PM, Simonsen AC, Khandelia H, Nylandsted J. Phenothiazines alter plasma membrane properties and sensitize cancer cells to injury by inhibiting annexin-mediated repair. J Biol Chem. 2021 Aug;297(2):101012. doi: 10.1016/j.jbc.2021.101012.
128. Boonnoy, P., Jarerattanachat, V., Karttunen, M. & Wong-ekkabut, J. Bilayer Deformation, Pores, and Micellation Induced by Oxidized Lipids. J. Phys. Chem. Lett. 6, 4884–4888 (2015).

129. Keynes RG, Karchevskaya A, Riddall D, Griffiths CH, Bellamy TC, Chan AWE, Selwood DL, Garthwaite J. N10 -carbonyl-substituted phenothiazines inhibiting lipid peroxidation and associated nitric oxide consumption powerfully protect brain tissue against oxidative stress. Chem Biol Drug Des. 2019 Sep;94(3):1680-1693. doi: 10.1111/cbdd.13572.
130. Keynes RG, Karchevskaya A, Riddall D, Griffiths CH, Bellamy TC, Chan AWE, Selwood DL, Garthwaite J. N10 -carbonyl-substituted phenothiazines inhibiting lipid peroxidation and associated nitric oxide consumption powerfully protect brain tissue against oxidative stress. Chem Biol Drug Des. 2019 Sep;94(3):1680-1693. doi: 10.1111/cbdd.13572.
131. Voronova O, Zhuravkov S, Korotkova E, Artamonov A, Plotnikov E. Antioxidant Properties of New Phenothiazine Derivatives. Antioxidants (Basel). 2022 Jul 14;11(7):1371. doi: 10.3390/antiox11071371